Radiotherapy in Practice: Imaging for Clinical Oncology

Radiotherapy in Practice
Imaging for Clinical Oncology

SECOND EDITION

Edited by

Peter Hoskin

Consultant in Clinical Oncology, Mount Vernon Cancer Centre, Northwood, UK; Professor of Clinical Oncology, University of Manchester, UK

Thankamma Ajithkumar

Consultant Clinical Oncologist, Cambridge University Hospitals NHS Foundation Trust, UK

Vicky Goh

Chair of Clinical Cancer Imaging, King's College London; Honorary Consultant Radiologist, Guy's & St Thomas' NHS Foundation Trust, UK

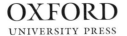

OXFORD
UNIVERSITY PRESS

UNIVERSITY PRESS

Great Clarendon Street, Oxford, OX2 6DP,
United Kingdom

Oxford University Press is a department of the University of Oxford.
It furthers the University's objective of excellence in research, scholarship,
and education by publishing worldwide. Oxford is a registered trade mark of
Oxford University Press in the UK and in certain other countries

Published in the United States of America by Oxford University Press
198 Madison Avenue, New York, NY 10016, United States of America

British Library Cataloguing in Publication Data
Data available

Library of Congress Control Number: 2021941848

ISBN 978–0–19–881850–2

DOI: 10.1093/med/9780198818502.001.0001

Printed in Great Britain by
Bell & Bain Ltd., Glasgow

Contents

Contributors

Helen Addley
Consultant Radiologist
Cambridge University Hospitals NHS
Foundation Trust
Cambridge, UK

Thankamma Ajithkumar
Consultant Clinical Oncologist
Cambridge University Hospitals NHS
Foundation Trust
Cambridge, UK

Luigi Aloj
Consultant Nuclear Medicine Physician
University of Cambridge School of
Clinical Medicine
Cambridge, UK

Victoria Ames
Consultant Radiologist
Norfolk and Norwich University
Hospitals NHS Foundation Trust
Norwich, UK

Gill Barnett
Consultant Clinical Oncologist
Cambridge University Hospitals NHS
Foundation Trust
Cambridge, UK

Bristi Basu
Academic Consultant Medical
Oncologist
Department of Oncology
University of Cambridge
Cambridge, UK

Gulshad Begum
Specialist Registrar in Clinical Oncology
Cambridge University Hospitals NHS
Foundation Trust
Cambridge, UK

David Bowden
Consultant Radiologist
Cambridge University Hospitals NHS
Foundation Trust
Cambridge, UK

Morag Brothwell
Specialist Registrar in Clinical Oncology
Cambridge University Hospitals NHS
Foundation Trust
Cambridge, UK

Nicholas Carroll
Consultant Radiologist
Cambridge University Hospitals NHS
Foundation Trust
Cambridge, UK

Anthony Chambers
Consultant Radiologist
Paul Strickland Scanner Centre
Mount Vernon Cancer Centre
Northwood, UK

Heok Cheow
Consultant Radiologist
Cambridge University Hospitals NHS
Foundation Trust
Cambridge, UK

Haesun Choi
Professor
Department of Abdominal Imaging
MD Anderson Cancer Center
Houston, Texas, USA

Ananya Choudhury
Chair and Honorary Consultant in
Clinical Oncology
The Christie NHS Foundation Trust
Manchester, UK

Katy Clarke
Consultant Clinical Oncologist
St James' University Hospital
Leeds, UK

Tom Crosby
Clinical Oncologist
Velindre Cancer Centre
Cardiff, UK

Michael Darby
Consultant Radiologist
St James' University Hospital
Leeds, UK

Tilak Das
Consultant Neuroradiologist
Cambridge University Hospitals NHS
Foundation Trust
Cambridge, UK

June Dean
Associate Radiotherapy Manager
Cambridge University Hospitals NHS
Foundation Trust
Cambridge, UK

Sara C. Erridge
Consultant Clinical Oncologist
Edinburgh Cancer Centre
Western General Hospital
Edinburgh, UK

Kieran Foley
Consultant Radiologist
Royal Glamorgan Hospital & Velindre
Cancer Centre
Cardiff, UK

Mark Gaze
Consultant in Clinical Oncology
University College London Hospitals
NHS Foundation Trust
London, UK

Emma-Louise Gerety
Consultant Musculoskeletal
Radiologist
Cambridge University Hospitals NHS
Foundation Trust
Cambridge, UK

Dinos Geropantas
Consultant Clinical Oncologist
Norfolk and Norwich University
Hospitals NHS Foundation Trust
Norwich, UK

Edmund Godfrey
Consultant Radiologist
Cambridge University Hospitals NHS
Foundation Trust
Cambridge, UK

Vicky Goh
Chair of Clinical Cancer Imaging
King's College London
Honorary Consultant Radiologist
Guy's & St Thomas' NHS Foundation
Trust
London, UK

Katy Hickman
Specialist Registrar in Radiology
Cambridge University Hospitals NHS
Foundation Trust
Cambridge, UK

Gail Horan
Consultant Clinical Oncologist
Cambridge University Hospitals NHS
Foundation Trust
Cambridge, UK

Peter Hoskin
Consultant in Clinical Oncology
Mount Vernon Cancer Centre
Northwood, UK;
Professor of Clinical Oncology
University of Manchester, UK

Paul Humphries
Consultant Paediatric Radiologist
University College London Hospitals
NHS Foundation Trust
London, UK

Pooja Jain
Consultant Clinical Oncologist
St James' University Hospital
Leeds, UK

N. Jane Taylor
Principal Clinical Scientist
Paul Strickland Scanner Centre
Mount Vernon Hospital
Northwood, UK

Rohit Kochhar
Consultant Radiologist
The Christie NHS Foundation Trust
Manchester, UK

Kate Lankester
Honorary Clinical Senior Lecturer
Sussex Cancer Centre
Royal Sussex County Hospital
Brighton, UK

Vivek Misra
Consultant Clinical Oncologist
The Christie NHS Foundation Trust
Manchester, UK

Carys Morgan
Clinical Oncologist
Velindre Cancer Centre
Cardiff, UK

Rebecca Muirhead
Consultant Clinical Oncologist
Oxford University Hospitals Trust
Oxford, UK

Francesca Peters
Consultant Radiologist
East and North Hertfordshire Trust
Stevenage, UK

Sarah Prewett
Consultant Clinical Oncologist
Cambridge University Hospitals NHS
Foundation Trust
Cambridge, UK

Marika Reinius
Specialist Registrar in Medical Oncology
Cambridge University Hospitals NHS
Foundation Trust
Cambridge, UK

Monique Shahid
Consultant Paediatric Radiologist
The Leeds Teaching Hospitals NHS Trust
Leeds, UK

Elizabeth C. Smyth
Consultant Oncologist
Cambridge University Hospitals NHS
Foundation Trust
Cambridge, UK

David Summers
Consultant Neuroradiologist
Western General Hospital
Edinburgh, UK

Simon Thomas
Consultant Clinical Scientist
Cambridge University Hospitals NHS
Foundation Trust
Cambridge, UK

Gerard Thompson
Senior Clinical Lecturer in Radiology
Department of Radiology
University of Edinburgh
Edinburgh, UK

Lavanya Vitta
Consultant Radiologist
Brighton and Sussex University
Hospitals NHS Trust
Brighton, UK

Huiqi Yang
Consultant Clinical Oncologist
Cambridge University Hospitals NHS
Foundation Trust Cambridge, UK

Connie Yip
Senior Consultant Radiation Oncologist
Department of Radiation Oncology
Singapore

Chapter 1

Introduction

Peter Hoskin and Vicky Goh

1.1 Introduction

Imaging is an essential component in the management of any patient with cancer. With perhaps the exception of a small superficial basal cell carcinoma all patients will require imaging evaluation of their malignancy. Therefore, it is essential that the principles of imaging and the specific requirements for each tumour site are clearly understood by those involved in the management of patients with malignant disease to enable optimum use of this essential modality.

1.2 The role of imaging

The role of imaging is extensive and integral to management at any point in the patient's journey. At their initial presentation imaging may have led to the discovery of a tumour, resulting in an image-guided or surgical procedure to confirm its malignant nature. It will then be essential to assess the full extent of that tumour and define the tumour stage by evaluating pathways of direct, lymphatic, and blood borne spread. The tumour stage is critical to subsequent management and it is therefore vital that full and appropriate imaging is undertaken at this point.

For the patient having radiotherapy, an accurate assessment of the tumour to be treated and of the surrounding organs at risk is critical to planning radiotherapy. Detailed evaluation with diagnostic imaging is essential for delivering optimal radiotherapy. The most important step in radiotherapy planning is tumour localization and, with the few exceptions of readily palpable and visible skin tumours, a full appreciation of the anatomical localization, involvement of surrounding structures, and proximity to critical organs is essential, and can only be provided through appropriate radiological investigations.

Following treatment, further management is based on response assessment and continued surveillance in which imaging will play a major part. It is important to have an understanding of the positive and negative predictive value of a test and the level of reliance that can be placed upon it. This is particularly the case in the setting of response assessment when patients having persistent disease may be subject to major salvage procedures on the basis of failure to achieve a radiological complete response.

1.3 **Imaging modalities**

X-ray imaging was available soon after the discovery of X-rays by Roentgen in 1895. It is remarkable that despite technical improvements in the production of plain X-ray images and increased understanding of the use of contrast materials it took almost 80 years for the next revolution in imaging to appear in the clinical setting with the introduction of computed tomography (CT).

Since then, there has been a major revolution in imaging, with ever more sophisticated and rapid CT imaging, and progressive integration of magnetic resonance imaging (MRI), and molecular imaging techniques—[18]F-flurodeoxyglucose positron emission tomography/computed tomography (^{18}F-FDG PET/CT)—in radiotherapy planning.

Simultaneously, radiotherapy techniques have evolved from two-dimensional planning to modern high-precision techniques such as intensity modulated radiotherapy (IMRT), image-guided radiotherapy (IGRT), tomotherapy, volumetric modulated arc therapy (VMAT), adaptive radiotherapy, and proton beam therapy. Imaging modalities such as stereoscopic X-ray, CT scan, and MRI are also integrated with the therapy machines to ensure accurate delivery.

The result of these dramatic technological changes is that a modern cancer centre has a sophisticated range of imaging modalities available for each patient, to provide detailed information on both the anatomical distribution and physiological characteristics of the tumour in question. The challenge in this setting is to optimize the use of each modality in order to obtain the most accurate and reliable information possible with the technology available.

1.4 **Integration into the radiotherapy department**

Modern radiotherapy is a complex multistep process, optimizing the many features of a modern linear accelerator and, recently, that of particle therapy machines in order to deliver a high dose of radiation to the tumour yet minimizing exposure to surrounding organs at risk, thus ensuring that patients receive accurate reproducible treatment. Imaging is an integral component of many of the stages through which a patient will pass in the radiotherapy department. The technological developments in imaging in recent years have also driven important changes in the radiotherapy department.

Currently, most radiotherapy departments use three-dimensional (3D) CT-based planning systems in which a CT scan is imported into a radiotherapy planning computer system and the treatment volume, together with the organs at risk (OAR), are defined on screen on sequential CT images. The use of intravenous contrast can be useful in radiotherapy planning to distinguish vessels from abnormal soft tissue structures such as lymph nodes. Large volumes of oral contrast to outline bowel are not used because large volumes of contrast can alter the absorption characteristics of the dosimetric calculations.

Four-dimensional (4D) CT scans are useful in situations where tumour movement during respiration is likely. Co-registration of MRI sequences is used where MR is superior to CT in demarcating tumour and normal tissue structures: particular examples would include the brain and pelvis (for prostate, bladder, and uterine tumours). ^{18}F FDG PET/CT images could improve further the accuracy of treatment volume delineation for lung and head and neck cancers and lymphoma.

During the treatment planning process, radiation physicists and dosimetrists derive an optimal beam arrangement based on the intended radiotherapy volume and delivery technique to achieve a homogeneous dose distribution within the planning target volume (PTV), whilst minimizing dose to OARs. Information from the planning CT scan is used for dosimetric calculations. Currently, MR is not used in radiotherapy dosimetry. This is because of the distortion characteristics at the edge of the MR field so that the patient outline is less accurate and also the fact that the information on X-ray absorption heterogeneities is not obtained in the process of MR scanning. With the evolution of the MRI-Linac, there are increasing efforts to incorporate MRI dosimetry for adaptive radiotherapy, but this remains investigational at present.

1.5 **Summary**

◆ Imaging is an integral component of patient care throughout the cancer journey, being required for diagnosis and staging, radiotherapy planning, and subsequent response evaluation and follow-up.

◆ The evolution of imaging in recent years with widespread availability of increasingly sophisticated CT, MR, and molecular imaging has driven major changes in radiotherapy practice.

◆ The precise requirements for individual tumours and tumour sites vary and a clear appreciation of the relative strengths and weaknesses of different imaging modalities for a given patient is essential.

◆ It is critical to bear in mind that increased use of ionizing-radiation based imaging exposes the patient to a higher concomitant radiation dose, the long-term sequelae of which are as yet to be fully evaluated.

◆ Clear justification based on sound evidence is essential in this setting for each diagnostic radiation exposure to ensure that the imaging tools are used optimally for each patient.

Chapter 2

Principles of imaging

Connie Yip, N. Jane Taylor,
Anthony Chambers, and Vicky Goh

2.1 Introduction

Imaging is fundamentally important to the management of the cancer patient. Anatomical imaging is the mainstay for patient evaluation; however, molecular, functional, and hybrid (combined molecular/functional–anatomical) imaging have acquired an increasing role.

To obtain the most accurate and reliable information possible with the most appropriate imaging modality the relative performance of the imaging test has to be defined. Commonly used measures of test performance include:

- *Sensitivity*: how good the test is at picking up disease (true positive (TP)/TP + false negative (FN)), expressed as a percentage.
- *Specificity*: how good the test is at excluding disease (true negative (TN)/TN + false positive (FP)), expressed as a percentage.
- *Accuracy*: how good a test is at picking up and excluding disease (TP + TN/TP + FP + TN + FN), expressed as a percentage.

Test performance is also affected by the prevalence of disease in the population: test performance will be lower if disease prevalence in the population is low, that is, the *positive predictive value* (TP/TP + FP) will be lower (Table 2.1). Other parameters that have been used include receiver operator curve (ROC) analysis, frequency of management change, and cost-benefit analysis.

2.2 X-ray

X-ray remains an important part of cancer management, for example for suspected lung cancer. Although it has poor sensitivity and specificity, it is widely available and cheap. Digital systems which have replaced conventional films have the advantage that images can be viewed and distributed with a higher patient throughput. Digital detectors also demonstrate increased dose efficiency and a greater dynamic range, potentially reducing radiation exposure to the patient.

Table 2.1 Effect of disease prevalence on the performance of a test with 90% sensitivity and 90% specificity in the population imaged (1000 independent tests)

Disease prevalence (%)	True positives	False positives	Positive predictive value (%)
75	675	25	96
50	450	50	90
10	90	90	50

2.2.1 Production of X-rays

X-rays are produced from an X-ray tube, a glass envelope vacuum with a wire element at one end forming the cathode, and a heavy metal target (e.g. tungsten or copper) at the other end forming the anode. Application of a high voltage at the cathode results in the formation of electrons which are drawn towards the anode. Collision with the heavy metal target produces X-rays.

2.2.2 X-ray quality and intensity

Quality describes the penetrating power of an X-ray beam. *Intensity* describes the quantity of radiation energy flowing in unit time. In practice an X-ray beam consists of a continuous spectrum of energies up to a maximum determined by the voltage applied between the cathode and the anode, for example a voltage setting of 120 kV will produce a range of X-ray energies up to a maximum of 120 keV.

Factors affecting X-ray tube output include:

- *Tube kilovoltage*: this affects both beam quality and intensity. The higher the kV, the greater the beam penetration: settings ranging from 28 kV to 30 kV are used for mammography, and 70–90 kV for body imaging.
- *Tube current*: this affects beam intensity only. In general, beam intensity is directly proportional to tube current.
- *Beam filtration*: filters are placed into the X-ray beam to improve beam quality by absorbing lower energy radiation, yet transmitting higher energy X-rays. Typical filters include aluminium, copper, molybdenum, or palladium.
- *Distance from source*: an X-ray tube produces a diverging beam, subject to a reduction in intensity with distance obeying the inverse square law.
- *Tube target material*: the proton number of the target affects the intensity of the beam produced. Beam quality is not affected.

2.2.3 Interaction of X-ray with matter

There are two main types of interaction between X-ray and matter at the photon energies produced for diagnostic radiology:

- *Photoelectric effect*: the interaction of X-ray photons with tightly bound electrons which absorb all the energy of the X-ray photon. The electrons are then ejected from the atom, a 'photoelectron'. Photoelectric interactions occur at lower energies (<1 MeV) and predominate in the diagnostic energy range. The degree of absorption is highly dependent upon the atomic number of the tissue.
- *Compton scattering*: the interaction of X-ray photons with loosely bound orbital electrons. The X-ray photons lose some energy and are deflected or scattered; this interaction predominates in the megavoltage energy ranges used for therapeutic radiation beams. The probability of interaction is independent of atomic number and varies with tissue electron density.

Different tissues in the body attenuate X-rays differently. Tube voltages between 20 kV and 65 kV provide the best contrast for body imaging, with excellent differentiation between soft tissue and bone as the photoelectric effect is dominant. At higher energies, when the Compton effect dominates, image contrast is predominantly due to tissue density.

2.2.4 Image generation and processing

Digital images consist of picture elements or *pixels*; the 2D representation of pixels in an image is called the *matrix*. Following exposure of digital detectors to X-rays, the energy absorbed is transformed into electric charges, which are then processed into a greyscale clinical image representing the amount of energy deposited. A digital header file containing patient information is added to the image generated.

The following factors influence image quality:

- *Spatial resolution*: in digital radiography, spatial resolution (the minimal resolvable separation of two high-contrast objects) is defined by minimum pixel size. This is in the order of 100–200 microns. The use of direct conversion detectors increases spatial resolution as the scatter of X-ray quanta and light photons within the detector influences spatial resolution.
- *Dynamic range*: this refers to the range of X-ray exposures over which a meaningful image can be obtained. Digital detectors have a wide and linear dynamic range in comparison to previously used screen-film combinations, so that differences in specific tissue absorption (e.g. bone versus soft tissue) can be displayed in a single image without the need for additional imaging.
- *Detective quantum efficiency*: this refers to the efficiency of a detector in converting X-ray energy into an image signal. It is dependent on radiation exposure, radiation quality, spatial frequency, modulation transfer function (the capacity of the detector to transfer the modulation of input signal at a given spatial frequency to its output), and detector material.

Post-processing is performed following exposure and readout to ensure images are optimized for viewing (Figure 2.1). Spatial resolution is dependent on the detector and cannot be altered by post-processing; however, manoeuvres including contrast optimization, noise reduction, and artefact removal can compensate for poorer spatial resolution. Different algorithms are generally applied to different anatomic regions in order to prevent inadvertent suppression of useful information.

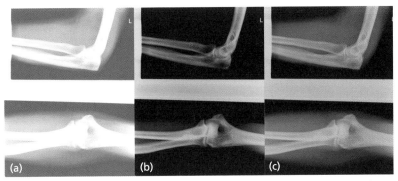

Fig. 2.1 Digital radiographs: images can be digitally processed to alter image quality. The effect of contrast enhancement (a), contrast reduction (b), and edge enhancement (c) is shown.

2.3 Computed tomography

CT is currently the most widely used imaging modality for cancer imaging. Since its introduction in 1971, CT technology has evolved rapidly. In general it is a sensitive and specific test, though values vary depending on the body part examined.

2.3.1 Basic principles

CT is an *X-ray tomographic technique* that provides non-superimposed cross-sectional images of the body. As the X-ray tube rotates around the patient, the X-ray beam passes through an axial section of the patient's body from different directions. Detectors around the patient measure the intensity of the attenuated radiation beam as it emerges from the body. Detectors convert the X-ray intensity into electric signals which are amplified and processed to compensate for inhomogeneities in the detector system and to correct for beam hardening effects. Data are then transformed into X-ray attenuation values producing the CT raw data. These are then reconstructed mathematically to yield the image dataset, for example using *filtered back projection*. Different *convolution kernels* can be applied enabling different types of images to be obtained (e.g. soft, smooth, sharp, edge enhanced). More recently, with the increasing use of low dose CT, advances in scanner hardware and increasing computing power, *iterative reconstruction* techniques are replacing *filtered back projection* to improve image noise and image characteristics.

During image reconstruction a *CT number* (Hounsfield unit) is assigned according to the degree of attenuation. This is defined as:

$$CT = 1000 \times (\mu - \mu_{water})/\mu_{water}$$

A CT number of -1000 represents air, 0 represents water, around 50 represents soft tissue, and >1000 represents cortical bone. There is no upper limit. Images are displayed as a greyscale image. The resulting CT image is composed of a square matrix ranging in size from 256 × 256 to 1024 × 1024 pixel elements. Each pixel represents a scanned voxel, each with its own CT number. Axial CT images can be manipulated further to produce reformatted images in any secondary plane and 3D images.

2.3.2 Computed tomography acquisition

CT is currently based on helical CT, which was made possible by the introduction of slip ring technology allowing for a continuously rotating CT gantry. Images are acquired using the continuously rotating X-ray tube by moving the table top on which the patient lies through the scan plane. This results in a helical scan pattern and acquisition of a data volume. Because of the helical acquisition, *interpolation* has to be performed during image reconstruction to generate a planar dataset for each table position and to produce artefact-free images. Images can be generated from any segment within the scanned volume by overlapping reconstructions as often as required. Different reconstruction intervals (spacing between sections) and section collimations (section thickness) can be used.

Multidetector helical CT, introduced in 1998, has resulted in a large gain in CT performance, including a shorter acquisition duration, longer scan ranges, and thinner sections with near isotropic resolution. Multidetector helical CT uses the radiation delivered more efficiently. The number of detector rows currently stands at 320 for state-of-the-art scanners. Dual-source CT with two X-ray tubes and two corresponding multidetector arrays has also been developed. The acquisition systems are mounted on a rotating gantry with a 90° angular offset. The gantry rotation time is <0.3 s, and dual-source CT can provide temporal resolutions one-quarter of the gantry rotation time.

Typical acquisition parameters for general imaging of the thorax, abdomen, and pelvis are summarized in Table 2.2.

◆ *Kilovoltage (kV)*: typically 120 kV is applied for diagnostic body imaging, although more recently kV modulation is possible according to patient habitus. Dual-energy imaging is performed on a dual-source CT using two different kV, for example 140 kV and 100 kV with beam filtration.

Table 2.2 Typical CT acquisition parameters for multidetector CT (64 rows and above)

	Thorax	Abdomen	Pelvis
Positioning	Thoracic inlet to below diaphragm	Above diaphragm to iliac crest	Iliac crest to symphysis pubis
kV	120	120	120
Effective mAs	200	280	300
Pitch	0.75	0.75	0.75
Detector collimation (mm)	0.6	0.6	0.6
Reconstruction increment (mm)	3–5	3–5	3–5
Reconstruction kernel	B30f medium smooth and B80f ultra sharp	B30f medium smooth	B30f medium smooth
Effective slice collimation (mm)	3–5	3–5	3–5

- *Milliampere second (mAs)*: this is the product of the tube current (e.g. 200 mA) and rotation time of the scanner (e.g. 0.6 s). With multidetector CT this is often quoted as *effective mAs* which is the product of the tube current and exposure time of one slice (rotation × collimation/feed per rotation). The mAs applied will depend on the body part examined. A higher mAs generally reduces image noise, thus improving the detectability of low-contrast structures, but has to be tempered by patient dose considerations. Current scanners use dose modulation techniques to reduce patient radiation exposure: the dose during each tube rotation is measured and altered depending on the attenuation level, making it possible to reduce the dose by as much as 56%.

- *Collimation*: the radiation beam emitted by the X-ray tube can be shaped using special diaphragms or 'collimators' positioned either directly in front of the X-ray source (to shape the emitted beam) or directly in front of the detectors (to reduce the effect of scattered radiation). The collimation and focal spot size determines the quality of the slice profile. Images can be reconstructed with slice thicknesses equal to or greater than the detector collimation.

- *Increment*: the distance between images reconstructed from a data volume. This should be selected as an overlapping increment to lower noise and improve image quality. An overlap of up to 90% can be achieved but an overlap of 30–50% is generally used in clinical practice. For example, if slice thicknesses of 10 mm are reconstructed with a 5 mm increment, slices will overlap by 50%.

- *Pitch*: this traditionally refers to table feed per rotation/collimation for single-slice CT. For multidetector CT, pitch is more complicated. Its value will depend on whether a single section collimation or total collimation of the detector array is used. Good image quality is obtained with a pitch between 1 and 2, defined as table feed per rotation/single section collimation.

2.3.3 Image processing

Multiplanar reformations (MPRs) are 2D reformatted images that are reconstructed secondarily from a stack of axial images, for example in the sagittal or coronal plane. Oblique and curved reformations can also be obtained but require interpolation between adjacent voxels. Curved reformations are needed for structures that pass through multiple axial planes, for example blood vessels and bronchi. Isotropic imaging is ideal for good quality MPRs. MPRs are generally the width of one voxel but can be produced with a greater section thickness to reduce image noise and further improve image quality. An example is shown in Figure 2.2.

Maximum (MIP) and minimum intensity projections (MinIP) are volume rendering techniques. Images are generated by displaying the maximum or minimum CT numbers encountered along the direction of the projection, known as the viewing angle. This ensures that contrast is optimized between high-contrast structures and surrounding tissue.

MIP views are generally used for CT angiography and for specialized pulmonary studies. MinIP images are used mainly for visualizing the central tracheobronchial

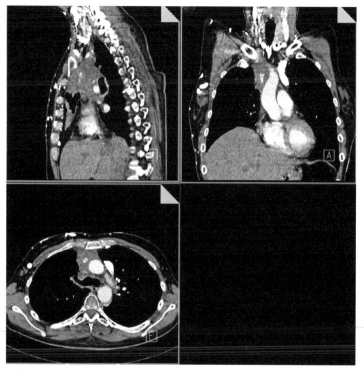

Fig. 2.2 CT Images of the thorax: multiplanar reformats can be obtained from manipulating the original data set, in this case demonstrating a lung tumour causing superior vena cava obstruction.

system. Volume rendering techniques have become the standard technique for CT angiography and for musculoskeletal imaging. Virtual colonography is a special type of volume rendered dataset giving a perspective view of 'flying through' the colon.

2.3.4 Radiation dose

Radiation exposure in CT is dependent on scan parameters, scanner, and patient characteristics. Radiation dose with CT is generally 5–10× higher than corresponding conventional radiography, hence the importance of the ALARA (As Low As Reasonably Achievable) principle in ensuring that the patient receives the lowest possible radiation dose without compromising diagnostic scan quality.

Parameters that are commonly used to describe dose are the volume CT dose index ($CTDI_{vol}$), the total scan dose (dose length product, DLP), and radiation risk (effective dose).

- $CTDI_{vol}$: this is the average local dose delivered to a phantom cross-section (in milliGray, mGy) and indicates the average local dose delivered to the patient. CTDI will underestimate the dose for children and slim patients, and overestimate this for obese patients.

♦ *DLP*: this is a measure of the cumulative dose delivered to the patient (in mGy.cm). It takes into account the average dose in the scan volume and the scan length (L).

$$DLP = CTDI_{vol} \times L$$

♦ *Effective dose*: this is an estimate of the radiation risk to patients (in millisieverts, mSv). Mathematical modelling is used to calculate effective dose appropriately weighted for individual organs for a standard male or female (of 70 kg). Again such estimates of E will underestimate the dose for children and slim patients, and over-estimate it for obese patients.

The European guidelines for quality in CT[1] and UK national reference doses for CT (2003)[2] provide reference doses for CT, indicating the $CTDI_{vol}$ and DLP that should not be exceeded (Table 2.3). The risk of death from radiation-induced cancer has been calculated from BEIR V and IRCP 60 data which extrapolate the risk estimates from accidentally or occupationally exposed groups, therefore reflecting high doses. The risk from diagnostic radiology (much lower doses) has to be extrapolated. The radiation-induced risk of death is approximately 0.5/10,000 persons, while the risk of fatal cancer is 3000/10,000 persons. The radiation-induced risk is age dependent (Table 2.4).

2.4 **Ultrasound**

US remains one of the most widely used imaging modalities worldwide as it offers real-time imaging, is inexpensive, safe, and portable. In general it has moderate sensitivity and specificity. High-frequency sound beams (usually >20 kHz) are used to generate high-resolution anatomical imaging. Modern US equipment still uses a pulse echo approach with a brightness mode (B-mode) display but performance has been improved by the introduction of tissue harmonic imaging, extended field of view imaging, coded pulse excitation, and electronic section focusing; 3D and 4D imaging is also possible. US can also provide functional information, for example assessment of tissue regional perfusion using Doppler or contrast-enhanced US.

2.4.1 **Basic principles**

US pulses are generated by an US transducer made from piezoelectric crystals. As an alternating electric voltage is applied, the crystal changes thickness and vibrates,

Table 2.3 National reference dose levels for multi-slice CT as indicated by UK 2003 national dose review

Body part	CTDIvol (mGy)	DLP (mGy/cm)
Brain	65	930
Chest	13	580
Abdomen	14	470
Abdomen and pelvis	14	560

Table 2.4 Calculated radiation-induced risk of dying from cancer (ICRP 60)

Age (years)	Risk (death per mSv)
0–10	14/100,000
10–20	18/100,000
20–30	7.5/100,000
30–40	3.5/100,000
60	2.0/100,000
80	1.0/100,000

generating a *mechanical wave*. These mechanical waves range in frequency of 2–15 MHz, travelling through biologic tissue at a velocity dependent upon the medium through which it is travelling. Sound travels more rapidly through tissues which demonstrate medium density and elasticity.

US wavelength (length of a single sine-wave cycle in a medium) is related to frequency and speed of sound as follows:

$$c = f\lambda$$

where c = speed of sound; f = frequency; and λ = wavelength.

As an US beam passes through tissue, it loses energy and amplitude. The following contribute to the attenuation of the US beam:

- Transfer of energy to tissue resulting in heating (*absorption*).
- Removal of energy by reflection and scattering.

The *attenuation*—measured in decibels per centimetre (dB/cm)—is proportional to path length and frequency. Longer path lengths and higher frequencies produce greater attenuation. Thus the depth of the field available when imaging at higher frequency is shorter than at a lower frequency: higher frequencies (>10 MHz) are used to image objects near to the skin surface, while lower frequencies (3–5 MHz) are used for tissue deeper within the body.

Echoes are produced from boundaries between tissues with different mechanical properties. The amount reflected from an interface between two tissues depends on the difference in *acoustic impedance* (Table 2.5), a measure of the tissue's resistance to distortion by US, in turn determined by the density and elasticity of the tissue. The intensity of the echo is proportional to the difference in acoustic impedance between the two tissues. For example, strong echoes are generated at a muscle:fat interface (intensity reflection coefficient = 1.5%). In most soft tissues, acoustic impedances are fairly similar, so the proportion of a sound pulse reflected at each interface is relatively small and most of the US energy is transmitted further into the body. If an US pulse encounters reflectors that have dimensions smaller than its wavelength (i.e. d < λ), then *scattering* occurs, with echoes reflected through a wide range of angles. For example, the *speckled* texture of organs like the liver is the result of interference between multiple

Table 2.5 Acoustic impedance values of various tissues

Tissue	Acoustic impedance (kg/m$^{(2)}$/s)
Air	$0.0004 \times 10^{(6)}$
Fat	$1.38 \times 10^{(6)}$
Water	$1.48 \times 10^{(6)}$
Liver	$1.65 \times 10^{(6)}$
Bone	$7.80 \times 10^{(6)}$

scattered echoes. The depth of any structure giving rise to an echo can be determined from the time taken for the sound pulse to reach it and the time for the echo to return to the surface, because the velocity of sound is very similar in all soft tissue. Echoes returning from greater depths must be amplified to compensate for the attenuation.

2.4.2 Image generation

US pulses required for image generation are produced by transducers consisting of piezoelectric elements which also receive the reflected US pulse producing real-time images. Transducers may be linear, curvilinear, or radial. Most modern US machines use transducers consisting of multiple arrays with as many as 196 elements. The US beam is not uniform, altering in configuration as it moves away from the transducer. Initially the beam converges after leaving the transducer. This corresponds to the near field and is narrowest at its focal distance; it then diverges. The US beam diameter is affected by:

- *US frequency*: higher frequency US provides better image resolution as the near field is longer than at lower frequencies, but it is more heavily absorbed.
- *Distance from the transducer.*
- *Transducer diameter*: the near field is longer with larger diameter transducers, thus image resolution is better.
- *Use of mechanical or electronic* focusing: focusing can only be achieved within the near field.

Amplification of received echoes is necessary for image generation. Immediately after echoes are received by the transducer, echoes are pre-amplified uniformly. Noise and clutter are reduced by removal of small signals and demodulation.

2.4.3 Ultrasound methods

Modern US scanners are based on B-mode imaging where echoes of differing magnitudes are displayed as a greyscale. However, different methods can be applied to further improve imaging or obtain functional information.

Tissue harmonic imaging is based on frequencies that are multiples of the frequency of the transmitted pulse (fundamental frequency). The second harmonic (twice the fundamental frequency) is most commonly used to generate an image. Artefacts and clutter from multiple pulse reflections in surface tissues are also rejected, thus tissue harmonic imaging is ideal for patients with thick body walls who would normally be challenging and sub-optimally imaged.

Spatial compound imaging is a method to reduce speckle. Electronic steering of the US beam is used to image the same tissue multiple times using parallel beams oriented along different directions. Echoes from these multiple acquisitions are then averaged into a single composite image with the effect of reducing speckle and improving contrast and margin definition.

Extended field of view imaging allows a single composite image with a large field of view to be obtained. By slowly translating the transducer laterally across the region of interest, multiple images are acquired which are registered relative to each other to generate a single composite image. This is useful to assess vessels, for example for deep venous thrombosis or stenotic disease.

2.4.4 Doppler ultrasound

The Doppler principle states that there is a shift in frequency of a sound wave as the source of the sound moves relative to an observer. This change in frequency is called the Doppler frequency shift (DFS) which can be depicted by:

$$DFS = (2 \times IF \times BF/c) \times cosine\ \theta$$

where BF = blood flow; IF = incident frequency; c = speed of sound; θ = angle between the US beam and vascular flow.

This can be exploited to demonstrate tissue or organ vascularity. Doppler techniques include:

- *Continuous wave (CW) Doppler*: velocity is portrayed as a function of time. The blood flow patterns in the arteries can be shown by a simple CW Doppler device with two transducers, one for transmitting and one for receiving.
- *Pulsed Doppler*: the spatial distribution of blood flow can be obtained from Doppler analysis of US pulses. Different velocities are portrayed in a range of colour in a 2D image. By convention, red represents flow towards and blue away from the transducer. Different intensities of colour represent velocity and turbulence.
- *Colour Doppler*: B-mode images with superimposed Doppler information in colour.

2.4.5 Imaging with ultrasound contrast agents

These consist of gas microbubbles, stabilized by a shell of albumin or lipid, that have very different acoustic impedances from soft tissue. As the US contrast agent is injected into a vein and passes through the tissues being imaged the microbubbles are broken up by the US waves. The large number of small bubbles increases scatter, producing more echoes, enabling areas that are well perfused to be identified. For example, microbubbles enable differentiation of a benign liver lesion such as haemangioma or focal nodular hyperplasia from a metastasis (Figure 2.3).

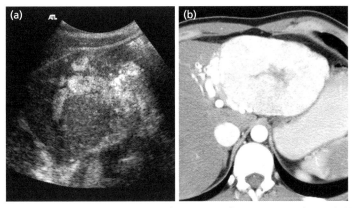

Fig. 2.3 Contrast-enhanced US images, with corresponding contrast-enhanced CT showing a benign focal nodular hyperplasia.

2.5 **Magnetic resonance imaging**

MRI is a versatile technique, capable of multiplanar high-definition imaging of soft tissues with a good sensitivity and specificity. Whilst it does not carry the same risks of ionizing radiation exposure, special precautions to remove all ferromagnetic materials from the patient and to assess prosthetic implants for imaging suitability on online databases is required, for example cardiac pacemakers. It is also important to relate risk to magnetic field strength since an implant safe at one field strength may not be safe at another.

2.5.1 **Magnetic resonance principles**

Three main types of magnet are used in clinical MRI installations: permanent ferromagnets, and resistive and superconducting electromagnets. The most commonly used superconducting MRI scanners work at a field strength of 1.5 tesla. Lower field strengths may be preferred for specialist applications such as extremity imaging and higher field strengths confer advantages in image signal-to-noise, speed of acquisition or resolution.

MR imaging is based on the principle that positively-charged protons in the body water line up with or against the magnetic field B_o, depending on their energy. A relatively small number of them line up predominantly with the field, and are termed the net magnetization, M_o. For most applications, this is taken to lie along the main (Z) axis of the scanner, and therefore along the patient. The individual protons do not actually line up: they rotate or spin around the Z axis with a frequency directly proportional to the field strength: this is termed the *Larmor frequency* and is given by the *Larmor equation*:

$$\omega_o = \gamma B_o$$

where ω_o is the angular frequency of rotation, γ is the gyromagnetic ratio (constant of proportionality: fixed for a given nucleus) and B_o the magnetic field strength in tesla

(T). Bold italic text indicates a vector quantity, that is, there is implied direction as well as magnitude. The nuclei are usually referred to as *spins*.

To acquire an image, a radiofrequency (RF) energy pulse with a bandwidth of frequencies centred around the Larmor frequency is produced using an RF power amplifier. It feeds currents to the RF transmit coil (usually the *body coil*), producing a circularly polarized magnetic field. This so-called B_1 field locally overcomes the main field B_0 and so the net magnetisation tips to rotate around the B_1 field direction instead, gaining energy as they do so. The RF pulses can either be given enough energy to flip the spins exactly orthogonal to their starting position (the RF pulse is then termed a 90° pulse), antiparallel to it (180° pulse), or any intermediate angle.

At the end of the RF pulse, the orientation of the spins returns to its base position giving off the energy they gained in an exponential decay, characterized by *relaxation times*, termed T1 and T2. The energy release is detected either by the same coil used to transmit the RF pulse, or a smaller, more sensitive *surface coil* which is much closer to the tissue of interest and can acquire higher resolution data. Most data are acquired via surface coils.

2.5.2 Image generation

A 'slice' of the patient is selected by applying a gradient, which changes the Larmor frequencies of spins along itself. This can be in any orientation, as the XYZ gradients can be used singly or in combination. An RF pulse with a given bandwidth of frequencies is applied, and only those spins in the patient with corresponding Larmor frequencies will be excited. The spins in the slice are then encoded using an orthogonal combination of gradients in Z (transverse, or axial), X (sagittal), and Y (coronal) orientations. For a typical axial image, X will be termed the 'frequency encoding' direction and Y the 'phase encoding' direction. However, this encoding takes time, and the *free induction decay* (FID, the exponential decay of the signal as the protons return to their original position), is usually much faster than the time it takes to perform the encoding. To compensate for this, more gradients and/or (usually) 180° RF pulses are used to form an *echo* of the initial signal, which is detected after the encoding. If the echo is formed by an RF pulse, it is termed a *spin echo*; if a gradient is used, it is a *gradient echo*. A diagram of spin echo formation (and associated T2* decay) is given in Figure 2.4.

Images are built up line by line using multiple *repetitions* of pulse + gradient sequences and the signal amplitudes of each line recorded by the computers in the scanner. At the end of a sequence, the images are reconstructed using a mathematical transformation called a *Fourier transform*. Usually, sequences can be designed to collect many image slices at once, in order to save time.

Variables which can be changed by the scanner operator include the echo time TE, repetition time TR, and flip angle, α. These cause the amount of relaxation in the spins to vary before signal readout, and a knowledge of the intrinsic relaxation times T1 and T2 for a given tissue allows the changing of image contrast between imaging sequences, allowing different physiological characteristics to be assessed. Most basic images are therefore termed T1-*weighted* or T2-*weighted* (Figure 2.5).

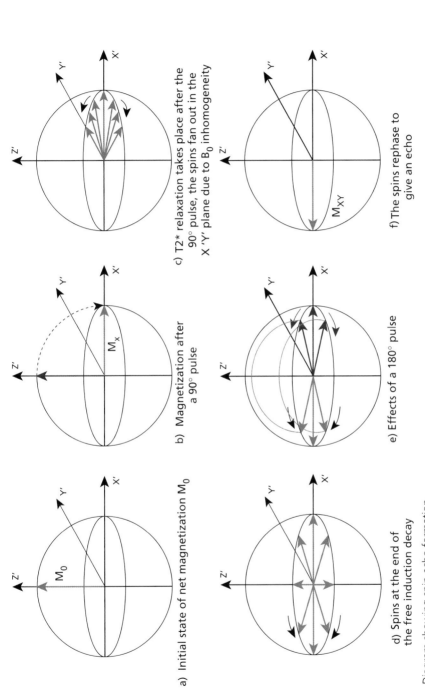

a) Initial state of net magnetization M_0

b) Magnetization after a 90° pulse

c) T2* relaxation takes place after the 90° pulse, the spins fan out in the X'Y' plane due to B_0 inhomogeneity

d) Spins at the end of the free induction decay

e) Effects of a 180° pulse

f) The spins rephase to give an echo

Fig. 2.4 Diagram showing spin echo formation.

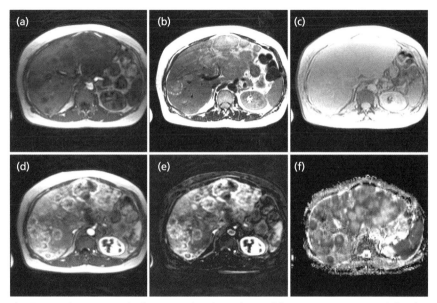

Fig. 2.5 MR images acquired at 1.5 T showing colorectal liver metastases: T1-weighted pre-contrast (a), T2-weighted (b), PD-weighted (c), T1-weighted postcontrast (d), T1 subtraction (e), and ADC map (f).

T1-weighted scans have short TE and short TR, and show long T1 tissues as dark and short T1 tissues as bright. Contrast agents such as gadolinium, which tend to shorten T1, therefore highlight tissues where it is taken up. Water, which has a long T1, appears relatively dark, and fat, with a short T1 is bright. T2-weighted scans have long TE and long TR. They show tissues with longer T2 as bright, as the shorter T2 tissues' signal will have decayed away at the long echo times used. This is very useful for showing fluid around tumours, for example gliomas, or tumours in prostate peripheral zones, where the tumour appears darker than the peripheral zone. Fat is less bright than water. Another common sequence used is termed *proton-density* (Figure 2.5) as it shows the relative proton densities within the slice. Gradient echo sequences bring in another relaxation time weighting called T2*, which allows magnetic field variations to be assessed.

In Figure 2.4, T2* is the decay constant of the FID. This can be refocused by a spin echo but not a gradient echo sequence, thus is only a significant contrast mechanism in the latter. A combination of T2* and T1-weighting is useful for looking at contrast agents such as ferromagnetic or gadolinium particles, which work by changing the local field around them, and therefore the tissue relaxation times. A post-contrast T1-weighted gradient echo image is shown in comparison with the pre-contrast (Figure 2.5).

2.5.3 Advanced imaging

Modern scanners permit more flexible scanning beyond basic spin and gradient echo sequences. This stems from technological developments including *parallel imaging* speeding up acquisition, increasing resolution, and reducing scan time. Another development is implementation of echo-planar imaging (EPI). This technique requires very fast gradient switching, but can acquire an entire image in <1 s. It enables measurement of physiological factors such as *water diffusion* in tissues: depending on the cellular organization and density, this can be predominantly in one direction (isotropic) or all (anisotropic), restricted (dense cellular structure) or unrestricted (loose structure) (Figure 2.5).

Dynamic contrast-enhanced (DCE) MRI (Figure 2.6) consists of injecting contrast, usually gadolinium-based, while rapid T1-weighted gradient echo or EPI scanning takes place. Permeability of the vasculature can be assessed both semi-quantitatively evaluating the initial area under the gadolinium concentration-time curve in the first minute ($IAUGC_{60}$) or by generating fully-quantitative data such as K^{trans} (the rate at which the contrast passes into the extracellular space), the extracellular space volume, v_e, the onset time at which the contrast arrives at a given region, and the rate at which it passes back out to the plasma again, k_{ep}.

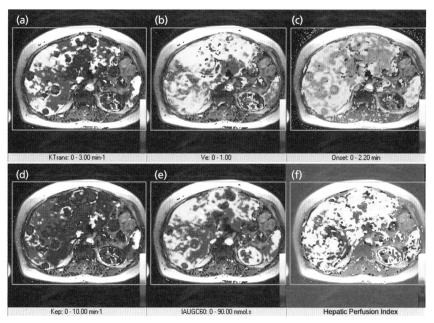

Fig. 2.6 Parametric images, all calculated from one DCE-MRI data set of 40 images: (a) K^{trans}; (b) v_e; (c) onset time; (d) k_{ep}; (e) $IAUGC_{60;}$ and (f) hepatic perfusion index.

2.6 **Radionuclide radiology**

This section deals with common investigative techniques that utilize the administration of a radiopharmaceutical, which is then imaged (or counted) with a gamma camera, concentrating on the management of patients with malignant conditions.

2.6.1 The radiopharmaceutical (radiotracer)

A radiopharmaceutical consists of a radionuclide bound to a pharmaceutical. The radionuclide provides the gamma radiation which forms the image and is chosen for its physical properties of half-life, gamma energy emitted (i.e. in the range of 100–250 keV which is best captured by a gamma camera), 'purity' of emission (i.e. no undesirable alpha or beta particles), and simplicity of production. It should also bind well to the bioactive compound or molecule, not dissociating under physiological conditions. The pharmaceutical enables the targeting of the particular physiological process of interest to the investigator. This can range from osteoblastic activity to left ventricular ejection fraction to specific peptide receptor expression.

Some physiological processes can be targeted by the radionuclide without a pharmaceutical. Iodine transport in the thyroid via the sodium iodine symporter can be imaged with radioisotopes of iodine, ^{123}I and ^{131}I. For imaging ^{123}I is preferred as it is a pure gamma emitter, whereas ^{131}I is also a beta emitter and therefore can be used for therapy. ^{123}I can only be produced in a cyclotron, limiting its availability and so benign thyroid disease is imaged with ^{99m}Tc-pertechnetate which follows a similar physiological pathway.

^{99m}Tc (an isomer of technetium) is the workhorse of the nuclear medicine department due to its ideal imaging properties. It emits a 140 keV gamma ray, giving good penetration of soft tissue, while causing minimal damage. This energy is ideal for imaging by the gamma camera crystal. Its half-life of 6.03 hours is convenient for the logistics of production, administration, and imaging over a few hours—and short enough to allow acceptable outpatient use (it does not linger, giving the patient and surroundings ongoing radiation exposure). The daughter isotope ^{99}Tc (a beta emitter) has a long half-life and is excreted in the urine before it decays. It is generated from molybdenum-99 which has a long half-life of 66 hours, allowing a generator to last a working week. It readily binds to a variety of pharmaceuticals.

2.6.2 The gamma camera

A gamma camera consists of crystals linked to photomultiplier tubes (PMTs). The crystals consisting of sodium iodide with added thallium capture the incident gamma photons emitted from the patient. The photon releases its energy to an electron, exciting it. The electron then falls back to a lower energy state and a light photon is emitted. The crystal is linked to a close fitting array of PMTs which amplify and locate the signal. The incident light photons from the crystal hit the entry window which is a photocathode. They liberate electrons—the photoelectric effect. These are accelerated and amplified via a series of dynodes through the tube to reach the end anode. This produces a current which gives a voltage which varies over time depending on the energy of the original gamma photon. Every incident gamma photon on the crystal will produce a scatter of light from the crystal into a group of PMTs at varying distances from the collision. The relative intensity of the signal from each neighbouring tube can be compared to give the location of each collision event.

As gamma photons leave the patient in random directions, a collimator is placed between the patient and crystal to exclude radiation that is not useful in forming the image, thus bringing the image into 'focus'. The collimator excludes radiation with an oblique incident angle (by absorption and scatter)—only allowing through gamma photons at a narrow angle useful in forming the image. The choice of collimator depends on the gamma energies involved and the particular examination. The most commonly used is a lead collimator with a series of parallel holes. A pinhole collimator is a cone which works like a camera obscura, giving a sharp image but with a small field of view and longer imaging time.

A computer system controls the operation of the camera, acquisition, and storage of acquired images. It is important for image quality to have the head as close as possible to the patient. A simple gamma camera has a single head and is static. A dual-headed camera can image a patient from two different angles simultaneously. Either can be used with a moving table. The heads can be positioned manually or automatically. Some have software and infrared sensors to adjust the position of the head according to the contours of the patient's body as it moves past. Pressure sensors stop the movement of the table if the gamma camera head is touched.

2.6.3 Single photon emission computed tomography

A single photon emission computed tomography (SPECT) camera is a type of gamma camera. It can acquire images tomographically. SPECT imaging is analogous to X-ray CT in that the image is acquired by rotating detectors around the patient, that is, gamma camera heads (usually two) then reconstructing an image in three planes. This localizes the focus of activity in 3D and improves the visualization of faint foci of activity. Very intense concentrations of activity (e.g. the bladder in a bone scan) will produce artefacts, obscuring activity in adjacent structures. SPECT acquisitions can be gated to an electrocardiogram (ECG) allowing imaging of the myocardium and definition of the left ventricular volume. Gamma camera images can also be co-registered with radiographs and CT images to further localize the physiological process to the anatomy.

2.6.4 Imaging

Once the radiopharmaceutical is administered then, depending upon the half-life, multiple subsequent images can be obtained with no further patient dose (unlike X-rays). This allows images of different phases of the radiopharmaceutical's progress through the patient, for example the perfusion, blood pool, and delayed skeletal images of a bone scan, or several views of the same body part from various projections.

Data can be acquired in dynamic or 'spot' modes. The dynamic mode measures activity level as it changes over time. It is used for physiological processes which operate in the time period of the scan, for example the passage of tracer through the kidneys in a MAG3 (mercaptoacetyltriglycine) renogram. The data can be displayed as a series of images or as a time-activity graph. The spot mode records the sum of all activity in a given time. It is used for activity which is more or less constant during the scan, for example renal cortical activity in a DMSA (dimercaptosuccinic acid) scan. The data can also be used to produce an image or as a number of total counts, giving the relative function in various defined regions of interest.

Thus the image produced is not directly of an organ or patient, but a map of the amount of the physiological process under study within the organ or patient. Therefore, on a DMSA study, an image of a fully functioning kidney will be kidney shaped but a damaged kidney will produce an irregular image, indicating the level of function within different parts of the kidney. Gamma camera images can be co-registered with radiographs and CT images to further localize the physiological process to the anatomy. In cardiac imaging, acquisitions can be gated to an ECG, allowing imaging of the myocardium or left ventricular volume.

The great strength of these techniques is that they complement the anatomical detail of radiological examinations with functional information. The target physiology can be highly specific, for example iodine uptake in a deposit of papillary thyroid carcinoma. Often, however, the physiological process targeted is a surrogate marker for malignancy. This can reduce the specificity, for example gallium uptake as a marker for metabolic activity and transferrin receptor status is increased in lymphoma, but also sarcoidosis.

An isotope bone scan uses osteoblastic activity as a marker for the presence of metastases and so produces false negatives if there are lytic deposits with a poor osteoblastic reaction and false positives due to osteoblastic reactions to other processes such as fractures or infection. This makes it essential to interpret results in conjunction with the complete clinical picture, particularly correlating functional and anatomical investigations.

The following are examples of the way in which radionuclide imaging contributes to the management of patients with malignancy.

2.6.4.1 The isotope bone scan

The radiopharmaceutical ^{99m}Tc MDP (methylene-diphosphonate) is taken up by active osteoblasts. Osteoblastic activity may be a marker for the presence of metastases but will produce false positives due to osteoblastic reactions in other processes such as fractures or infection and false negatives with lytic deposits with a poor osteoblastic reaction. Causes of apparent increased activity on a ^{99m}Tc MDP bone scan include:

♦ True increased osteoblastic activity.

♦ Increased arterial supply to a body part, for example inflammation.

♦ Impaired venous drainage of a body part, for example deep vein thrombosis.

♦ Excretion of radiopharmaceutical, for example in urine.

♦ Distance from gamma camera head, for example iliac crests appear more active on anterior images, sacroiliac joints appear more active on posterior images.

♦ Lack of intervening soft tissue, for example the pectoral muscles attenuate gamma photons from the ribs but not the sternum.

♦ Thickness of bone, for example the distal humerus has a greater volume of bone than the shaft, producing a difference in apparent activity.

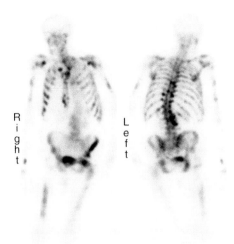

Fig. 2.7 99mTc MDP bone scan: patchy diffuse foci of increased activity throughout the central axial skeleton and proximal long bones with low background and renal activity indicates a metastatic 'superscan'. This results from the osteoblastic response to the widespread skeletal malignant deposits typical of prostate carcinoma metastases.

True osteoblastic activity can be in response to many processes, from malignancy to infection, Paget's disease to fractures. Thus the art of interpretation is to pay attention to the pattern of activity and correlation with the clinical picture and other imaging techniques (Figure 2.7). Lytic deposits without osteoblastic reactions will produce photopenic 'holes' in the normal bone activity. The isotope bone scan can also demonstrate paraneoplastic processes such as hypertrophic osteoarthropathy (Figure 2.8).

2.6.4.2 The multi-gated acquisition scan

Multi-gated acquisition (some companies use analysis) (MUGA) is a technique used as a method of measuring left ventricular ejection fraction in a reproducible manner. This is important in oncology for monitoring patients undergoing therapies with cardiotoxic side effects such as trastuzumab.

To assess the left ventricular luminal volume the radiotracer must stay within the intravascular space, thus red blood cells are the ideal 'tracer'. In order to label the red cells with the radionuclide (^{99m}Tc), the patient is injected with a stannous (tin) salt. Later the pertechnetate is injected, enters the red cell, is reduced by the stannous salt, and then cannot diffuse back out again. A more laborious *in vitro* labelling method is described but not often used in clinical departments.

The camera head is put in an oblique position to throw the left ventricle into relief, free of overlapping structures, and the number of radioactive counts obtained over about 10–15 min. This data acquisition is gated to an ECG, so the software can divide the counts into those acquired during different phases of the cardiac cycle, plotting a graph of activity versus phase of cardiac cycle. The total activity in all the time points

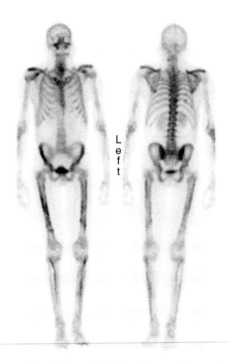

Fig. 2.8 Irregular increased cortical activity in both femora in a patient with lung cancer, typical of HOA.

in end systole is compared to those in end diastole. This activity is proportional to the volume of the ventricle and so an ejection fraction can be calculated.

The final report includes a summated image acquired in end systole and end diastole to demonstrate the regions of interest have been accurately sited over the left ventricle and area of lung for background correction and that there is no overlapping activity from adjacent structures, such as the spleen. There is also a diagram showing the wall motion divided into segments, but the oncologist will generally be interested in the overall percentage figure and any change in the value over the course of treatment.

2.7 Positron emission tomography

Positron emission tomography (PET) is used for detecting and localizing cancers, distinguishing benign from malignant tumours, staging, and monitoring response to treatment. It is generally more sensitive than anatomical imaging for cancer detection, and may be more specific.

2.7.1 Basic principles

PET relies upon the administration of positron-emitting radio pharmaceuticals, of which the most common in routine use is the glucose analogue ^{18}F-fluorodeoxyglucose (^{18}F-FDG). The ^{18}F molecule is unstable and decays via emission of a positron and neutrino to form stable non-toxic ^{18}O. Energetic emitted positrons scatter with electrons in tissue before combining to annihilate, creating two 511 keV photons emitted ~180° apart that are detected in PET scanners.

These two emitted 511 keV photons travel through tissue before being recorded in rings of detectors surrounding the patient. The detectors consist of scintillator crystals coupled to photo multiplier tubes where interacting photons create pulses of light that are converted to electrical signals. If two signals are recorded within a small time window (nanoseconds) in the detection circuitry then a coincidence event has potentially occurred, creating a line-of-response (LOR) that defines the relative position of the event for use in image reconstruction.

Typical crystal scintillators employed today are based on bismuth germanate (BGO), lutetium oxyorthosilicate (LSO), and gadolinium oxyorthosilicate (GSO). Required characteristics for PET crystals are high detection efficiency for good sensitivity, fast speed to reduce random noise, and good energy resolution to reduce scatter. Some scanners can be operated in 2D or 3D acquisition mode. In 2D scanning, physical septa are placed between detector rings to accept relatively parallel LOR in order to reduce interplane scatter (~20%) and enable simple and speedy image reconstruction at the expense of detection sensitivity. In 3D scanning, septa are retracted and all LOR are accepted, resulting in approximately five times the sensitivity compared with 2D. However, scatter increases by up to 50%, as do random events, thus requiring superior timing and scatter compensation in hardware and software compared with 2D. In 3D more bed positions are also scanned due to the non-uniform axial sensitivity encountered. Modern scanners utilize 3D-list mode data acquisition for increased versatility with iterative image reconstruction and recent fast time-of-flight systems offer superior signal-to-noise ratio.

2.7.2 Fundamental limitations

Positron range depends upon its kinetic energy and Table 2.6 illustrates this for different radiopharmaceuticals and tissues. The residual kinetic energy of the positron before annihilation translates into an angular variation of ~0.5° for photons created post annihilation. FDG positron range and photon non-collinearity are limitations to image resolution.

Table 2.6 The effect of energy on positron range in different tissues

Radioisotope	Max energy (KeV)	Cortical bone FWHM (mm)	Soft tissue FWHM (mm)	Lung tissue FWHM (mm)
^{18}F	633	0.18	0.19	0.37
^{11}C	959	0.22	0.28	0.52
^{13}N	1197	0.26	0.33	0.62
^{15}O	1738	0.33	0.41	0.86
^{68}Ga	1900	0.36	0.49	0.98
^{82}Rb	3350	0.56	0.76	1.43

FWHM, full width at half-maximum.

2.7.3 **Imaging**

FDG is phosphorylated intracellularly into FDG-6-phosphate and trapped, taking no further part in the glycolytic pathway, and the image therefore represents a map of glucose utilization in the scanned area. Typically scanning is performed at least one hour after intravenous injection, which allows for sufficient FDG uptake to achieve good signal-to-noise ratio for imaging lesions.

Modern imaging combines PET with CT to give added topographical information on the distribution of FDG. Initially a full helical CT image set is acquired, then the couch moves into the PET component where individual bed positions, typically about 16 cm in length, are scanned to cover the entire body length required; this may take up to 30 min (Figure 2.9). In fused images the registration accuracy of ~1 mm arises from precise mechanical alignment in scanners. Artefacts arising from respiratory motion and attenuation correction are known pitfalls and can be minimized with experience and by using gating techniques.

Malignant cells typically have a higher glucose metabolism compared with normal cells and hence may be identified on PET; however, increased glucose metabolism is not unique to malignancy and hence false positive scans may occur in areas of infection and inflammation. Additional functional information is available by performing kinetic investigations in PET with dynamic scanning techniques.

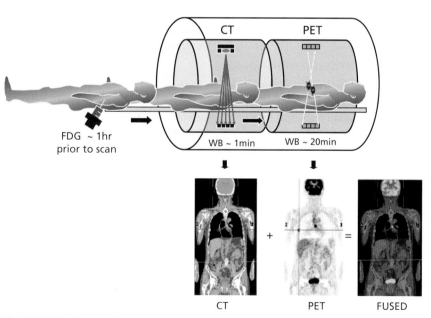

Fig. 2.9 Clinical PET/CT depicting transmission scanning in CT and emission scanning in PET leading to fused whole body images.

2.8 **Imaging in clinical oncology**

Imaging is an integral part of clinical oncology and continues to play an essential role in the diagnostic and therapeutic pathways of our patients. Over the past few decades, we have seen an evolution in radiotherapy treatment planning from the use of 2D planning to the advent of CT simulators and more recently, the introduction of multileaf collimators and inverse planning, leading to the introduction of intensity-modulated radiotherapy (IMRT) and image-guided radiotherapy (IGRT). These technological advancements have improved tumour control and reduced treatment-related toxicities with the delivery of more focused and targeted radiation. However, these advancements have placed an even greater emphasis on the need of good quality imaging tools to guide radiation therapy. In this section, we will explore the use of imaging in clinical oncology.

2.8.1 **Diagnostic role**

2.8.1.1 Diagnosis

Tumour biopsy under US or CT guidance are commonly used now as an alternative to more invasive procedures such as bronchoscopy or laparoscopy. However, the ultimate goal is to have an imaging tool that could replace tissue diagnosis. Unfortunately, this is still beyond what the current imaging technology can achieve. Nonetheless, a unique tumour that may be diagnosed based on radiological and clinical features is hepatocellular carcinoma (HCC). A liver tumour which shows the classical imaging features of arterial hypervascularity and venous or delayed phase washout on a background of liver cirrhosis can be diagnosed as HCC without the need for biopsy prior to definitive treatment. However, this does not apply in other tumours. The American College of Radiology has introduced standardized imaging reporting datasets to categorize radiological features into risk categories of increasing malignant potential in breast (Breast Imaging Reporting and Data System [BI-RADS]), prostate (Prostate Imaging Reporting & Data System [PI-RADS]), and liver cancers (Liver Imaging Reporting & Data System [LI-RADS]) in order to help clinicians to identify suspicious tumours for further evaluation.

2.8.1.2 Staging

Cross-sectional imaging such as CT and MRI are routinely used to diagnose and stage cancers. CT remains the standard staging modality in most cancer types, particularly in less developed countries, due to its widespread availability, ease of access and cost. However, its limited soft tissue contrast makes it less ideal for local tumour (T) staging in certain tumours such as prostate and rectal cancers. In these cancer types, MRI has played an important role in stratifying patients for treatment based on its superior soft tissue characterization for T staging and additional physiological information derived from DCE and diffusion-weighted (DWI) sequences compared to standard CT. In addition to cross-sectional imaging, endoscopic ultrasound (EUS) is also an important tool for tumour staging. EUS has superior T staging accuracy compared to cross-sectional imaging for oesophageal cancer coupled with its ability to sample suspicious lymph nodes. Despite this, EUS is still underutilized in oesophageal staging because of its user dependency and the lack of trained endoscopists.

With regards to nodal and distant tumour staging, ^{18}F-FDG PET/CT is now widely accepted as part of the standard staging pathway for melanoma, lymphoma, head and neck, lung, breast, and upper gastrointestinal cancers. It has improved staging accuracy, leading to tumour stage migration which has influenced subsequent patient management and ultimately improved patient survival. In non-small cell lung cancer (NSCLC), ^{18}F-FDG PET has shown superior sensitivity and specificity in mediastinal nodal staging compared to CT. In addition, up to a third of patients with conventionally staged locally advanced NSCLC initially suitable for radical chemoradiation were found to have occult metastatic disease (20%) and locoregional disease too extensive for radical irradiation (10%) following PET staging.[3] Similar findings were also found in other tumour types.

Ideally, all patients should have equal access to the different types of staging modalities but this is not feasible in the real world. Hence, the choice of any imaging modalities in cancer staging will depend on a number of factors such as intent of treatment, affordability, ease of access and patient suitability (e.g. presence of contraindications to MRI).

2.8.1.3 Prognosis

Imaging may also have a role in risk stratifying and prognosticating patients. The prognostic value of TNM staging, lymphovascular/perineural invasion, and extramural/capsular extension is well established. In recent years, there is growing interest to identify additional qualitative and quantitative imaging features that may portend poor prognosis. Functional imaging holds great promise in this regard as it could provide surrogates for aggressive tumour phenotypes, for example cellular metabolism, proliferation, and hypoxia.

Pre-treatment ^{18}F-FDG PET parameters such as maximum standardized uptake values (SUV_{max}) and metabolic tumour volume (MTV) were shown to be associated with overall survival in various cancers including lung, head and neck, oesophageal, pancreatic, endometrial, ovarian, and cervical cancers. Early evidence also suggests that DWI parameters such as apparent diffusion coefficient (ADC) may be associated with aggressive pathological features in prostate, rectal, and gynaecological cancers. However, it is important to remember that most of these findings although promising, cannot be reliably used to direct patient management at present due to unresolved issues regarding standardization of image acquisition and analysis protocols, as well as the unknown impact of intra- and intertumoral heterogeneity.

2.8.2 Therapeutic role

2.8.2.1 Tumour volume delineation

With the shift from 2D to 3D planning and now IMRT, there is a need to accurately define target volumes and organs at risk (OARs) in order to improve local tumour control and decrease treatment-related toxicities, resulting in a surge of interest in the use of PET and MRI in target volume delineation. ^{18}F-FDG PET has shown potential in improving the contouring accuracy in clinical practice. Its role in lung cancer radiation planning has been the most extensively studied, differentiating lung tumours from adjacent atelectasis although experience in other tumour types has also been reported.[4,6] The use of ^{18}F-FDG PET may significantly alter the treatment volumes compared to the use of planning CT alone. PET may also identify suspicious metabolically active mediastinal/supraclavicular nodal disease and is increasingly used in oesophageal, lymphoma, and head and neck radiation planning. In oesophageal cancer, PET is commonly fused with planning CT to assist with the definition of the craniocaudal extent of primary tumours. In lymphoma and head and neck cancers, it is predominantly used for nodal volume delineation. In most head and neck cancers, MRI is commonly fused with the planning CT for primary tumour delineation due to its superior soft tissue definition compared to CT or PET. Most studies have shown that GTV using CT or MR tends to overestimate the actual tumour extent, with ^{18}F-FDG PET-defined GTVs showing the best pathological correlation, although these correlations are modest at best.

Furthermore, there are many complexities associated with the use of MRI/^{18}F-FDG PET in radiation planning which remains CT based. In most cases, these scans are performed at different time points relative to simulation and are not done in the radiotherapy treatment positions which create problems with subsequent co-registration of the diagnostic and simulation images for radiation planning purpose. Rigid image registration using bony anatomy is commonly used in intracranial and prostate cancers where tumour motion is negligible, but this has limited utility in mobile thoracic or intra-abdominal tumours. Non-rigid or deformable registration, where the pixel-to-pixel relationships within the diagnostic images are changed to adapt to the reference planning CT, was introduced to overcome these issues by improving the mapping of tumour volumes between the two datasets. However, there are limited validation studies to support the routine use of non-rigid registration in clinical practice due to the uncertainties regarding the accuracy of such image deformation algorithms. Where possible, the MRI or PET scans that are used for radiation planning should be performed in the treatment positions, and the interval between these scans and CT simulation should be kept as short as possible.

Hence, although MRI and PET have the potential to help oncologists to better define tumour volumes, we should be aware of the limitations associated with each imaging modality and its use in different tumour types. The advances in anatomical and functional imaging have huge potential to improve radiotherapy volume delineation when they are used appropriately.

2.8.2.2 Image-guided radiotherapy

The introduction of cone beam CT (CBCT) on the linear accelerator allows interfraction tumour localization, which greatly increases the precision of radiation delivery and enables hypofractionated treatment in the range of 8–30 Gy per fraction in extracranial sites. This led to the surge in the adoption of stereotactic ablative/body radiotherapy (SABR/SBRT) in various tumour types due to its superior local control and favourable toxicity profile. However, the image quality of CBCTs remains suboptimal, especially of intra-abdominal or pelvic tumours.

In addition, the use of MRI-guided brachytherapy has improved outcomes in cervical and prostate cancers.[7,8] This allowed for more refined dose distribution and encouraged dose escalation to dominant tumours, hence increasing the therapeutic ratio.

However, widespread adoption of this technique is still limited, particularly in countries with limited resources as it requires rigorous imaging protocols and intensive manpower.

2.8.2.3 Response assessment

A pertinent use of imaging is in the assessment of treatment response following non-surgical therapy. Radical (chemo)radiation is a standard treatment in unresectable or locally advanced lung, head and neck, and upper gastrointestinal cancers. Discerning residual or recurrent tumours from radiation-related CT changes can be difficult. Standardized reporting guidelines such as Response Evaluation Criteria in Solid Tumours (RECIST) was established to provide a reproducible objective quantitative volumetric assessment to evaluate treatment response. In those with suspicious CT findings, the use of follow-up ^{18}F-FDG PET has helped oncologists to identify patients for salvage therapy. Significant FDG uptake in treated tumours will raise suspicion of residual or recurrent disease, provided that there is an adequate interval between the end of radiation and PET scan (typically at least 3–6 months, with improved accuracy as the interval increases). Similarly, PET Response Criteria in Solid Tumours (PERCIST) is also used to quantify changes in SUV_{peak} for response assessment.

Early interim ^{18}F-FDG PET has been shown to have prognostic value in oesophageal cancer and lymphoma treated with chemotherapy. This identifies early non-responders for treatment intensification or triggers a switch in therapy. In contrast, a watch and wait strategy is an attractive option as it allows patients with complete response to avoid the morbidities of surgery and is currently being evaluated in rectal cancer and N2/N3 nodal metastases in head and neck cancers. This strategy requires intensive imaging follow-up to detect disease relapse early to allow timely salvage treatment without compromising on survival.

Identification of patients at risk of radiation toxicities is still an evolving field. Pre-treatment ^{18}F-FDG PET uptake in normal lungs (SUV_{95}) is postulated to predict for risk of radiation pneumonitis in NSCLC and oesophageal cancer.[9,10]

2.9 **Future directions**

Imaging will continue to play an important role in the practice of clinical oncology. Technological advances in imaging hardware and software will increase its utility in cancer management, with strong emphasis in functional imaging that offers glimpses of *in vivo* intratumoral physiology which are also targets of novel therapies. MRI/PET simulators and MRI-linear accelerators are now available and may soon be ready for clinical use. This will improve tumour delineation and localization, and ultimately treatment outcomes. Last but not least, intertumoral genetic heterogeneity is well established which may affect the intrinsic tumour radiosensitivity. Imaging has the ability to assess intertumoral phenotypic heterogeneity in a non-invasive manner. The combination of genomics and radiological features termed 'radiogenomics' has potential to improve clinical decision making and patient outcomes.

References

1. **European Commission (1999)**. *European Guidelines on Quality Criteria for Computed Tomography. EUR 16262 EN*. Luxembourg: Office for Official Publications for the European Communities.
2. **Shrimpton PC, Hillier MC, Lewis MA, et al.** (2003). *Doses from Computed Tomography (CT) Examinations in the UK 2003 review. NRPB-W67*. Chiltern: National Radiation Protection Board, UK.
3. **MacManus MP, Hicks RJ, Ball DL, et al.** (2001). F-18 fluorodeoxyglucose positron emission tomography staging in radical radiotherapy candidates with non-small cell lung carcinoma: powerful correlation with survival and high impact on treatment. *Cancer.* **92**(4): 886–895.
4. **Konert T, Vogel W, MacManus MP, et al.** (2015). PET/CT imaging for target volume delineation in curative intent radiotherapy of non-small cell lung cancer: IAEA consensus report 2014. *Radiother Oncol.* **116**(1): 27–34.
5. **MacManus M, Nestle U, Rosenzweig KE, et al.** (2009). Use of PET and PET/CT for radiation therapy planning: IAEA expert report 2006–2007. *Radiotherapy and Oncology.* **91**(1): 85–94.
6. **Even AJG, van der Stoep J, Zegers CML, et al. (2015).** PET-based dose painting in non-small cell lung cancer: Comparing uniform dose escalation with boosting hypoxic and metabolically active sub-volumes. *Radiother Oncol.* 116(2): 281–6.
7. **Albert JM, Swanson DA, Pugh TJ, et al.** (2013). Magnetic resonance imaging-based treatment planning for prostate brachytherapy. *Brachytherapy.* **12**(1): 30–37.
8. **Tanderup K, Viswanathan AN, Kirisits C, Frank SJ.** (2014). Magnetic resonance image guided brachytherapy. *Semin Radiat Oncol.* **24**(3): 181–91.
9. **Petit SF, van Elmpt WJC, Oberije CJG, et al.** (2011). [18F]fluorodeoxyglucose uptake patterns in lung before radiotherapy identify areas more susceptible to radiation-induced lung toxicity in non small-cell lung cancer patients. *Int J Radiat Oncol.* **81**(3): 698–705.
10. **Castillo R, Pham N, Castillo E, et al.** (2015). Pre-radiation therapy fluorine 18 fluorodeoxyglucose PET helps identify patients with esophageal cancer at high risk for radiation pneumonitis. *Radiology.* **275**(3): 822–31.

Additional resource

Information on specific CT scanning protocols can be found on websites such as http://www.CTisus.org.

Chapter 3

MRI and functional imaging in radiotherapy planning, delivery, and treatment

Huiqi Yang and Thankamma Ajithkumar

3.1 Introduction

Over the decades, continuous technological advances and developments have led to considerable evolution in the way in which radiotherapy is being planned and delivered. The confidence in the anatomical representation of CT-based planning has paved the way for intensity-modulated radiotherapy (IMRT) across a range of tumour sites, where radiotherapy dose is sculpted in great adherence to the underlying anatomy. Better visualization of soft tissue with magnetic resonance imaging (MRI) and the capability of positron emission tomography (PET) scan in accurately measuring biological function have led to the application of these modalities in radiotherapy planning.

3.2 Computed tomography

Current clinical practice of radiotherapy planning of lesions at depth is predominantly CT-based.

Typically, dedicated CT planning scans are acquired at the start of the radiotherapy planning process with the patient in the treatment position in order to maintain geometric accuracy throughout planning process. It is used in radiotherapy volume delineation, dose calculation, treatment verification, and image-guided radiotherapy (IGRT) systems. Although 3D images are commonly used, 4D scans can combat motion issues relevant to body sites such as the thorax.

Use of CT-alone for radiotherapy planning has numerous pitfalls. The presence of metallic implants such as hip replacements and dental fillings arise in streak artefacts in the acquired CT images, which can be substantial relative to the size of the implants. Although the soft tissue contrast of CT images is generally good across a range of body sites, which could be enhanced with intravenous (IV) contrast, on many occasions the visualization is suboptimal (e.g. differentiation between lung tumour and adjacent atelectasis/collapse). Large inter- and intra-observer variation in CT-based volume delineation has been reported for several tumour sites, which can potentially lead to marginal misses and/or suboptimal sparing of normal tissues. For these reasons there has been a drive to adopting other modalities in the radiotherapy treatment pathway.

3.3 **Magnetic resonance imaging**

MRI images are being increasingly used for radiotherapy delineation, primarily due to superiority in soft-tissue contrast compared to CT. The absence of radiation exposure during image acquisition, is particularly preferred for the younger population. The gadolinium-based contrast used in MRI has less risk of nephrotoxicity compared with iodinated CT contrast agents. Additionally, unlike CT scanning, where data acquisition is performed in the axial plane, MR images can be obtained in any orientation, thereby having greater scope in functionality, which can be tailored and aligned according to the tumour and anatomy.

3.3.1 Magnetic resonance workflow in radiotherapy systems

Electron density obtained from CT-based imaging is required for tissue dose calculations. Thus, MRI-only radiotherapy planning workflows are restricted in their capability for estimating dose distributions as image intensity in MRI does not directly correlate with electron density. Currently, most institutions are acquiring separate MRI and CT planning scans which are then used together in the radiotherapy planning process.

Ideally, MRI scans should be performed with patients immobilized in the same position as treatment delivery. Historically, the physical size of the MRI bore limited the use of immobilization devices and, unlike planning CT scan, most diagnostic MRI scanners employ different set-up that focus on patient comfort. Due to the increasing demand for MRI use in radiotherapy processes and with larger bore scanners, commercial systems are developing products and solutions compatible with radiotherapy use.

Co-registration of MRI with CT planning images is commonly done using rigid fusion algorithms based on bone anatomy. It is crucial to ensure that the quality of image alignment is satisfactory to avoid a systematic geometric error during treatment. Despite the presence of multiple fusion algorithms, errors are inherently introduced in this process, especially if there are marked differences in patient position between the scans. Not only can matching be poor with inadequate soft tissue contrast information, differences in the tissue contrast between multimodality imaging can lead to poorer accuracy as compared to single modality registration. The lack of robust measures for quality assessment of co-registration increases the complexity of the problem. The deficiencies of image registration are well recognized, and there remains a continuous pursuit for rigorous solutions to address this issue, such as deformable registration algorithms.

3.3.2 Contrast and soft tissue visualization/artefacts

The use of higher field strengths with higher signal-to-noise ratios (SNRs) results in greater contrast and improved soft tissue resolution. The enhanced visualization of the anatomy for both tumour and organs at risks (OARs) is hugely advantageous as it allows greater accuracy in volume delineation, which is desired in highly conformal treatment delivery such as IMRT. Furthermore, delineation accuracy is imperative in stereotactic treatment techniques where the precision of the delivery allows larger doses per fraction to be used safely whilst minimizing the dose to normal tissues. There are many developments in treatment boosts and dose escalation with MRI-based planning capitalizing on its edge over CT-only systems.

However, there is conflict between obtaining MRI images of high SNR with high spatial resolution in a short time. Due to the different tumour and tissue constituents for a given body site, multiple MRI sequences are often required in order to elicit images with clinically useful contrast characteristics. Together with the acquisition of further functional sequences, execution of MRI workflows is usually more complex due to the tailoring of several different sequences according to the specific site and pathology.

Many metal implants in current clinical use are MRI compatible. During the scan, local currents within metal implants induced by the radiofrequency and gradient fields disrupt the homogeneity of the magnetic field and result in susceptibility artefacts, which cannot be completely eliminated in spite of image distortion minimization techniques. This results in images with residual regions of signal loss and accumulation, which can compromise the radiotherapy planning process. Specialist techniques such as the use of high image gradients to minimize signal loss often come at a cost of increase in acquisition time. Nonetheless, the impact of these artefacts is generally of a much smaller magnitude in MRI as compared to CT.

3.3.3 Treatment position/motion

Ordinarily, CT acquisition takes place over seconds compared to tens of minutes for multiple MRI sequences, where the former is more reflective of the timescales for radiotherapy delivery.

Longer duration for image acquisition is often required in order to obtain images with higher spatial resolution and sufficient image quality, especially of larger body sites such as the pelvis. This augments the risk of subject motion which can jeopardize image quality through blurring. Physiological motion of particular body organs can result in 'ghost' appearances from the reproduction of the object along the phase-encode direction. It may not be possible to match physiological motion (e.g. free breathing) that is captured on MRI examinations directly to radiotherapy delivery, and planning margins for motion assessment may have to be performed separately.

Time-sensitive 4D MRI images can be obtained through the capture of several motion cycles which is then averaged according to the specific phase of motion, in comparison to 4D CT where a single motion cycle is typically acquired. However, irregular physiological motion can give rise to errors in the estimate of 4D MRI which can in turn compromise image quality. Further advances in faster sampling techniques, parallel imaging, and computation can improve this.

3.3.4 Geometric accuracy

The geometric accuracy of MRI images is dependent on the uniformity of the static magnetic field and gradient linearity. Any warping of the field and gradient can lead to distorted images that affect the portrayal of anatomical features in their respective locations.

Due to the trade-off between magnet size and gradients of high magnitude with high slew rates, most MRI images are highly accurate geometrically in the centre of the field of view, which become increasingly distorted towards the periphery, up to a few centimetres at the edges. Thus, this phenomenon has greater impact on larger body sites such as the pelvis, compared to the head. The presence of a subject can also disturb the magnetic field and, depending on the presence of implants and curvature of structures, result in patient-based distortion to varying degree. The differences in distribution of ^{1}H nuclei between fat and water in body tissues also result in signal readouts at frequencies that are slightly offset (i.e. chemical shift).

In the setting of radiotherapy planning where geometric integrity is paramount, careful selection of pulse sequence parameters to achieve high SNR through the balance of high gradient amplitude and high receiver bandwidth is required to mitigate both system- and patient-related geometric distortion. Although post-processing corrections are often applied to limit geometric distortion, this can affect image quality. Additionally, the choice of MR sequences applied to radiotherapy planning has to be circumspect, especially as some uncorrected functional MRI imaging techniques are known to produce significant warping near air interfaces.

3.3.5 Electron density estimation

Various methods have been used to establish an MR-only radiotherapy planning process to simplify the planning pathway, minimize radiation exposure of CT scanning, and eliminate the uncertainties associated with multi-modality image registration.

This involves the construction of MR-based CT equivalent images (i.e. substitute or synthetic CT (s-CT)) generated from MRI data. Although a good approximation of dosimetry can be achieved through bulk electron density assignment, where either single or multiple electron densities are designated according to specific tissue types, this has not taken off due to the time-consuming process of tissue segmentation. Specialized MRI techniques such as ultra-short echo time sequences, which can distinguish and therefore separate tissue types, have been explored that allow the assignment of electron densities to be performed on a voxel-wise basis. Other methods include atlas-based techniques, where a most representative series is selected from a library of pre-existing MRI images and warped to fit the acquired patient images. The resulting deformation field is then applied to the CT associated with the selected pre-existing MRI, to create a series of CT images in the same frame of the acquired MRI. Although this has also been shown to produce good estimation of dosimetric calculations, it suffers from the inadequacies associated with registration-based approaches, including poor results where the anatomy is vastly different to the datasets in the repository.

Despite a number of solutions to MRI-only workflows, none of the approaches have routinely been adopted in clinical practice as yet, owing to their drawbacks and lack of clinical validation.

3.4 **Positron emission tomography**

All clinical PET/CT systems acquire whole-body PET and standard multi-slice CT images within a single gantry. The maximum displacement error of co-axial imaging using combined PET/CT has been demonstrated to be in the region of 0.5 mm, thereby offering complementary functional and anatomical imaging that can be clinically useful.

Due to the presence of both metabolic and structural information of PET/CT images, as well as the availability of electron density maps, they are ideally suited for the radiotherapy planning process. However, most departments worldwide commonly acquire diagnostic PET/CT imaging with different patient set-up to that of radiotherapy treatment. Unless dedicated radiotherapy PET/CT scans are performed, the PET/CT images typically serve as a visual guide in the volume definition process, with separate radiotherapy planning scans for dose calculation purposes.

3.4.1 Positron emission tomography settings

One recognized drawback of PET/CT imaging is the lack of uniformity in image acquisition and reconstruction protocols across different institutions. Non-standardized procedures and settings can affect the quality of the data and limit its generality, as this can result in considerable differences between different centres. Not only does this present as an issue with the accuracy of target delineation and dose modulation, but validation studies will also be difficult to conduct. Although qualitative interpretation of the functional imaging is commonplace, quantitative readings (e.g. standardized uptake value (SUV) for ^{18}F-FDG tracer) allows objective comparison. Guidelines have also been published with the aim of standardizing and improving the robustness of the procedures for image acquisition and interpretation to ensure consistency and reduce data variability.[1]

3.4.2 Sensitivity and specificity of positron emission tomography tracers

The value of PET imaging is also limited by the sensitivity and specificity of PET tracers administered. For example, ^{18}F-FDG provides a measure of glucose metabolism, considered to be a good surrogate for tumour-cell density, which tends to be high for most but not all cancers. Additionally, regions of necrosis in large cancers with high cellular turnover may not be adequately identified (Figure 3.1). Conversely, false positivity from tissues with an inflammatory component can result in overestimation of the tumour extent. Physiological factors also typically result in increased uptake, which includes the urinary tract containing the excreted tracer, and metabolically active tissue such as the brain, myocardium, brown fat, and contracting walls of the gastrointestinal tract. Thus, it is recommended that target delineation using PET/CT imaging should be carried out with the support of nuclear medicine experts to correctly identify tumours and avoid the inclusion of non-disease ^{18}F-FDG-avid areas.

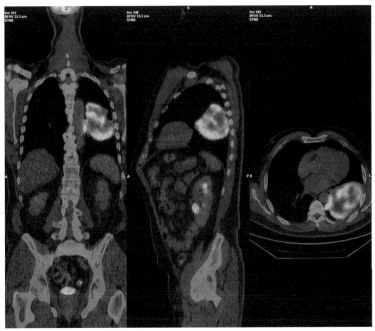

Fig. 3.1 Fused coronal, sagittal, and axial FDG PET-CT images show a heterogeneous tracer uptake in a large left lower lobe lung mass. Areas of low grade activity (dark grey) suggest tissue necrosis.

3.4.3 Motion

The duration of a PET scan is typically around 20–30 min., making it susceptible to significant subject and physiological motion. Organ motion is particularly relevant for structures in the chest which, in free breathing, often causes indistinct edges with an inhomogeneous appearance. It has been demonstrated that respiratory misalignments between CT and PET data within a single PET/CT scan can lead to significant under-estimation of the SUV of the attenuation-corrected PET.

Dedicated PET/CT imaging for radiotherapy planning should ideally adopt motion management strategies such as deep inspiration breath-hold to minimize the blurring and improve the inhomogeneity due to movement artefact. Gating schemes can also be employed where data at the corresponding portion of the respiratory cycle can be extracted and processed, thereby increasing the spatial-temporal match. For instance, 3D PET/CT has been shown to underestimate target volume of lung cancers, giving rise to potential geometrical miss compared to 4D PET/CT. In the absence of such respiratory adaptations where treatment is delivered in free breathing, verification of the PET/CT data should be performed in order to ensure accurate representation of the target volume. Errors secondary to misalignments should be corrected to improve the match prior to application of the attenuation correction.

3.4.4 Implementation of PET/CT for radiotherapy purposes

Recently, multiple advances in PET technology have been implemented to harness its capabilities in PET/CT-guided management in radiation oncology. Examples of this include faster detector electronics which can increase the SNR in PET images, smaller detector size resulting in improved spatial resolution by reducing partial volume effect, retrospective correction for point spread function to gain uniform image resolution and improve image quality, as well as the addition of PET detectors in the z-direction which can improve the volume sensitivity and reduce the scan time through the extended axial field-of-view. Some units have adopted radiotherapy treatment positioning through the installation of big-bore PET/CT systems that allow increased versatility in the use of immobilization equipment and customizable pallets to ensure reproducible patient set-up.

3.5 Applications of advanced imaging techniques in radiation oncology

In this section, the scope and purposes that MRI and PET/CT imaging can serve in the radiotherapy treatment process are illustrated through examples of their use across different tumour sites.

3.5.1 Target/organ at risk volume delineation

Volume delineation is one of the key reasons for the increasing use of advanced imaging techniques in the radiotherapy planning process. This is mainly through MRI images, which provide improved contrast resolution over CT across a multitude of tumours and OARs, resulting in better anatomical definition. Functional imaging using PET has also been adopted in some tumour sites, and the application of multi-parametric MRI is being increasingly explored.

3.5.1.1 Central nervous system

One of the earliest body sites to adopt the use of MRI for volume delineation is the brain. Contrast-enhanced MRI provides superior visual discrimination of brain tumours from surrounding oedema over CT images, resulting in reduced intra- and inter-observer tumour delineation variation. Moreover, there are many intra-cranial structures there are poorly seen on CT as compared to MRI. Many of these constitute OARs that are commonly required to be outlined for dosimetric purposes, including the optic apparatus, pituitary gland, brainstem, and hippocampus (Figure 3.2).

The use of MRI for the brain also suffers less drawbacks as compared to other body sites. For instance, the head is less affected by field inhomogeneity due to its relative smaller size. Additionally, co-registration of MRI to planning CT of the head is subject to less set-up errors due to the rigidity of the bony skull.

^{18}F-FDG is typically unhelpful as a radiotracer for visualization of structures within the brain due to the high glucose metabolism by normal brain tissue resulting in high uptake. Instead, metabolic activity is better reflected through amino acid tracers,

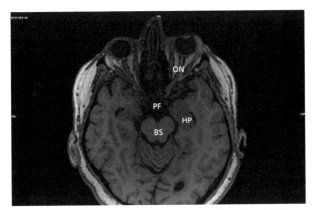

Fig. 3.2 Axial reconstructed MR brain image at the level close the skull base. PF: pituitary fossa; ON: optic nerve; HP: hippocampus; BS: brain stem

where tumour definition has been reported to be significantly larger on PET appearances than MRI. Navarria et al. compared CTVs generated from ^{11}C-MET PET to those from MRI and found that part of the biological target volume (BTV) was exterior to the T1-based high dose region in 50% of the high grade glioma cases.[2] In all cases, relapse corresponded to the BTV regions, suggesting that PET imaging can complement MRI in radiotherapy planning.

3.5.1.2 Head and neck cancer

MRI has been shown to be superior to CT in detecting intracranial infiltration, orbital invasion, and perineural tumoural spread for nasopharyngeal and sinonasal cancers. Oropharyngeal tumours have been reported to appear larger on MRI than CT, where MRI detects disease regions not picked up on CT. Also, diffusion-weighted imaging (DWI) MRI has higher correlation with pathological findings than conventional imaging for the detection of lymph node metastases. Other advantages of MRI-based planning include the reduction of signal degradation with MRI in the presence of dental amalgams which are often close to the regions of interest, as well as improved visualization of OARs such as the spinal cord, brainstem, and parotid glands.

^{18}F-FDG PET/CT has an established role in disease identification in head and neck cancers. In high-risk disease, modification of high-dose radiotherapy volumes occurs in about 10% of cases through the detection of ^{18}F-FDG positive neck nodes. It has also been reported that smaller tumour volumes are derived in up to a third of cases where PET-guidance is used.

3.5.1.3 Lung cancer

^{18}F-FDG PET/CT is the standard of care for staging of lung cancer for patients being considered for treatment with radical intent. The International Atomic Energy Agency (IAEA) has also published a set of consensus guidelines on the visualization and use of PET/CT imaging for target volume delineation of radically treated non-small cell lung cancer (NSCLC).[3]

It has been demonstrated that PET/CT imaging contributes to an alteration in radical radiotherapy plans in a third of cases. Tumour control probability is higher with PET/CT-based planning than conventional CT planning through improved target coverage. Moreover, dose to normal tissue can also be minimized through avoidance of non-tumour regions. For instance, ^{18}F-FDG uptake in tumours can help distinguish adjacent regions of lung collapse or atelectasis, which is a classically difficult task based solely on CT appearances. Not only can PET/CT imaging decrease inter-observer variation in radiotherapy treatment planning, a dedicated radiotherapy treatment PET/CT has been shown to reduce the inter-observer differences even further beyond that of a diagnostic scan. Additionally, integration of 4D PET/CT and 4D CT using a respiratory tracking system to correlate with the breathing cycle can improve the accuracy of SUV quantification for a moving lung tumour.

3.5.1.4 Breast cancer

MRI can aid planning in partial breast irradiation, where MRI-derived volumes have been shown to be smaller than CT-based delineation. Inter-observer contouring variation of tumour bed volumes has been demonstrated to be significantly reduced through MRI use.

3.5.1.5 Rectal and anal cancers

The depiction of rectal tumours with anal or sigmoid involvement is superior on MRI, resulting in better delineation accuracy than based on CT only. MRI-derived volumes of rectal cancers also tend to be smaller and shorter, allowing the potential for dose escalation. Interestingly, both MRI and PET/CT, especially automatic PET/CT delineation, have been significantly correlated with pathological findings, whilst CT-derived volumes did not. Some studies also demonstrated that ^{18}F-FDG PET/CT guidance result in smaller volumes than MRI. Other tracers displaying different functional characteristics such as ^{18}F-FLT and ^{18}F-FMISO are being explored for their value in radiotherapy planning.

^{18}F-FDG PET is being routinely used in the staging of locally advanced anal cancers due to its greater sensitivity in the detection of primary, nodal, and distant spread of disease as compared to conventional imaging. It is an invaluable tool in radiotherapy planning, where contours are modified to ensure that node positive disease is encompassed within the treated volume. Studies evaluating its role in dose escalation for locally advanced disease are currently under way.

3.5.1.6 Prostate cancer

Multiple studies have shown that MRI is more reliable than CT for radiotherapy planning as the prostate gland is overestimated on CT appearances. MRI use has improved accuracy and decreased inter-observer variability in delineation of both prostate gland and OARs, which corresponded with a reduction of dose to normal tissues compared to CT. The ESTRO ACROP guidelines summarize how MRI adds integral information for delineation.[4] In addition to bolstering the identification of seminal vesical invasion and extracapsular extension, MRI allows better approximation of the prostate apex and enhanced discrimination of the prostate from OARs especially in the presence of hip prostheses.

Radio-labelled choline PET has been proven to be a reliable biomarker for staging of prostate cancer. Not only have there been reports on the value of choline-PET on BTV definition for tumoural extra-prostatic extension, it has been demonstrated that it can help define the sub-volume for delivering an integrated boost to prostate which can improve tumour control rates. Newer radiotracers targeting prostate-specific membrane antigen (PSMA) have been shown to be beneficial following radical prostatectomy by playing a pivotal role in staging and determining the volume in salvage radiotherapy. It has been demonstrated that whilst the target can be underestimated if based solely on the widely adopted RTOG (Radiation Therapy Oncology Group) contouring guidelines,[5] coverage of lymph node regions at risk of occult relapse is improved when PSMA PET is used. Its utility in volume definition of dominant intraprostatic lesions for dose boosts is being explored in association with multi-parametric MRI.

3.5.1.7 Gynaecological

MRI guidance for brachytherapy in cervix cancer has been shown to be superior to radiograph/CT-based planning, and is recommended by the GEC-ESTRO guidelines for volume definition.[6] The enhanced visualization of tumours on MRI allows brachytherapy cervical boost to be individually tailored according to the appearances of the residual tumour volume following external beam radiotherapy (EBRT). The most widely adopted technique is the acquisition of MRI images following applicator insertion for contouring and planning purposes, with T2-weighted sequences in the orientation of the applicator being the gold standard for target definition. In addition to the use of concomitant chemotherapy and improved staging, MRI-guided brachytherapy has contributed to improved overall survival by up to 30%, whilst significantly reducing morbidity when compared to historical controls. Major improvement in local control was most marked in large tumours through the use of dose escalation and interstitial needles.

^{18}F-FDG PET/CT has also influenced the coverage of EBRT treatment fields, where extended field irradiation has been shown to improve the survival rate in the presence of ^{18}F-FDG PET/CT positive para-aortic nodal disease.

3.5.1.8 Lymphoma

The incorporation of ^{18}F-FDG PET/CT in treatment planning to target metabolically active disease has led to the development of involved-site and involved-nodal radiotherapy techniques.

3.5.1.9 Oesophageal

The target definition of oesophageal cancer runs a risk of disease underestimation in the cranio-caudal plane. Several reports have demonstrated that ^{18}F-FDG PET/CT can reduce geographical miss in the delineation of the primary tumour, and has been found to be complementary to endoscopic ultrasound in determining the cranio-caudal extent of disease.

3.5.2 **Dose escalation and dose painting**

The addition of MRI and/or PET/CT have led to smaller target volumes, giving rise to the potential for radiotherapy dose escalation. Dose modulation based on the biological characteristics of the tumour (i.e. dose painting) can be applied up front or during the course of the treatment. To date, most dose painting studies have been PET/CT-based.

3.5.2.1 Head and neck cancers

Despite the ability of DWI and dynamic contrast-enhanced (DCE) MRI to discriminate regions within head and neck tumours and the link between low perfusion with poorer outcomes, their use in dose painting has been sparsely reported. On the other hand, most developments in dose painting of head and neck cancers are based on PET/CT imaging. ^{18}F-FDG PET/CT has been shown to provide prognostic information, and it has been estimated that up to a 30% higher dose is required in order to achieve similar local tumour control for cancers with FDG-avidity compared to lesions with lower uptake. ARTFORCE is a phase III international clinical trial on adaptive high-dose radiotherapy for advanced head and neck cancer where the impact of dose modulation based on ^{18}F-FDG PET/CT is being evaluated.[7] The utility of other PET tracers that detect hypoxia (e.g. ^{18}F-FAZA, ^{18}F-FMISO, and ^{64}Cu-ATSM) is being investigated for its role in dose intensification of intra-tumoural regions displaying hypoxic features. Similarly, ^{18}F-FLT, a measure of tumour proliferation, has been used to identify boost regions for dose escalation, although its association with tumour control has yet to be fully established.

3.5.2.2 Lung cancer

Biologically equivalent dose has been highly correlated with overall survival and loco-regional, relapse-free survival in locally advanced NSCLC, establishing the efficacy of dose escalation in this setting. There have been several reports on personalizing dose escalation based on pre-treatment ^{18}F-FDG and ^{18}F-FMISO PET metrics in locally advanced NSCLC. Additionally, dose adaptation based on the interim response of ^{18}F-FDG PET to treatment is also being evaluated, by exploiting its ability to detect the resistant sub-volumes in the middle of the course of radiotherapy.

3.5.2.3 Rectal cancer

There are multiple reports on dose escalation for rectal cancers through simultaneous integrated boost which allows increased dose to be delivered to the tumour volume without extension of the overall treatment time. Although simultaneous integrated dose boost as guided by ^{18}F-FDG PET has been described, further investigation into boost strategies incorporating MRI and PET guidance are awaited.

3.5.2.4 Prostate

In the setting of whole prostate gland low dose rate (LDR) brachytherapy for early stage disease, the superiority in anatomical definition that MRI provides improves the confidence in dosimetric parameters for plan assessment. Moreover, it offers unparalleled views of intraprostatic characteristics, and has an established role in the planning of high dose rate (HDR) brachytherapy boosts for higher risk, localized, and/or recurrent disease. Multiparametric imaging, including T2-weighted, apparent diffusion coefficient (ADC) maps from DWI and K^{trans} maps from DCE sequences are being used to localize tumour targets. The role of partial gland irradiation where additional dose is delivered to focal regions of the prostate in combination with EBRT is being investigated in the PIVOTAL boost trial.[8]

3.5.3 Image-guided radiotherapy: MRI-LINAC

The management of tumour and organ motion is one of the key challenges in radiotherapy delivery. Although planning target volumes encompass the error associated with this, large margins increase the risk of clinically significant toxicity, especially near critical organs. Image-guided radiotherapy allows the delivery to be reproducible through the visualization of the tumour and surrounding anatomy at the time of treatment. There is a range of solutions which is dependent on the treatment location, including tracking systems and devices, electronic portal imaging devices (EPID), as well as kV and MV CT imaging platforms. Fiducial markers can also be placed for selected tumour sites and used as surrogates for visualization.

Recently, there is growth in the installation of MRI-guided treatment systems, which encompasses an MRI scanner and a LINAC (linear particle accelerator) treatment delivery facility all within the same unit. This has advantages over EPID and CT-based verification systems through improved soft-tissue contrast, enabling better visualization of the more challenging body sites such as the oesophagus, pancreas, and rectum. Online adaptive radiotherapy (ART) can then be applied to correct for the differences seen in the anatomy. A number of solutions exist for this: (1) shifting the patient to match the relative anatomy seen on the day; (2) selection of a treatment plan from a pre-prepared library with the best fit to the anatomy acquired at the time of treatment; (3) applying translational and rotational shifts to the dose distribution to suit the patient position; (4) applying a deformation field where the original dose distribution is warped based on image of the day; (5) online/real-time re-planning with generation of new target outlines and dose calculations.

With no radiation exposure, MRI-guided systems are ideally suited for continuous visualization of the tumour during treatment delivery in real-time, permitting the tracking of intra-fractional motion of soft tissues. The technology also enables implementation of other techniques such as gating in treatment delivery, which is useful for tumours that are subjected to respiratory motion. The MRI-LINAC platform is also highly applicable in stereotactic treatment, which capitalizes on the precision of treatment to employ the use of hypofractionated dose schedules, as well as in re-irradiation to ensure the safety of the dose delivery.

Moreover, this presents the opportunity for biomarker discovery studies from the wealth of potentially minable data on the response to treatment. With the scope for performing functional sequences, this allows the potential for personalized adaptation of therapy according to the biological images acquired at the time of treatment.

3.6 **Future work**

The incorporation of MRI and PET/CT imaging has dramatically altered radiotherapy planning practices recently. The landscape is continuing to evolve with multiple promising avenues on the horizon.

There is ongoing research into the exploitation of information acquired through multi-parametric MRI and PET imaging for advancing dose delivery techniques, especially where there is strong evidence of a biological rationale and improved outcomes. For many institutions further adaptations and upgrades to systems need to be carried out, with the increasing demand for their incorporation in radiation practice.

Another field of work includes radiomics, which has recently become an actively explored domain with an increasing number of groups working on the extraction of radiomic signatures from functional imaging to derive prognostic information. This involves the harvesting of mathematical descriptions from particular regions of interest which serve as imaging biomarkers. Apart from its promise in disease prognostication, other uses warrant future developments, including its application with MR and PET data.

There is great interest with advent of machine learning algorithms as a tool for data mining and for addressing issues that have been historically performed by humans. Its application and validity in autosegmentation of images including MRI and PET is being actively explored across a range of body sites, with early indicators of success.

Hybrid imaging with combined PET/MRI is an emerging technology which allows the unique opportunity for assessing the functional and biological characteristics of tumours within a single examination. The benefits of a fully integrated imaging system allowing simultaneous assessment of multiple pathophysiolotanal parameters may further improve radiotherapy treatment planning and dose painting.

References

1. **Boellaard R, Delgado-Bolton R, Oyen WJG, et al.** (2015). FDG PET/CT: EANM procedure guidelines for tumour imaging: version 2.0. *European Journal of Nuclear Medicine and Molecular Imaging*, **42**(2): 328–354.

2. **Navarria P, Reggiori G, Pessina F, et al.** (2014). Investigation on the role of integrated PET/MRI for target volume definition and radiotherapy planning in patients with high grade glioma. *Radiotherapy & Oncology*, **112**(3): 425–429.

3. **Konert T, Vogel W, MacManus MP, et al.** (2015). PET/CT imaging for target volume delineation in curative intent radiotherapy of non-small cell lung cancer: IAEA consensus report 2014. *Radiotherapy & Oncology*, **116**(1): 27–34.

4. **Salembier C, Villeirs G, De Bari B, et al.** (2018). ESTRO ACROP consensus guideline on CT-and MRI-based target volume delineation for primary radiation therapy of localized prostate cancer. *Radiotherapy and Oncology*, **127**(1): 49–61.

5. **Michalski J M, Lawton C, El Naqa I, et al.** (2010). Development of RTOG consensus guidelines for the definition of the clinical target volume for postoperative conformal radiation therapy for prostate cancer. *International Journal of Radiation Oncology. Biology. Physics*, **76**(2): 361–368.

6. **Haie-Meder C, Potter R, Limbergen EV, et al.** (2005). Recommendations from Gynaecological (GYN) GEC-ESTRO Working Group (I): concepts and terms in 3D image based 3D treatment planning in cervix cancer brachytherapy with emphasis on MRI assessment of GTV and CTV. *Radiotherapy & Oncology*, **74**(3): 235–245.

7. **Heukelom J, Hamming O, Bartelink H, et al.** (2013). Adaptive and innovative Radiation Treatment FOR improving Cancer treatment outcomE (ARTFORCE); a randomized controlled phase II trial for individualized treatment of head and neck cancer. *BMC Cancer*, **13**(1): 84.

8. **London: BioMed Central.** ISRCTN80146950, A phase III randomised controlled trial of prostate and pelvis versus prostate alone radiotherapy with or without prostate boost. Available from: http://www.isrctn.com/ISRCTN80146950

Chapter 4

Breast

Dinos Geropantas and Victoria Ames

4.1 Clinical background

4.1.1 Incidence

Breast cancer is the most common cancer in women in the UK, with an estimated lifetime risk of 1 in 7 (15%) for all women born after 1960. There were nearly 55,000 new cancer diagnoses in 2015, accounting for 15% of all new cancer cases, though only 1% of these cancers were in men. Since the early 1990s, there has been a steady increase in breast cancer incidence rates, reflecting the changing risk factor profiles as well as the improving diagnostic techniques and the more accurate data recording.

Breast cancer incidence remains strongly associated with age, with over 25% of new cases in 2013–15 in people aged over 75. Hereditary factors only account for about 25% of breast cancer risk. Although the genetic mutations of BRCA1 and BRCA2 confer a high risk of developing breast cancer (45–65% by age 70), as they are uncommon (affecting approximately 1 in 450 women) they only account for about 2% of breast cancers overall. It is estimated that 23% of breast cancer cases are preventable, with risk factors such as obesity and alcohol each accounting for up to 8% of cases diagnosed.

Up to 87% of cancer cases in the UK are at an early stage (I or II) at the time of diagnosis, with only 7% of cases having evidence of metastatic disease at presentation. A late stage of disease at diagnosis is associated with older age (over 80) and social deprivation.

Breast cancer mortality rates in the UK have fallen dramatically since 1971, with a decrease of 38% in females and 45% in males. The reduction in breast cancer mortality rates is likely to have several different causes, including screening, increasing availability of standardized specialist care, and advances in diagnostic methods and therapies.

4.1.2 Screening

In 2017–18, the UK NHS breast screening programme (NHSBSP) screened 2.1 million women aged over 45 years, seeing a 34% increase in the uptake of screening in the ten years preceding, with over 70% taking up their invitation to be screened. Of the 2.1 million women screened, 18,001 women were diagnosed with cancer, providing a cancer detection rate of 8.4 cases per 1000 women screened. There is a notable spike in overall breast cancer incidence at around 50 when routine breast screening starts.

Screening of those individuals with a documented increased risk of breast cancer, is well established and is predominantly performed with a combination of mammography and/or contrast-enhanced magnetic resonance imaging (MRI). The imaging modality and screening interval is dictated by the individual's risk category (e.g. BRCA carrier status, TP53, supradiaphragmatic radiotherapy irradiated below 30), and age. Although standard practice in many parts of Europe and the USA, routine screening or surveillance with ultrasound (US) is not recommended in the UK.

Non-invasive and micro-invasive disease accounts for approximately 20% of screen-detected cancers. Ductal carcinoma *in situ* (DCIS) registrations have increased markedly since the introduction of breast screening, because it is a condition that is not usually palpable and therefore is mostly diagnosed by mammography. Critics of the breast screening programme have voiced concerns that identifying DCIS can lead to unnecessary diagnosis of breast tumours, as the low- to intermediate-grade histological subtypes may never progress or threaten the woman's life. Small studies have reported progression to invasive disease rates of 39–53%. These series included patients diagnosed with invasive disease who had a history of an incorrectly labelled 'benign' excisional biopsy in the past which on review appeared positive for DCIS. Of interest, low-grade pathology did not predict a benign course. Autopsy studies suggest a median prevalence of DCIS of 8.9%. However, the majority of screen-detected DCIS is high grade and necrotic and given that this is the histological subtype that develops into high-grade invasive cancer, its early detection and treatment aims to improve the prognosis for these more aggressive tumours.

4.2 Diagnosis and staging

4.2.1 Radiological diagnosis

Despite advances in imaging techniques over the last two decades, in particular MRI, the main diagnostic tools used radiologically in the diagnosis of breast cancer remain mammography and US. In women younger than 40 years of age mammography is not routinely performed in the assessment of a breast lesion, as the breasts are radiographically dense and therefore difficult to interpret mammographically. As a result, US remains the primary imaging modality for this group.

4.2.1.1 Mammography

In women of 40 years and over, a mammogram is the first-line investigation, often accompanied by a focused US of the area of clinical concern. The routine use of full field digital mammography has improved diagnostic accuracy when compared to film-screen mammography, with the additional benefits of image manipulation and electronic image transfer.

The most common mammographic feature of breast cancer is a dense mass with an ill-defined border; though a spiculate irregular mass has a pathognomonic appearance (Figure 4.1). Usually, a well-marginated mass on a mammogram represents a benign entity such as a simple cyst, a fibroadenoma, or an intramammary node. However, some invasive cancers can mimic these entities. Therefore, histological confirmation

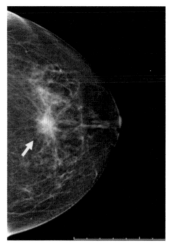

Fig. 4.1 Left craniocaudal mammogram confirming a spiculate mass in the central breast with associated architectural distortion (arrow).

via US-guided biopsy is usual practice for a new solid lesion in women over 25 years, or of any age if atypical.

Another mammographic sign of cancer is an architectural distortion of the breast tissue. This may be seen on only one mammographic view and can be very subtle. Post-surgical scarring, fat necrosis, radial scar, and sclerosing adenosis are all benign entities that show distortion or sometimes even a spiculate mass and hence can be indistinguishable mammographically from cancer and require US correlation. The emergence of techniques such as digital breast tomosynthesis has enabled improved accuracy in the assessment of these more diagnostically challenging lesions, as well as asymmetrical densities—the latter is usually secondary to composite shadowing from normal breast parenchyma (Figure 4.2). Digital breast tomosynthesis is a mammographic technique in which an arc of images is taken in both planes of the breast. The images obtained are then post-processed to provide a 3D-like reconstructed image of the breast parenchyma. This has the objective of overcoming the effects of summation artefact present in conventional 2D mammography, with the aim of improving diagnostic sensitivity and specificity.

Another mammographic feature of cancer is calcification. This is a common mammographic finding associated with both benign and malignant pathology. Unfortunately, due to the poor mammographic specificity and sonographic sensitivity, most presentations remain indeterminate on imaging. As such, when calcification is indeterminate or suspicious, a mammographically-guided stereotactic biopsy is usually performed. Many units now use a vacuum-assisted biopsy technique with large 10 G needles to increase the volume of tissue retrieved. This optimizes the chance of providing a definitive diagnosis as compared to standard 14G biopsy devices. With improving imaging techniques, more subtle findings are being identified and targeted for sampling under imaging guidance. As a result, there has been an increased

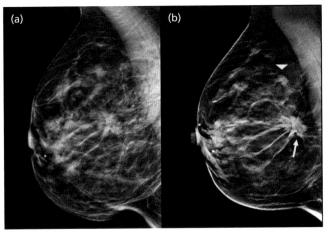

Fig. 4.2 Single mediolateral oblique view right breast digital tomosynthesis confirming the known spiculate mass within the central breast (arrow) but also identifying a second lesion within the upper half of the breast (arrowhead).

interest in homogenizing the management of these histologically indeterminate (B3) lesions, some of which confer a significant malignancy (B5) upgrade rate (Table 4.1). For this reason, the practice of vacuum-assisted excision of B3 lesions under either US or stereotactic guidance has become a well-established technique in the UK, with the publication of NHSBSP guidelines on the same.

Over the last five years, contrast-enhanced spectral mammography (CESM) has grown as a technique, becoming integrated into the standard imaging pathway for many units for those patients presenting with a clinically suspicious mass, replacing the use of conventional four-view mammography. The technique utilizes intravenous iodinated contrast medium to provide a more accurate assessment of disease extent. However, as with the use of iodinated contrast in general radiology, there are contra-indications that require recognition and which need to be carefully managed. The use

Table 4.1 Core biopsy reporting categories

B1	Normal tissue
B2	Benign lesion
B3	Lesion of uncertain malignant potential
B4	Suspicious
B5	Malignant
B5a	*In situ*
B5b	Invasive
B5c	Not clear if invasive or *in situ*

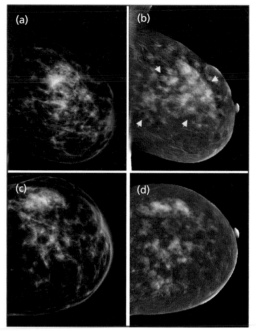

Fig. 4.3 Contrast-enhanced spectral left breast mammography, low kV (a) and (c) and recombined view (b) and (d) demonstrating multicentric enhancing malignancy (arrowheads) within complex heterogeneous breast parenchymal background.

of CESM aims to streamline the staging pathway for patients with breast cancer, particularly those with poorly marginated or multifocal/multicentric disease (Figure 4.3), with the aim of negating the need for MRI staging studies, and the frequently encountered sequelae examinations.

4.2.1.2 Ultrasound

On US, cancers are typically solid, low-echogenicity masses with irregular margins. Other features such as acoustic shadowing are present to a varying extent dependent on the make-up of the tumour (Figure 4.4). It is this variability in the sonographic appearance of breast cancers that strengthens the argument to maintain a low threshold for percutaneous sampling of new or atypical solid masses. The role of other US techniques such as colour doppler and elastography remain under debate and have not yet become generally established into routine practice.

It is standard practice to assess the ipsilateral axillary nodes with US for size and morphology at the time of the initial breast assessment. However, US has significant limitations, with one third of morphologically normal lymph nodes being confirmed metastatic at histology. Despite this, given the absence of an alternative technique, it remains the gold standard for preoperative axillary assessment. If a node is indeterminate or abnormal, then percutaneous sampling with US-guided fine needle aspiration (FNA) or biopsy is indicated.

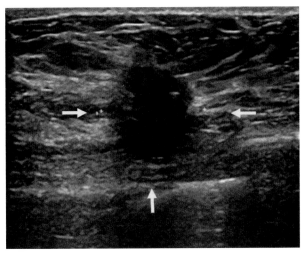

Fig. 4.4 Breast US confirming an irregular hypoechoic mass with some posterior acoustic shadowing, typical of a breast carcinoma (arrows).

The internal mammary nodal chain (IMC) is usually involved by spread from superior and medial tumours, although axillary disease is still more common in patients with tumours at those sites. Due to the parasternal location of the nodes, they are not usually suitable for assessment with US and are therefore not standardly assessed unless further imaging with MRI, CT, or PET-CT (positron emission tomography) is undertaken.

4.2.1.3 MRI

Dynamic contrast-enhanced breast MRI (Figure 4.5) has been shown to have a high sensitivity for the detection of invasive breast cancer, but traditionally at the expense of a variable specificity. There is also increasing evidence that high-grade necrotic DCIS, which is often non-calcified and therefore mammographically invisible, can be detected with MRI but this is not always reliable. The high detection rate is underpinned by the tendency of breast cancer (like other malignant tumours) to develop malignant angiogenesis. When gadolinium-DTPA contrast is administered intravenously, on T1-weighted images, there is an intense peak with subsequent washout (reflecting leaking capillaries). Lesion morphology as well as its time intensity curve aims to help risk stratify enhancing lesions. However, this remains relatively non-specific, with a resulting reliance on second-look US, MRI guided biopsy, or MRI follow-up to provide guidance on clinical significance.

Breast MRI has a well-established role in screening for breast cancer in those patients identified to be at high risk, following the publication of National Institute for Health and Clinical Excellence (NICE) guidance. This guidance was evidenced by trials such as the UK MARIBS and advised a screening protocol involving annual MRI +/- mammography at differing schedules dictated by the individual genetic risk.

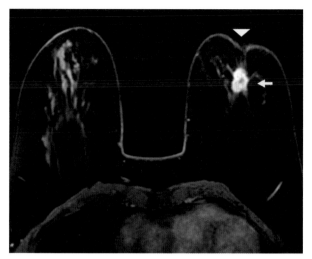

Fig. 4.5 Contrast-enhanced dynamic breast MRI study confirming a centrally necrotic left breast carcinoma (arrow) with associated nipple retraction (arrowhead).

4.2.1.4 PET/CT

^{18}F-fluorodeoxyglucose positron emission tomography (^{18}F-FDG-PET) imaging utilizes functional data to detect malignancy and has been shown to be able to detect breast carcinoma. When fused with computed tomography (PET/CT), the functional-anatomical detail provides a sensitive map for malignancy. However, the poor spatial resolution limits its sensitivity for primary breast carcinoma when comparing it with conventional mammography and MRI. The introduction of positron emission mammography (PEM) overcomes this issue but has the disadvantages of cost, availability of the technique, and radiation dose.

PET/CT has been found to be useful in the assessment of silicone-laden nodes in the context of breast cancer with ruptured breast implants. Silicone-laden nodes cannot be formally assessed with US due to the obscuration of the nodal anatomy by the echogenic silicone. ^{18}F-FDG PET/CT can demonstrate differential FDG-avidity between non-metastatic silicone nodes and those with co-existent metastatic disease (Figure 4.6).

4.2.1.5 Other considerations

The breast radiologist routinely uses excision or mastectomy specimen radiography to assess for the presence of tumour within the specimen as well as the apparent extent of disease relative to the specimen margins. Specimen radiographs are used not only at the time of percutaneous biopsy but also in the peri-operative setting.

The use of hydrophilic localization clips is standard practice within all breast imaging units in the UK. They are implanted percutaneously and provide multiple functions, including cross-correlation of biopsy sites between different imaging techniques and marking tumour sites prior to neoadjuvant chemotherapy to aid pre-surgical localization in the presence of significant disease response.

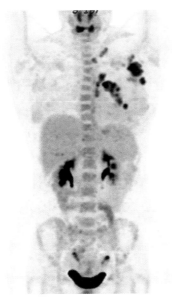

Fig. 4.6 ¹⁸F-FDG PET/CT confirming differential avidity in enlarged silicone laden nodes in the right axilla and enlarged metastatic nodes in the left axilla.

Artificial intelligence (AI) and other deep learning technologies continue to gain traction in breast cancer diagnostics. Algorithms can be applied either to a digital mammography unit or an MRI workstation with the aim to flag abnormal areas on the mammogram (or MRI) by producing electronic markers on the image at the touch of a button. It aims to provide a system that has benchmark screen reading indicators at least as good as trained film readers so as to provide a solution to the current UK workforce shortages. Work continues to develop in this area with no systems currently in standard practice within the UK.

4.2.2 Radiological staging

The eighth edition of the AJCC TNM (tumour, node, metastasis) system has been widely adopted, and is being increasingly influenced by imaging techniques. Primary disease radiological staging continues to be performed routinely by mammography and US, which although reasonable in accuracy when correlated to final pathology are not perfect. Conventional imaging techniques have significant limitations in assessing disease extent in the context of dense parenchyma, poorly marginated lesions, non-calcified *in situ* disease, and multifocal tumours. Some tumour subtypes are more difficult to locally stage: lobular carcinoma is classically very difficult to measure as it often grows by infiltrating along normal tissue planes without forming a mass.

Dynamic contrast-enhanced MRI has improved accuracy at assessing local staging in these more challenging cases and identifies additional cancer in 16% of patients. However, the relatively poor specificity (positive predictive value 66%) has been blamed for unnecessarily increasing the extent of breast surgery for some women.

These factors, coupled with the cost, the need to assess any indeterminate additional findings with targeted US, and the limited availability of MR-guided biopsy services act to disadvantage this technique.

CESM demonstrates a comparable sensitivity to MRI for staging of local disease, but with some published papers suggesting a slightly improved false positive rate. Given the easy access to mammography and contrast, the low relative costs and potential for time-saving in the patient pathway, CESM is an attractive imaging alternative for locoregional staging in some breast units.

CT with or without isotope bone scan remains the standard imaging modality to assess for metastatic disease. However, the increasing experience with PET/CT in breast cancer patients has enabled formal guidance to be published. Although it has limitations in characterizing sub-centimetre lesions, development of the techniques including increased experience, fusion with other imaging modalities and novel tracers are improving this issue. In 2016, the Royal College of Radiologist (RCR)/Royal College of Physicians (RCP) provided a set of accepted indications for PET/CT in breast cancer:

1. Assessment of multi-focal disease or suspected recurrence in patients with dense breasts.

2. Differentiation of treatment-induced brachial plexopathy from tumour infiltration in symptomatic patients with an equivocal or normal MRI.

3. Assessment of extent of disease in selected patients with disseminated breast cancer before therapy.

4. Assessment of response to chemotherapy in patients whose disease is not well demonstrated using other techniques; for example bony metastases (Figure 4.7).

There is much interest in the use of other tracers such as ^{18}F-flouride for bony disease as they provide a fine-tuning role in the development of PET/CT. However, their place in breast cancer management in the NHS will require evidence to support their cost effectiveness.

Metastatic disease can present either *de novo* or usually within 2–5 years after diagnosis (within 2–3 years in triple negative breast cancers—TNBC). Differences in patterns of spread among various histological types of breast cancer and among various biological profiles of the tumour need to be taken into account when imaging is considered. ER-positive/Her2-negative tumours are more likely to metastasize to bones, but can also spread to lungs, liver, and brain. TNBC has a tendency to metastasize primarily to lung, liver, and brain. HER2-positive breast cancer can involve the CNS more frequently, particularly in patients treated with anti-HER2 targeted therapies. Invasive lobular tumours can exhibit a distinct pattern of metastatic spread and compared with ductal tumours they have a higher likelihood of gastrointestinal, ovarian, and omental involvement. Radiological investigations in patients with known metastatic disease should be guided by symptoms.

Bone metastases are classified as lytic, sclerotic, or mixed. Bone scan is a sensitive imaging modality routinely used in their diagnosis and it commonly demonstrates increased uptake in the affected areas (hotspots), while in cases of extensive skeletal involvement a 'superscan' can be observed. Large lytic lesions can sometimes appear as photopenic areas (cold spots) (Figure 4.8). CT can demonstrate pathological fractures

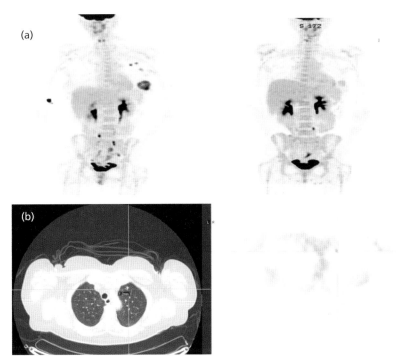

Fig. 4.7 (a) PET/CT images demonstrating response to neo-adjuvant chemotherapy in a patient with subtle indeterminate distant findings in the lungs and bones. (b) PET/CT study performed to characterize an incidental sub-solid lung mass in the right lower lobe identified on CT staging for breast cancer. Images confirmed that bilateral sub-centimetre nodules thought to be intrapulmonary nodes on conventional CT were actually pulmonary metastases.

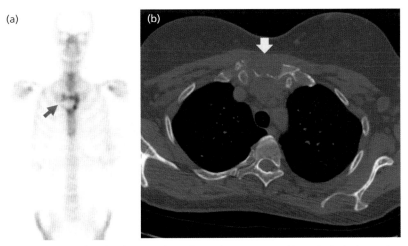

Fig. 4.8 Bone scan showing increased uptake at the sternum with central photopaenia in keeping with a metastasis (red arrow). CT scan confirms a 45 mm x 26 mm destructive bone lesion in the upper sternum (yellow arrow).

and provide detailed information on the structural integrity of the spine, but MRI is better at identifying epidural and bone marrow infiltration and describing the extent of extraosseous soft tissue component.

Chest radiography can help diagnose pleural effusions but a CT scan is required to identify lung and pleural metastases, and mediastinal nodes. Multidetector CT involves thin slice imaging, also providing an excellent opportunity for detecting other processes such as lymphangitis carcinomatosa.

Liver metastases can be seen as hypoechoic lesions on US and sometimes appear as 'target' lesions. They will usually present as low attenuation lesions on CT, with variable enhancement in the portal venous phase of scanning. Occasionally a more diffuse pattern of infiltrative disease is observed, which makes the liver appear cirrhotic-like or 'pseudocirrhotic'. MRI can be used if there is equivocation.

A CT scan of the head is usually employed first to investigate symptoms suggestive of brain metastases, but contrast-enhanced MRI can provide a more definitive diagnosis and much improves sensitivity for leptomeningeal disease.

4.3 **Radiotherapy planning**

Most patients treated with breast conservation surgery (BCS) and a good proportion of those having a mastectomy (e.g. those with involved margins, T3–T4 tumours, node positive disease) will be considered for postoperative radiotherapy (RT). Usually the whole breast is treated, but in low-risk cases partial breast radiotherapy may be considered.

In addition to breast and/or chest wall, the supraclavicular fossa (SCF) with or without the infraclavicular fossa (ICF) might need to be irradiated if there is increased risk of spread to this areas (e.g. always consider if ≥4 positive axillary nodes and sometimes if 1–3 positive nodes). Treatment to the axilla can be avoided in patients with a negative sentinel node. The same is true for patients with ITCs or micrometastasis in the sentinel node and for those with macrometastases in one or two nodes and otherwise T1, ER-positive, HER2-negative, grade 1–2 tumours, treated with BCS. Traditionally, patients requiring further axillary treatment would undergo a surgical clearance, but in recent years, axillary radiotherapy has been considered a safe alternative in order to reduce the risk for lymphoedema (AMAROS study eligible patients—T1/T2). The IMC nodes should be targeted when involved; however, new evidence suggest that prophylactic IMC RT can be considered in those with T4 and/or N2–3 disease and perhaps even in those with N1 disease and central or medial tumours. A radiotherapy boost is considered in patients treated with BCS for invasive cancer and <50 years of age or those ≥50 years with high-risk features (grade 3, etc.).

In the era of 2D conventional RT, a fluoroscopic simulator was used to plan the treatment and bony landmarks were used to define the field borders. In the era of 3D-Conformal Radiotherapy (3DCRT) and more recently in that of Intensity Modulated Radiotherapy (IMRT) the target areas are carefully contoured on a RT planning CT scan. This is performed with the patient in supine position on a breast board either lying flat or slightly inclined with the arms abducted. A maximum slice thickness of

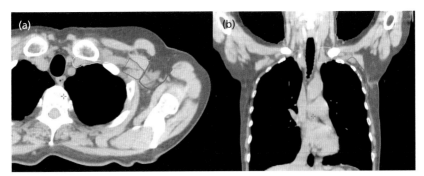

Fig. 4.9 Axial and coronal images of radiotherapy planning CT scan. From medial to lateral CTVn_L4, CTVn_L3, CTVn_L2, CTVn_L1 can be seen in both images. CTVn_interpectoralis can be seen anterior to CTVn_L2 on the axial image (between pectoralis major and pectoralis minor muscles).

2–3 mm should be aimed for, and IV contrast should be administered in order to better visualize the axillary, low neck, and internal mammary vessels.

The European Society for Radiotherapy and Oncology (ESTRO) has published a consensus guideline on target volume delineation for elective radiation therapy of early stage breast cancer, describing in detail the anatomical borders of breast/chest wall and nodal clinical target volumes (CTVs) (Figure 4.9) (Table 4.2).

ESTRO has also published a consensus guideline for target volume delineation in the setting of postmastectomy radiation therapy after implant-based immediate breast reconstruction (IBR) for early stage disease. It is suggested that after IBR with a pre-pectoral implant, the CTV includes the ventral part between skin and implant, which contains the subcutaneous lymphatic plexus and possible residual glandular tissue. The dorsal part between the implant and the pectoral muscle/chest wall, containing any residual glandular tissue can be either partially or completely incorporated in the CTV depending on the presence of adverse factors. These include large tumours (pT3), locally advanced breast cancer (LABC) in the absence of a pathological complete response to induction systemic anti-cancer therapy, and invasion of the major pectoral muscle and/or the chest wall. In cases of IBR with a retro-pectoral implant, if the dorsal fascia is not involved with tumour the CTV encompasses the subcutaneous lymphatic plexus but largely excludes the implant. In the presence of adverse factors as described above or in caudal breast tumours located adjacent to the dorsal fascia and not covered by the major pectoral muscle, clips can be used to demarcate the area and a separate dorsal CTV can be drawn.

A uniform margin is added to the CTV for the planning target volume (PTV) in order to account for set-up errors. Two tangential fields are used to encompass the breast/chest wall PTV and a third vertical field is matched to the tangential fields superiorly when the SCF (with or without the ICF) need to be irradiated. Wider tangential fields are required when the axilla and/or IMC is targeted. Inverse planning IMRT or arc RT (e.g. volumetric modulated arc therapy, rapid arc) can offer increased conformity and might be required for complex anatomy cases (e.g. when tangential

Table 4.2 ESTRO delineation guidelines for the CTV of lymph node regions, breast, and postmastectomy thoracic wall for elective irradiation in breast cancer

Border per region	Axilla level 1 CTVn_L1	Axilla level 2 CTVn_L2	Axilla level 3 CTVn_L3	Lymph node level 4 CTVn_L4	Internal mammary chain CTVn_IMN	Interpectoral nodes CTVn_interpectoralis	Residual breast CTVp_breast	Thoracic wall CTVp_thoracic wall
Cranial	Medial: 5 mm cranial to the axillary vein Lateral: maximally up to 1 cm below the edge of the humeral head, 5 mm around the axillary vein	Includes the cranial extent of the axillary artery (i.e. 5 mm cranial of axillary vein)	Includes the cranial extent of the subclavian artery (i.e. 5 mm cranial of subclavian vein)	Includes the cranial extent of the subclavian artery (i.e. 5 mm cranial of subclavian vein)	Caudal limit of CTVn_L4	Includes the cranial extent of the axillary artery (i.e. 5 mm cranial of axillary vein)	Upper border of palpable/ visible breast tissue; maximally up to the inferior edge of the sternoclavicular joint	Guided by palpable/ visible signs; if appropriate guided by the contralateral breast; maximally up to the inferior edge of the sterno-clavicular joint
Caudal	To the level of rib 4–5, taking also into account the visible effects of the sentinel lymph node biopsy	The caudal border of the pectoral muscle If appropriate: top of surgical ALND	5 mm caudal to the subclavian vein. If appropriate: top of surgical ALND	Includes the subclavian vein with 5 mm margin, thus connecting to the cranial border of CTVn_IMN	Cranial side of the 4th rib (in selected cases 5th rib)	Level 2's caudal limit	Most caudal CT slice with visible breast	Guided by palpable/ visible signs; if appropriate guided by the contralateral breast
Ventral	Pectoralis major and minor muscles	Minor pectoral muscle	Major pectoral muscle	Sternocleidomastoid muscle, dorsal edge of the clavicle	Ventral limit of the vascular area	Major pectoral muscle	5 mm under skin surface	5 mm under skin surface
Dorsal	Cranially up to the thoraco-dorsal vessels, and more caudally up to an imaginary line between the anterior edge of the latissimus dorsi muscle and the intercostal muscles	Up to 5 mm dorsal of axillary vein or to costae and intercostal muscles	Up to 5 mm dorsal of subclavian vein or to costae and intercostal muscles	Pleura	Pleura	Minor pectoral muscle	Major pectoral muscle or costae and intercostal muscles where no muscle	Major pectoral muscle or costae and intercostal muscles where no muscle

Medial	Level 2, the interpectoral level and the thoracic wall	Medial edge of minor pectoral muscle	Junction of subclavian and internal jugular veins >level 4	Includes the jugular vein without margin; excluding the thyroid gland and the common carotid artery	5 mm from the internal mammary vein (artery in cranial part up to and including first intercostal space)	Medial edge of minor pectoral muscle	Lateral to the medial perforating mammary vessels; maximally to the edge of the sternal bone	Guided by palpable/visible signs; if appropriate guided by the contralateral breast
Lateral	Cranially up to an imaginary line between the major pectoral and deltoid muscles, and further caudal up to a line between the major pectoral and latissimus dorsi muscles	Lateral edge of minor pectoral muscle	Medial side of the minor pectoral muscle	Includes the anterior scalene muscles and connects to the medial border of CTVn_L3	5 mm from the internal mammary vein (artery in cranial part up to and including first intercostal space)	Lateral edge of minor pectoral muscle	Lateral breast fold; anterior to the lateral thoracic artery	Guided by palpable/visible signs; if appropriate guided by the contralateral breast Usually anterior to the mid-axillary line

ALND = axillary lymph node dissection.

Reproduced with permission from Offerson, B.V. et al. 'ESTRO consensus guideline on target volume delineation for elective radiation therapy of early stage breast cancer'. *Radiotherapy and Oncology.* Volume 114, Issue 1, pp. 3–10. Copyright © 2015 Elsevier.

fields cannot cover the IMC and spare the heart at the same time or in patients with corpus excavatum). A potential downside with these techniques is the irradiation of a larger area of lung, heart, and contralateral breast. In mastectomy patients, chest wall targeting can be aided by placing radio-opaque wires where it is clinically felt that the borders of the breast were located prior to surgery. A separate radio-opaque wire should be placed on the mastectomy scar to ensure it is fully encompassed in the chest wall CTV when possible.

Surgical clips should be placed in the tumour bed during the operation to facilitate targeting of the area for the breast boost. The boost CTV encompasses the tumour bed and all visible clips on planning CT and then a margin (usually 1 cm) is added to this for the boost PTV. The boost PTV should be treated with photons using a conformal technique (3DCRT or IMRT) unless electrons are felt more appropriate (e.g. in the case of a very superficial tumour bed). Defining the tumour bed on CT can prove difficult in mammoplasty cases as often the clips have been pulled in different directions during this surgical procedure.

Image-guided radiotherapy (IGRT) is employed for treatment verification and positional correction. IGRT techniques include the 2D megavoltage (2D-MV) portal imaging, the 2D kilovoltage planar imaging (2D-kVPI), the megavoltage CT (MV-CT) and the kV cone beam CT (CBCT). The bony anatomy and titanium surgical clips are used for the verification.

Radiation dose to the heart has been associated with increased risk of cardiac damage. For this reason, cardiac sparing techniques such as deep inspiration breath holding (DIBH), or active-breathing control (ABC) should be used in left breast/chest wall RT to minimize the dose to the heart.

4.4 **Therapeutic assessment and follow-up**

4.4.1 Local control

For primary breast cancer that has been treated curatively, standard radiological follow-up is annual mammography for five years followed by discharge to the NHSBSP. For those patients who are less than 45 years at diagnosis, they are advised to have annual mammography until breast screening age. For patients who have had mastectomy, mammographic surveillance is for the contralateral side only, with clinical assessment providing the mainstay for screening the affected side.

Scar tissue can be difficult to assess mammographically. As it is heterogeneous, it can take a varying time to involute and may appear quite different between mammograms due to subtle differences in the way the breast is compressed. If there is clinical or mammographic suspicion of local scar recurrence at any time, then a focused US is appropriate. With the advent of MRI breast screening, those high-risk patients that develop a cancer should, post-treatment, continue with their annual MRI as well as annual mammography as per the NICE guidelines. The exception is the patient who has undergone bilateral mastectomy where no imaging surveillance is necessary. Contrast-enhanced MRI has the advantage of being highly sensitive in detecting recurrent disease, though the previously discussed limitations of this technique remain.

4.4.2 **Toxicity and complications**

A common early side-effect of radiotherapy is breast lymphoedema. On mammogram this appears as diffuse skin and trabecular thickening with interstitial oedema (Figure 4.10). Breast fat necrosis after surgery and radiotherapy needs to be differentiated from local tumour recurrence. Mammographically, it can present as a round oil cyst or as a subcutaneous asymmetric opacity with or without microcalcifications, while on US, subcutaneous tissue hyperechogenicity and/or a cyst can be demonstrated. Nonetheless, imaging cannot always provide a definite diagnosis and a biopsy might be required to exclude recurrent breast cancer. An uncommon effect of the combination of surgery and radiotherapy is benign dystrophic calcifications seen on a mammograph, but this rarely translates into actual clinical symptoms. Significant late breast fibrosis is not common, but when present the breast gland appears smaller, dense, and fibrotic on mammography as a result of the atrophy.

A small strip of lung (usually <2 cm) underlying the treated breast or thoracic wall is commonly included in the tangential fields and receives substantive doses of radiation. Similarly, the lung apex receives the exit dose from the vertical field used to treat the SCF/ICF. However, only a small percentage of patients will develop radiation pneumonitis within six months of breast radiotherapy or radiation-induced lung fibrosis after six months. The lung changes on imaging will commonly follow the radiation beam path. A chest X-ray can show dense opacification but high-resolution computed tomography (HRCT) has better sensitivity and its findings can include ground glass attenuation, linear opacities, thickened septum, areas of atelectasis, and in more severe cases 'honeycomb' changes.

Ribs included in radiotherapy fields can appear slightly sclerotic on CT and a post-radiotherapy rib fracture can be identified on CT, bone scan, or even X-ray.

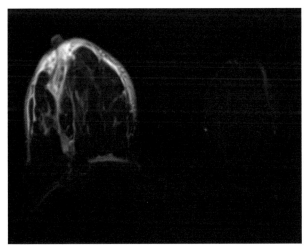

Fig. 4.10 Axial turbo inversion recovery MRI sequence showing skin thickening and parenchymal oedema in the treated right breast.

Brachial plexopathy is a rare late complication of SCF irradiation and has a peak onset at 1–2 years from treatment. An MRI (or PET/CT) can sometimes help exclude obvious recurrent tumour that might be pressing on the brachial plexus. Radiation-induced plexopathy can present in the acute phase as symmetric nerve thickening with occasional T1 enhancement and increased nerve, muscle, and fat intensity on T2. In the late phase, contrast enhancement is absent but there is more thickening of nerves and reduced intensity on T2-weighted images.

4.4.3 Metastases

Metastatic patients staged with CT and started on systemic treatment can have a follow-up CT at three months to assess response to treatment. Bone scans are not as reliable in assessing treatment response in patients with bone metastases. Follow-up PET/CT scan can be used in those initially staged with PET/CT. The Response Evaluation Criteria in Solid Tumours (RECIST) v1.1 is often used in clinical trials to assess response to systemic anti-cancer treatment on CT scans. Similar criteria have been developed for PET/CT (PET Response Criteria in Solid Tumours—PERCIST v.1.0).

4.5 Summary

- Mammography and US remain the primary diagnostic tools for breast cancer, though CESM and digital breast tomosynthesis are being utilized increasingly.
- Secondary disease staging is performed typically with contrast enhanced CT and isotope bone scan, though PET/CT may have a role in advanced or complex disease.
- Mammography and US are still performed for assessment of local recurrence, though MRI and PET/CT may have a role.
- Modern conformal radiotherapy (3DCRT, IMRT) requires careful contouring of clinical target volumes with a contrast-enhanced CT scan.

Further reading

Brierley JD, Gospodarowicz MK, Wittekind C (eds) (2017). Breast in: *TNM Classification of Malignant Tumours* (eighth edition). Oxford: Wiley-Blackwell.

Cancer Research UK. Available at: cancerresearchuk.org.

Department of Health (2016). Clinical guidelines for breast cancer screening assessment: fourth edition. NHSBSP Publication No 49; PHE publications gateway number: 2016426. Retrieved from: https://assets.publishing.service.gov.uk/government/uploads/system/uploads/attachment_data/file/567600/Clinical_guidance_for_breast__cancer_screening__assessment_Nov_2016.pdf.

Donker M, van Tienhoven G, Straver ME, et al. (2014). Radiotherapy or surgery of the axilla after a positive sentinel node in breast cancer (EORTC 10981-22023 AMAROS): a randomised, multicentre, open-label, phase 3 non-inferiority trial. *Lancet Oncology*, **15**(12): 1303–1310.

Fallenberg EM, Schmitzberger FF, Amer H, et al. (2017). Contrast-enhanced spectral mammography vs. mammography and MRI—clinical performance in a multi-reader evaluation. *European Radiology*, **27**(7): 2752–2764.

Kaidar-Person O, Vrou Offersen B, Hol S, et al. (2019). ESTRO ACROP consensus guideline for target volume delineation in the setting of postmastectomy radiation therapy after implant-based immediate reconstruction for early stage breast cancer. *Radiotherapy & Oncology*, **137**: 159–166.

Kuhl CK (2007). Current status of breast MR imaging. Part 2. Clinical applications. *Radiology*, **244**(3): 672–691.

Leach MO, Boggis CR, Dixon AK, et al. (2005). Screening with magnetic resonance imaging and mammography of a UK population at high familial risk of breast cancer: a prospective multicentre cohort study (MARIBS). *Lancet*, **365**(9473): 1769–1778.

National Institute for Health and Care Excellence (2013). Familial breast cancer: classification, care and managing breast cancer and related risks in people with a family history of breast cancer. Clinical guideline [CG164]. Published: June 2013 Last updated: March 2017. Available at: https://www.nice.org.uk/guidance/cg164/resources/familial-breast-cancer-classification-care-and-managing-breast-cancer-and-related-risks-in-people-with-a-family-history-of-breast-cancer-pdf-35109691767493.

Offersen BV, Boersma LJ, Kirkove C, et al. (2015). ESTRO consensus guideline on target volume delineation for elective radiation therapy of early stage breast cancer. *Radiotherapy & Oncology*, **114**(1): 3–10.

The Royal College of Radiologists; Royal College of Physicians of London; Royal College of Physicians and Surgeons of Glasgow; Royal College of Physicians of Edinburgh; British Nuclear Medicine Society; Administration of Radioactive Substances Advisory Committee (2016). Evidence-based indications for the use of PET-CT in the United Kingdom 2016. *Clinical Radiology*, **71**(7): e171–188.

The Royal College of Radiologists. Postoperative radiotherapy for breast cancer: UK consensus statements. London: The Royal College of Radiologists. Available at: https://www.rcr.ac.uk/system/files/publication/field_publication_files/bfco2016_breast-consensus-guidelines.pdf.

Chapter 5

Lung and thorax

Pooja Jain, Katy Clarke, and Michael Darby

5.1 Lung cancer

5.1.1 Clinical background

Lung cancer remains the most common cause of cancer death, accounting for 21% of all cancer deaths, in the UK. There are approximately 47,000 new cases per annum and 36,000 deaths. With the reduction in tobacco use in men since the 1990s, lung cancer incidence rates have decreased by almost 10%, broken down into a decrease in men of 31% but conversely an increase in women of 28%. However, it is estimated that nearly 80% of lung cancers are still considered preventable.

If diagnosed at its earliest stage, more than a 35% of people with lung cancer will survive their disease for five years or more compared to around 5% when diagnosed at a later stage. Unfortunately the majority (72–76%) of patients are diagnosed at stage III or IV.[1]

With this in mind, lung cancer screening programmes have come to the forefront. Two large studies looked at low dose computed tomography (CT) screening for high-risk patients and both showed a significant reduction in mortality (26% at ten years) from lung cancer in favour of screening.[2,3] Local screening programmes are now being implemented in the UK and this will have a positive impact on the number of patients referred for radical treatments and to a lesser extent on systemic therapies. As yet there is no national screening programme.

Histologically the majority of cases are classified as non-small cell, NSCLC (85–90%), further subtyped into adenocarcinoma, squamous cell carcinoma, and large cell carcinoma. The remaining lung cancers are small cell carcinoma, SCLC (10–15%). Worldwide there has been a decline in small cell lung cancer but an increase in adenocarcinoma which has now become the most common histopathologic type.[4]

SCLC disseminates early beyond the thorax and will often present with rapid onset symptoms of systemic disease such as weight loss, poor appetite, and deterioration in performance status.

Adenocarcinoma is often the slowest growing lung cancer and can be present as a peripheral lesion for years prior to diagnosis and is often asymptomatic until advanced. Squamous cell and large cell tumours are more rapidly growing, invading locally initially and early tumours often present with haemoptysis. Alternatively, patients who present later with nodal spread may demonstrate locally compressive symptoms such as dysphagia, superior vena cava or airway obstruction before developing systemic symptoms.

Previously the limiting factor for survival, even when diagnosed with early stage disease, depended on a patient's comorbidities, particularly cardio-respiratory and performance status. With the improvement in surgical techniques and the evolution of stereotactic ablative body radiotherapy and intensity modulated radiotherapy the morbidity and mortality from radical treatments has significantly improved and patients who previously would have been denied curative treatment can be safely and effectively treated.

5.1.2 Diagnosis and staging

5.1.2.1 Diagnosis

Radiological imaging is fundamental in the diagnosis, staging, and follow-up of lung cancer. Most patients still present to lung cancer services with an abnormal chest X-ray, but chest X-ray alone is inadequate for the diagnosis and staging of the disease. Contrast enhanced CT of the chest and upper abdomen, to include liver and adrenals, and ^{18}F-fluorodeoxyglucose positron emission tomography (^{18}F-FDG PET) are the mainstays of imaging early in the patient pathway (Figure 5.1). Other imaging modalities such as ultrasound (US), magnetic resonance imaging (MRI), and bone scans are used as problem-solving tools in individual cases where staging is still not certain with initial imaging.

Although CT and ^{18}F-FDG PET are highly sensitive in the detection of lung cancer both modalities have relatively low specificity (56–63%). Tissue confirmation is important, although in some cases biopsy is not possible and treatment is based on radiological features alone. Bronchoscopy and biopsy of abnormal tissue is the usual approach; otherwise as a general principle it is best to obtain tissue from the site that will confirm the highest stage of disease (i.e. biopsy metastatic disease before nodal disease before the primary).

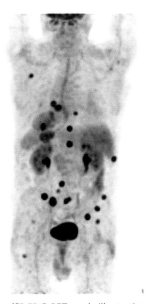

Fig. 5.1 Coronal images from a ^{18}F-FDG PET study illustrating avid uptake of FDG in a right upper lobe nodule along with distant nodal metastases.

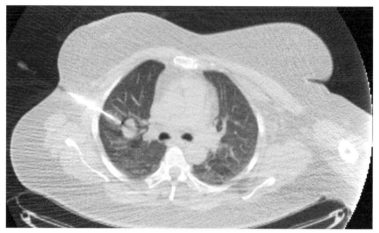

Fig. 5.2 CT guided biopsy of right upper lobe nodule.

Metastatic disease is often accessible with US guidance. US guided FNA of neck nodes is a quick and easy procedure which is positive in up to 20% of patients with N2 mediastinal disease, upstaging these patients to N3.

Endobronchial ultrasound (EBUS) has largely replaced mediastinoscopy in the diagnosis of mediastinal nodal disease, although surgical biopsy is sometimes still necessary if the nodes are inaccessible. Endoscopic transoesophageal US may be used for accessing nodes below the level of the carina and occasionally the left adrenal (Figure 5.2). If there is no accessible metastatic or nodal disease CT guided biopsy of the lung primary is performed (Figure 5.3).

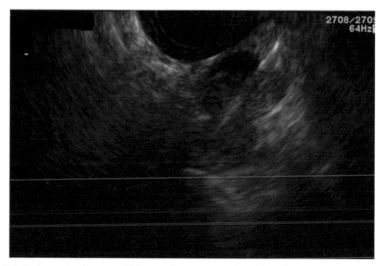

Fig. 5.3 Endoscopic ultrasound biopsy of a paraoesophageal node.

Occasionally in a patient who is felt unfit to undergo biopsy, characteristic imaging features and growth in the suspicious lesion over time may be taken as a surrogate marker of malignancy.

5.1.2.2 Staging

Accurate staging of lung cancer is vital for both prognostic and therapeutic decision making.

The current staging system is TNM 8[5] for both SCLC and NSCLC. In order to reflect prognostic and therapeutic similarities various TNM subsets are further characterized in stages I–IV (see Tables 5.1 and 5.2 below).

Table 5.1 TNM staging of lung cancer

T primary tumour	
TX	Primary tumour cannot be assessed or tumour proven by the presence of malignant cells in sputum or bronchial washings but not visualized by imaging or bronchoscopy
T0	No evidence of primary tumour
Tis	Carcinoma *in situ*[a]
T1	Tumour 3 cm or less in greatest dimension, surrounded by lung or visceral pleura, without bronchoscopic evidence of invasion more proximal than the lobar bronchus (i.e. not in the main bronchus)[b]
T1mi	Minimally invasive adenocarcinoma[c]
T1a	Tumour 1 cm or less in greatest dimension[b]
T1b	Tumour more than 1 cm but not more than 2 cm in greatest dimension[b]
T1c	Tumour more than 2 cm but not more than 3 cm in greatest dimension[b]
T2	Tumour more than 3 cm but not more than 5 cm; or tumour with any of the following features[d] ◆ Involves main bronchus regardless of distance to the carina, but without involvement of the carina ◆ Invades visceral pleura ◆ Associated with atelectasis or obstructive pneumonitis that extends to the hilar region either involving part of or the entire lung
T2a	Tumour more than 3 cm but not more than 4 cm in greatest dimension
T2b	Tumour more than 4 cm but not more than 5 cm in greatest dimension
T3	Tumour more than 5 cm but not more than 7 cm in greatest dimension or one that directly invades any of the following: parietal pleura, chest wall (including superior sulcus tumours) phrenic nerve, parietal pericardium; or separate tumour nodule(s) in the same lobe as the primary
T4	Tumour more than 7 cm or of any size that invades any of the following: diaphragm, mediastinum, heart, great vessels, trachea, recurrent laryngeal nerve, oesophagus, vertebral body, carina; separate tumour nodule(s) in a different ipsilateral lobe to that of the primary

(continued)

Table 5.1 Continued

N regional lymph nodes

Nx	Regional lymph nodes cannot be assessed
N0	No regional lymph node metastasis
N1	Metastasis in ipsilateral peribronchial and/or ipsilateral hilar lymph nodes and intrapulmonary nodes, including involvement by direct extension
N2	Metastasis in ipsilateral mediastinal and/or subcarinal lymph node(s)
N3	Metastasis in contralateral mediastinal, contralateral hilar, ipsilateral, or contralateral scalene, or supraclavicular lymph node(s)

M distant metastasis

M0	No distant metastasis
M1	Distant metastasis
M1a	Separate tumour nodule(s) in a contralateral lobe; tumour with pleural or pericardial nodule(s) or malignant pleural or pericardial effusion[e]
M1b	Single extrathoracic metastasis in a single organ[f]
M1c	Multiple extrathoracic metastases in a single or multiple organs

Notes

[a] Tis includes adenocarcinoma *in situ* and squamous carcinoma *in situ*.

[b] The uncommon superficial spreading tumour of any size with its invasive component limited to the bronchial wall, which may extend proximal to the main bronchus, is also classified as T1a.

[c] Solitary adenocarcinoma (not more than 3 cm in greatest dimension), with a predominantly lepidic pattern and not more than 5 mm invasion in greatest dimension in any one focus.

[d] T2 tumours with these features are classified T2a if 4 cm or less, or if size cannot be determined and T2b if greater than 4 cm but not larger than 5 cm.

[e] Most pleural (pericardial) effusions with lung cancer are due to tumour. In a few patients, however, multiple microscopic examinations of pleural (pericardial) fluid are negative for tumour, and the fluid is non-bloody and is not an exudate. Where these elements and clinical judgment dictate that the effusion is not related to the tumour, the effusion should be excluded as a staging descriptor

[f] This includes involvement of a single non-regional node.

Reproduced with permission from Sobin LH, Gospodarowicz MK, Wittekind CH. *UICC TNM Classification of Malignant Tumours*. 8th ed. © 2017 Wiley Blackwell.

T stage T stage depends upon the size of the primary tumour and any sites of local invasion. Both of these are most accurately assessed with CT scanning due to its higher spatial resolution compared to PET or MRI.

The primary tumour should be measured on CT lung windows setting across its largest possible diameter. Although distinguishing T1 from T2 tumours is unlikely to have any impact upon treatment, the various subdivisions have been shown to have prognostic importance. Accurately identifying T3 and T4 tumours can have important ramifications, and although CT is the mainstay in some specific circumstances other modalities are used in addition. US may be useful in possible direct chest wall invasion,

Table 5.2 Summary of TNM staging with respect to stage groups

	No	N1	N2	N3
T1	IA	IIB	IIIA	IIIB
T2a	IB	IIB	IIIA	IIIB
T2B	IIA	IIB	IIIA	IIIB
T3	IIB	IIIA	IIIB	IIIC
T4	IIIA	IIIA	IIIB	IIIC
M1a	IVA	IVA	IVA	IVA
M1b	IVA	IVA	IVA	IVA
M1c	IVB	IVB	IVB	IVB

Source: data from Amin MB et al. (Eds.) *AJCC Cancer Staging Manual* (8th edition). Springer International Publishing: American Joint Commission on Cancer; 2017.

and MRI is used in the assessment of superior sulcus tumours due to its superior soft tissue characterization when compared to CT.

CT should be interpreted with caution in cases of suspected direct mediastinal invasion where it has been shown to have a false positive rate of up to 33%, and direct surgical inspection is still occasionally necessary in this situation.

N stage CT assessment of mediastinal nodal disease is based on size, with a cut-off of 1 cm in the shortest axis, traditionally taken as the boundary between normal and abnormal. This is a very blunt tool, however, with sensitivity and specificity estimated at 60% and 77% respectively.

PET/CT, which relies on the uptake and concentration of the radioactive tracer ^{18}F-FDG by cancer cells, is a much more accurate way to assess the mediastinal nodes, with sensitivity and specificity of 79% and 91% respectively. ^{18}F-FDG PET/CT is therefore now routinely used for mediastinal nodal staging in all cases other than those with obvious metastatic disease on the original CT scan. Although high, the specificity of ^{18}F-FDG PET/CT is not 100%, however, and other inflammatory processes in the mediastinum, such as infection, can result in a positive PET scan. Tissue confirmation of malignancy, usually via endobronchial or endoscopic US, is therefore still necessary in cases of ^{18}F-FDG avid mediastinal nodes.

Conversely, in cases where there are visible but ^{18}F-FDG non-avid mediastinal nodes it is wise to sample these to confirm that they are not involved before putting a patient through surgery.

The gold standard for staging the mediastinum has traditionally been mediastinoscopy. Paratracheal (stations 2R, 2L, 4R, 4L), pretracheal (stations 1 and 3), and anterior subcarinal (station 7) nodes are accessible. Although invasive, it can be done as an outpatient procedure with minimal morbidity (2.3%) and mortality (0.05%). The average false negative rate of mediastinoscopy is 9%. Many papers have shown similar accuracy with EBUS-TBNA (transbronchial needle aspiration) and recent American College of

Chest Physician guidelines have recommended EBUS-TBNA as the best first test for nodal staging in patients with radiologically suspicious nodes.[6]

M Stage Lung cancer can metastasize to anywhere in the body, but the most common sites are elsewhere in the lung, the pleura, liver, adrenals, bone, and brain. The latest version of the TNM staging system for the first time distinguishes intrathoracic metastases from those outside the chest as well as single from multiple metastases.

As with nodal metastases ^{18}F-FDG PET/CT has been shown to be considerably more sensitive than CT in the detection of distant metastases (Figure 5.4). Combining nodal and distant metastatic disease together PET will upstage up to 18% of patients with localized disease on CT scanning alone. ^{18}F-FDG PET/CT has therefore become routine in the assessment of patients who are found on CT to have radically treatable disease.

Due to the high background levels of glucose uptake in the brain, ^{18}F-FDG PET/CT is not as accurate for brain metastasis. There is still much debate as to the role of routine brain imaging in asymptomatic patients prior to treatment but current NICE recommendations suggest considering brain imaging (either CT or MRI) in patients with N2 or T3 disease being considered for radical treatment.

Imaging for patients with known lung cancer and symptoms suggesting metastatic disease is performed on an individual basis. MRI spine is usually recommended for the investigation of new onset back pain as it allows assessment of not just the vertebrae but also any threat to the cord. Plain film is usually adequate for those with appendicular bone pain, but DMSA bone scan, CT, and MR are all more sensitive should further investigation be felt necessary.

5.1.3 Imaging for radiotherapy planning

5.1.3.1 Radical radiotherapy

Radiotherapy has a major role in the treatment of lung cancers both in curative and palliative settings, and can be useful in all stages regardless of histology. High doses are essential for local control and cure. According to the NLCA 2017 report there has

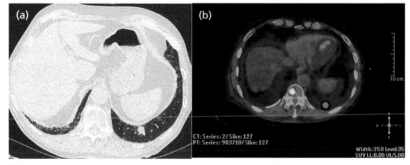

Fig. 5.4 Axial images from a ^{18}F-FDG PET/CT study showing avid uptake of FDG in a left upper lobe non-small cell bronchial carcinoma and uptake in the adjacent vertebral body upstaging the disease advanced stage.

been a significant increase in treatment with curative intent for NSCLC, with 81% of patients with stage I-II disease and PS 0-2 receiving either surgery or radiotherapy.[4]

High-dose radiation therapy delivered either as SABR,[8] accelerated in the CHART schedule or conventional fractionation is used as the primary management for medically inoperable stages I and II NSCLC. Radical radiotherapy is also delivered alongside chemotherapy as part of combined modality treatment, in suitable stage III NSCLC, in both concurrent and sequential settings. Adjuvant radiotherapy in patients with positive resection margins is used to reduce the risk of local recurrence. This can be particularly challenging as it can be difficult to reliably identify the area at risk, using pre- and postoperative images. Radical radiotherapy, especially SABR to extracranial metastases, has also been shown to improve survival in patients with oligometastatic stage IV disease.[9]

Delivery of modern radiotherapy requires 4DCT for advanced planning and verification techniques. These techniques help improve local control by: (1) improving target volume definition; (2) capturing respiratory motion accurately; (3) improving conformality of treatment with the ability to create steep dose gradients between tumour and organs at risk (OAR); and (4) improved accuracy of treatment delivery by better verification to minimize geographical misses. Radiotherapy with palliative intent is less reliant on these technological advances.

5.1.3.2 Treatment planning process

Patients are scanned in a supine position with their arms supported above their heads. Techniques for immobilizing the patient vary, including polystyrene bead-filled bags shaped by vacuum suction or boards with fixed armrests attached to support the patient. An arm down position, with immobilization for the shoulders provided with a five-point fixation mask of the head and upper thorax maybe preferred in patients with superior sulcus or apical tumours or in patients who are unable to maintain a reproducible position with their arms up due to loss of shoulder mobility.

A CT scan of the whole lung from apex to diaphragm is taken with the patient in the treatment position. For modern treatment planning systems the slice width should ideally be 2 mm. For patients with hilar or lower lobe tumours which can move significantly with respiration a 4D CT is recommended to take into account individual specific tumour motion and avoid the use of generic planning margins. Intravenous contrast administered for planning scans allows better definition of tumours close to the hilum.

PET based tumour delineation can improve the accuracy of tumour outlining, especially when there is adjacent collapse or consolidation. Trials are underway to boost PET avid areas to reduce the risk of local recurrence. However, fusion of images is complicated by differences in position of the patient between the scans and by respiratory movement which may be significant in a PET image series which has taken 20 min. to obtain during tidal breathing compared with a helical CT series done rapidly in a single breath hold.

5.1.3.3 Respiratory motion

Tumour motion from breathing during treatment is a major challenge in planning lung radiotherapy. With multidetector CT imaging there is a quick 'snapshot', with the

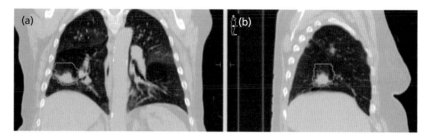

Fig. 5.5 Right lower zone cancer as seen on a standard planning scan, In blue is the ITV contour capturing respiratory motion based on 4D CT scan. (a) Shows coronal view. (b) Shows sagittal view.

result that the extent of respiratory motion is not captured so that the target volume derived from this single point in time may geographically miss the tumour as it moves with respiration (Figure 5.5).

Studies measuring real time tumour motion describe a complex motion 'hysteresis' which is a combination of motion in all three axes, rather than a simple longitudinal motion.[10] Generally tumours in the lower lobes and nodes around the hilum and subcarina tend to show more respiratory motion than in upper lobes. Voluntary breath-holding techniques, deep inspiration breath- hold, and active breath control are physical techniques which theoretically help in limiting tumour motion but have not been very successful as all rely on patient compliance and require levels of breath control which tends to be difficult for the majority of lung cancer patients.

It is usually easier to incorporate respiration in planning using a 4D CT. CT images are acquired over the whole respiratory cycle and sorted into 'bins' for each phase of respiration, so that the position of the tumour can be pinpointed for each phase. With a 'gating' radiotherapy technique the linear accelerator is set to function in an on-off mode coordinated with the phase of respiration for which the radiotherapy plan has been produced. With 'tracking' techniques there is continuous delivery throughout the breathing cycle of a 4D treatment plan which takes account of the varying position of the tumour over time.

5.1.3.4 Contouring for radiotherapy planning

Contouring of the target volume and OAR is performed on each axial slice of the planning CT.

The gross tumour volume (GTV) is delineated, using both lung and soft tissue windows to define the tumour volume accurately (Figure 5.6). When 4D CT is used for planning, the tumour needs to be contoured on all individual phases to incorporate the respiratory motion accurately. In some cases a maximum intensity projection (MIP) scan can be created from all the phases. It is essential that the tumour contours are checked against individual phases to ensure there is no geographical miss, especially as MIPs are not very reliable when the tumour motion is large or close to the diaphragm. In these cases the internal margin is incorporated within the GTV contour and this is called internal target volume (ITV).

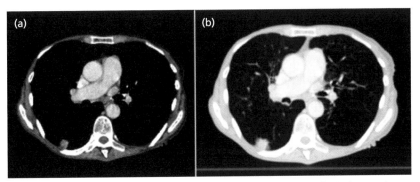

Fig. 5.6 (a) Peripheral tumour with GTV outline marked on mediastinal window setting. (b) The same peripheral tumour: this will often appear larger on lung window settings.

The GTV is then grown by a margin of 5–8 mm depending on histology, to a clinical target volume (CTV). As CTV margin is for microscopic extension, if a tumour is known not to invade nearby OAR, this should be amended manually. Growth of the volume to produce planning target volume (PTV) is usually achieved by an algorithm in the planning system to permit 3D growth in accordance with preset margins which must never be edited even if it is going into an OAR such as spinal cord or air as this margin is used to account for set-up variation (Figure 5.7).

Shielding conforming to the PTV is achieved by using multileaf collimation (MLC). To ensure optimal positioning of the beams the planning system uses a beam's eye view (BEV) which allows the reconstructed image of the patient to be rotated on the computer screen. In this way the MLC can be set up to conform closely to the PTV, for each individual beam, while viewing proximity to OARs such as spinal cord (Figure 5.8).

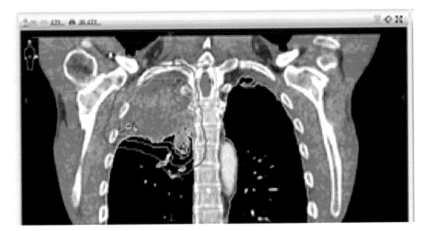

Fig. 5.7 Coronal view.

It is also important to outline OARs on the planning scan. The entire organ is contoured if a volumetric dosimetric constraint is used such as V20, volume of lungs getting 20 Gy or more. If a point or max dose is used then the OARS can be contoured 3–5 cm above and below the PTV as long as a coplanar beam arrangement is used. This is essential for IMRT/VMAT planning as detailed later.

5.1.3.5 Dose-limiting factors in lung radiotherapy

For lung radiation the dose-limiting factors traditionally are pneumonitis, oesophagitis, and spinal cord tolerance. However, as demonstrated by the dose escalation RTOG 0617 trial, there is increasing evidence of the importance of cardiac irradiation and the morbidity it can cause.[11] Contouring OARs enables dose volume histograms (DVHs) to be generated that can be used to compare alternative radiotherapy plans with regard to not only the radiation dose to PTV but also the relative volumes of OAR receiving radiation doses approaching defined tolerance levels (Figure 5.9). Other OARs such as brachial plexus, airways, and main vessels (aorta, superior vena cava) should be contoured when planning SABR.

Symptomatic radiation pneumonitis occurs in 5–15% of patients treated with radical radiotherapy doses and depends upon total dose, volume of lung irradiated,

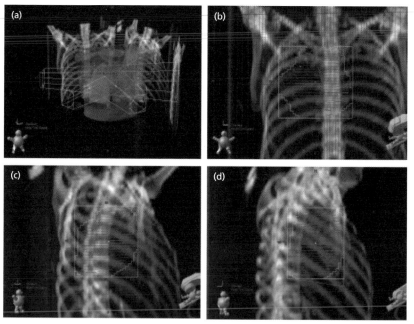

Fig. 5.8 Radiotherapy plan. (a) Three beam's eye view (BEV) images projected onto body showing orientation of fields. (b) Digitally reconstructed radiograph (DRR) of anterior field. PTV on each slice is marked in red. Blue lines show how multileaf collimator (MLC) conforms to target volume. (c) DRR for right anterior oblique field without MLC markings. (d) DRR for right posterior oblique filed without MLC markings.

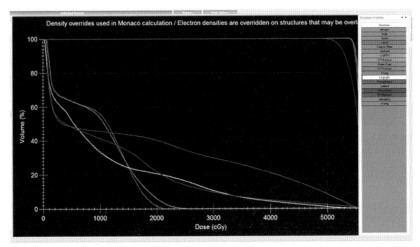

Fig. 5.9 Dose volume histogram for a patient receiving prescribed dose of 55 Gy. The volume of remaining lung (whole lung subtract PTV) receiving 20 Gy (V20) is approximately 20%.

fraction size, and use of chemotherapy. Presence of pulmonary fibrosis, particularly UIP, increases the risk of pneumonitis. Refinement of data on normal tissue complication probabilities over the past decade has led to the use of specific parameters to assess the risk of pneumonitis and guide decisions about radiotherapy.[12] The higher the percentage of lung volume receiving >20 Gy (V20), and mean lung dose (MLD), the higher the risk of pneumonitis.

Acute oesophagitis is another commonly recognized complication of radical radiation doses to the chest although with lower risk of fatal toxicity or long-term sequelae than lung damage. In practice increasing the length of the oesophagus, within the treatment field, increases the risk of symptomatic oesophagitis, especially for lengths >12 cm.

For spinal cord, maximum point doses are used as it is essential not to exceed tolerance dose at any single level within the cord. The aim is to stay below 44 Gy in 2-Gy fractions although tolerance may be lowered with altered fractionation.

5.1.3.6 Intensity modulated/volumetric arc radiation therapy

This approach to planning involves specifying objectives such as desired dose to PTV and dose constraints for OARs which is used by a planning algorithm to derive the optimal plan. Invariably the plans can achieve tight dose constraints around OARs by modulating the intensity of the radiation beam (Figure 5.10).

Functional imaging with PET and perfusion MRI scans can provide information on the distribution of functional lung tissue as many lung cancer patients will have emphysematous destruction or poorly perfused areas of lung which are therefore less important to spare. IMRT/VMAT planning can theoretically help in creating plans that can differentially spare irradiation of healthy lung. This opens the way for more

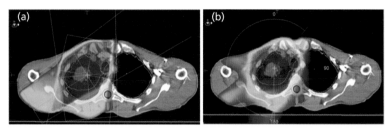

Fig. 5.10 (a) 3-D plan with fixed beam angles for an apical tumour (b) same tumour planned with VMAT showing better conformality of higher isodoses to tumour (red and orange colour-wash) with better sparing of cord (turquoise and indigo colour-wash).

sophisticated analysis of lung DVHs than is currently available where all lungs are assumed to be equal.

The drawbacks of lung IMRT, however, are that: (1) a larger total volume of lung may receive low dose radiation and (2) there are often sharp dose gradients. This is a particular problem with tightly conforming fields such that the respiratory motion may cause geographical miss in the absence of advanced treatment verification techniques like cone beam CT (CBCT).

5.1.3.7 Treatment verification

Treatment verification is essential to confirm that the treatment is delivered as planned. Modern linear accelerators have the capability of obtaining CBCT imaging which provides detailed anatomical information. This represents a significant advance on treatment verification. The planning scan is matched to the CBCT for treatment verification. Depending on doses to OARs, the match can be to the critical OAR such as spine, chest wall (surrogate for plexus), or the tumour itself (Figure 5.11).

CBCT can be converted to 4D CBCT, similar to 4D CT, and can provide a check of tumour motion during treatment. Sometimes when 4D CT cannot be acquired at the time of planning due to issues such as erratic or slow breathing, then 4D CBCT is useful in creating an appropriate ITV, thereby avoiding geographical miss and/or inappropriately large margins.

With improved anatomical verification it is easy to identify changes in the lung parenchyma during treatment such as reinflation of a collapse, development of a pleural effusion, or tumour shrinkage (Figure 5.12). Identifying such changes avoids geographical miss and gives an opportunity to readjust the treatment plan if there are dosimetric consequences for the tumour or OARs.

5.1.4 Therapeutic assessment and follow-up

The objectives of follow-up imaging after radiotherapy for lung cancer are threefold: to assess response to treatment; to monitor toxicity (both acute and late in onset); and to detect progression or relapse when it occurs.

In trials RECIST criteria for response assessment usually require two CT scans, a month apart, with the first done a minimum of six weeks following completion of

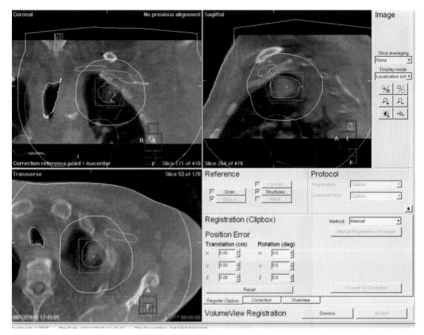

Fig. 5.11 Cone beam CT taken prior to radiotherapy delivery to match accurately to tumour as the tumour location is close to brachial plexus (green).

radiotherapy, although outside of clinical trials, usually, a single investigation is undertaken. Reduction in tumour or nodal mass can be measured but it is often difficult in the presence of pneumonitic changes, or associated collapse or consolidation, to categorize response definitively. There continues to be debate about the need for and frequency of further follow-up scans which should be determined on an individual patient basis, influenced by whether second-line therapy would be feasible in case of progressive disease or relapse.

The radiological changes of acute pneumonitis commonly peak at about three months and as well as monitoring clinical symptoms and pulmonary function it may be worth repeating imaging with chest X-ray, keeping CT in reserve for concerns, several months later to assess resolution of this toxicity (Figure 5.13).

Tumour response after treatment assessed by PET is much more powerfully correlated with survival than response measured by CT.[13] This has raised the potential role of PET in early monitoring of patients to allow response adapted therapy similar to approaches being developed in lymphoma.

5.2 **Other thoracic malignancies**

This chapter has thus far focused on radiotherapy planning for non-small cell lung cancer; however, the same principles can be applied to treating other thoracic malignancies.

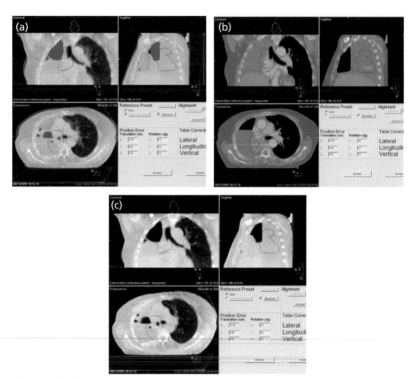

Fig. 5.12 (a) CBCT overlayed over planning scan showing changes in post pneumonectomy fluid space during treatment (purple represents changes seen on CBCT and green represents planning scan). Change in post pneumonectomy space is causing a lateral shift on the airways (green) which is likely to impact on PTV position. (b) Planning CT scan. (c) Cone beam CT.

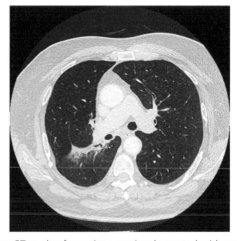

Fig. 5.13 Image from CT study of a patient previously treated with radical radiotherapy for a right upper lobe bronchial carcinoma. The scan demonstrates changes in lung parenchyma consistent with radiation fibrosis.

5.2.1 Small cell lung cancer

SCLC is characterized by an aggressive disease course with development of early meta-static disease despite often apparently limited thoracic disease. Combination chemo/radiotherapy remains the mainstay of treatment using a concurrent chemoradiotherapy protocol.[14]

There is also a benefit from consolidation thoracic radiotherapy in advanced disease, with a significant improvement in two-year survival and progression free survival.[15]

Because of the high rates of brain metastases the role of prophylactic cranial irradiation has been investigated in both limited and extensive stage small cell lung cancer. Doses varied from 20 Gy/5 fractions to 30 Gy/10 fractions within the studies. Initial studies did show improvement in both survival and reduction in the occurrence of brain metastases in patients both in the palliative and radical setting. However, this comes with significant toxicities such as severe fatigue, short-term memory loss, and alopecia, and recent studies have shown that this could be detrimental to patients in the extensive stage setting.

5.2.2 Thymoma

Thymoma is a rare tumour arising from the epithelial cells of the thymus and is most commonly seen as a mass in the anterior mediastinum. Pathologically this represents a spectrum of disease ranging from the relatively benign type A thymomas which take many years to grow and have very low recurrence rates, to a type C which often be-haves more like NSCLC.

The main stay of treatment remains surgical resection. However, adjuvant radio-therapy may be indicated when resection margins are positive, for higher stage disease and for the more aggressive pathological subtypes of thymoma. Radical radiotherapy and chemoradiotherapy, concurrent or sequential, are also used when thymomas are localized but surgically unresectable. In metastatic disease chemotherapy is the main treatment option.

Radiotherapy to the anterior mediastinum can be challenging both in terms of achieving adequate dosing and avoiding OAR. Traditional beam arrangements such as anterior oblique fields or APPA fields with a lateral beam often lead to plans exceeding safe lung tolerance parameters. However, using the advanced planning techniques de-scribed earlier in the chapter we can now avoid this.

5.2.3 Pleural mesothelioma

Malignant pleural mesothelioma continues to increase in incidence and presents with diffuse pleural involvement for which treatment is palliative rather than curative.

Systemic chemotherapy with a platinum and pemetrexed doublet remains the only treatment that has shown a survival benefit in phase three randomized controlled trials in the mesothelioma population.

5.3 Summary

- Lung cancer is the commonest cause of cancer death.
- Radical radiotherapy can potentially cure lung cancer, especially in early stage disease.

- Local control rates following radical radiotherapy are related to the dose delivered and for early lung cancers can be in excess of 80–90% especially if treated with SABR.

- Functional imaging with PET and 4D imaging with CT should contribute to improved target volume definition with reduced risk of geographical miss.

- Accurate defined target volumes and OAR are essential for advanced planning techniques such as IMRT/VMAT.

- Continued monitoring of normal tissue complication rates will better inform the use of DVH parameters to guide decisions about radiotherapy plans.

- Improved treatment verification techniques are evolving rapidly, with real-time electronic portal imaging, kV imaging on LINACs, and CBCT; these minimize geographical miss and allow the use of smaller planning margins.

References

1. **Statistics from Cancer Research UK** https://www.cancerresearchuk.org/health-professional/cancer-statistics/statistics-by-cancer-type/lung-cancer

2. **The National Lung Screening Trial Research Team (2011).** Reduced lung-cancer mortality with low-dose computed tomographic screening. *New England Journal of Medicine*, **365**(5): 395–409.

3. **De Koning H, Van Der Aalst C, Ten Haaf K, et al.** (2018). Effects of volume CT lung cancer screening: mortality results of the NELSON randomised-controlled population based trial. *Journal of Thoracic Oncology*, **13**(10): S185.

4. **Alberg AJ, Ford JG, Samet JM.** (2007). Epidemiology of lung cancer: ACCP evidence-based clinical practice guidelines, 2nd ed. *Chest*. **132**: 29S–55S.

5. **Goldstraw P, Chansky K, Crowley J, et al.** (2016). The IASLC Lung Cancer Staging Project: Proposals for Revision of the TNM Stage Groupings in the forthcoming (eighth) edition of the TNM classification for lung cancer. *Journal of Thoracic Oncology*, **11**(1): 39–51.

6. **Silvestri GA, Gonzalez AV, Jantz MA, et al.** (2013). **Methods for staging non-small cell lung cancer: diagnosis and management of lung cancer.** 3rd ed: American College of Chest Physicians evidence-based clinical practice guidelines. *Chest*, **143**(Suppl 5): e211S–e250S.

7. **National Lung Cancer Audit annual report** (2017) (for the audit period 2016): *National Lung Cancer Audit Report* (2014) Report for the audit period 2013.

8. **Chang J, Senan S, Paul M, et al.** (2015). Stereotactic ablative radiotherapy versus lobectomy for operable stage I non-small-cell lung cancer: a pooled analysis of two randomised trials. *Lancet Oncology*, **16**(6): 630–637.

9. **Juan O, Popat S** (2017). Ablative therapy for oligometastatic non-small cell lung cancer. *Clinical Lung Cancer*, **18**(6): 595–606.

10. **Seppenwoolde Y, Shirato H, Kitamura K, et al.** (2002). Precise and real-time measurement of 3D tumor motion in lung due to breathing and heartbeat, measured during radiotherapy. *International Journal Radiation Oncology. Biology. Physics*, **53**(4): 822–834.

11. **Chun S, Hu C, Choy H, et al.** (2017). Impact of intensity-modulated radiation therapy technique for locally advanced non–small-cell lung cancer: a secondary analysis of

the NRG oncology RTOG 0617 randomized clinical trial. *Journal of Clinical Oncology*, **35**(1): 56–62.

12. **Seppenwolde Y, Lebesque JV, de Jaeger K, et al.** (2003). **Comparing different NTCP models that predict the incidence of radiation pneumonitis.** Normal tissue complication probability. *International Journal Radiation Oncology. Biology. Physics*, **55**(3): 724–735.

13. **Patz EF, Connolly J, Herndon J** (2000). Prognostic value of thoracic FDG PET imaging after treatment for non-small cell lung cancer. *American Journal of Roentgenology*, **174**: 769–774.

14. **Turrisi AT, Kim K, Sause WT, et al.** (1999) Twice-daily compared with once-daily thoracic radiotherapy in limited small-cell lung cancer treated concurrently with cisplatin and etoposide. *New England Journal of Medicine*, **340**(4): 265–271.

15. **Slotman BJ, van Tinteren H, Praag JO, et al.** (2015). Use of thoracic radiotherapy for extensive stage small-cell lung cancer: a phase 3 randomised controlled trial. *Lancet*, **385**(9962): 36–42.

Chapter 6

Lymphoma

Heok Cheow, Peter Hoskin, and
Thankamma Ajithkumar

6.1 Introduction

Lymphoma covers a broad spectrum of disease entities which is reflected in a wide range of imaging involved in its diagnosis and management. It can be unifocal or multifocal, affecting lymph nodes or other organs. The two main groups, namely Hodgkin lymphoma (HL) and non-Hodgkin lymphoma (NHL), have very different patterns of disease distribution which can influence imaging strategies; however, the pathological subtypes, whilst important in disease management, do not greatly influence the staging processes for which imaging is used.

Contrast-enhanced computed tomography (CT) has a central role in the diagnosis, staging, and follow-up of lymphoma. In addition, extra nodal lymphoma is common, seen in approximately 40% of NHL, and these sites may have specific imaging requirements. However, lymphoma is one of the first conditions where molecular imaging with positron emission tomography/computed tomography (PET/CT), using ^{18}F-fluorodeoxyglucose (^{18}F-FDG) as the tracer, has been incorporated in international criteria for response.

The most common feature of lymphoma is lymph node enlargement. The central role of diagnostic imaging is therefore to identify pathological lymph nodes and distinguish these from normal nodes which can be enlarged due to physiological reactive change. The anatomical cross-sectional imaging modalities of computed tomography (CT), ultrasound (US), and magnetic resonance imaging (MRI) examine nodal architecture, whereas molecular imaging with ^{18}F-FDG PET/CT demonstrates alteration in physiology following neoplastic invasion. Both anatomical and molecular imaging techniques require a substantial degree of nodal involvement before a convincing abnormality can be identified; in early disease, imaging may be falsely negative.

Normal nodes are ovoid in morphology with a long-short axis ratio of around 1.5–2.1. They have a fatty hilum, smooth cortex, and well-defined margins. When a node becomes involved in a neoplastic process such as lymphoma, it enlarges, particularly in the short axis, resulting in a more rounded contour, and a reduction in the long-short axis ratio. The cortex may become irregular and there can be loss of the fatty hilum as neoplastic displaces normal nodal tissue. The margin of the cortex may be breached, which results in poor definition of the nodal margins on imaging.

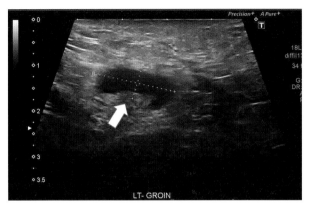

Fig. 6.1 Illustration of a normal lymph node: the lymph node has ovoid morphology with smooth cortex shown in grey and central hilar fat in white (arrow). The minimum short axis diameter (a) is measured at the widest point of the node, at 90° to the long axis (b).

The minimum short-axis diameter is the standard measurement criteria in lymph node for most malignancies. This is the minimum diameter of the node when measured at its widest point along the short axis, taken at 90° to the long axis (Figure 6.1). Nodes which measure >1 cm in minimum short-axis diameter are generally considered likely to be involved in a neoplastic process, with a sensitivity and specificity of 70%. The long-axis measurement is generally not as good an indicator for presence of disease as normal nodes may be long and slender. By consensus, the International Working Group for Lymphoma has, in 2007, defined an abnormal lymph node as >1.0 cm in short axis and >1.5 cm in long axis diameter. These criteria are still used in many international lymphoma trials.

6.2 **Diagnosis and investigations**

6.2.1 Diagnosis

HL and NHL have different patterns of disease spread and distribution; these determine the imaging modalities which are most frequently involved in making the first step towards the diagnosis. Lymphoma is the great clinical and radiological pretender and frequently mimics other aggressive conditions, such as solid neoplasms, infection, and sarcoid. It is only after biopsy and pathological assessment that a confident diagnosis can be established. Imaging is frequently used to guide core biopsy to obtain tissue for pathological diagnosis in non-palpable cases.

HL spreads via the lymphatics, resulting in a disease distribution which is contiguous along lymphatic pathways. It is more common above the diaphragm and generally involves lymph nodes within the mediastinal (70%), cervical (70%) and paraaortic (30%) groups, and the spleen (30%). Patients may present with respiratory symptoms or B symptoms which prompt a chest X-ray as part of baseline investigations, which may demonstrate mediastinal lymphadenopathy (Figure 6.2). Alternatively, cervical lymphadenopathy will result in referral to a head and neck surgeon who may request

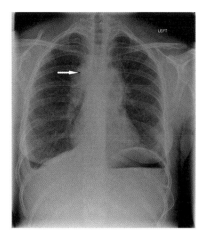

Fig. 6.2 Hodgkin lymphoma: chest x-ray showing mediastinal lymphadenopathy.

US and/or MRI to establish the origin of the palpable mass. US and MRI are particularly useful imaging modalities for the definition of neck anatomy; they have higher tissue contrast than CT and do not suffer from beam-hardening artefact due to dental amalgam which frequently degrades images of the upper neck.

NHL consists of a spectrum including B and T cell lymphoma which have their distinct characteristics. NHL can undergo haematological spread, resulting in a more diverse and discontinuous pattern of disease distribution than HL. It is commonly found on both sides of the diaphragm, with para-aortic (50%), mesenteric (50%), and mediastinal (30%) lymphadenopathy. There is also a high propensity for extra-nodal disease compared to HL, including bone marrow (30%), bowel (10%), renal tract (7%), central nervous system (2%), and lung parenchyma (3%). This is reflected in the wider range of imaging techniques used for diagnosis, including MRI for marrow and neurological lymphoma, and US for testicular lymphoma. Gastrointestinal mucosa associated lymphoma (MALT) most commonly involving the stomach or large bowel can be indistinguishable on imaging from adenocarcinoma, with irregular thickening of the wall and shouldering at the interface with normal anatomy. Lymphomatous involvement of the bowel can be suggested by longer segment involvement and better preservation of lumen than is generally seen with carcinomas, and involvement of the terminal ileum is more frequent with lymphoma.

Essential investigations for lymphoma would include the following:

- Excision biopsy or core needle biopsy for histological diagnosis, including full immunohistochemical profile, flow cytometry, and cytogenetic analysis when necessary.
- CT imaging from base of skull to femoral regions.
- Peripheral blood count, erythrocyte sedimentation rate, serum lactate dehydrogenase (LDH), serum albumen, and markers of renal and hepatic function.
- Immunoglobulin profile and protein electrophoresis.

◆ Bone marrow examination: no longer indicated for the routine staging of HL after PET/CT and most DLBCL. If there is uncertainty regarding bone marrow involvement in these situations or other lymphomas where involvement of bone marrow might alter treatment (e.g. early stage low-grade NHL), a bone marrow examination is indicated.

◆ Cerebrospinal fluid in NHL patients with high-risk features, in particular lymphoma affecting the paranasal sinuses and testes.

6.2.2 Anatomical imaging

6.2.2.1 Computed tomography

CT remains the mainstay of imaging for the staging of lymphoma. Modern helical multi-slice scanners now allow sub-millimetre imaging through the neck, chest, abdomen, and pelvis to be obtained in seconds, with isotropic axial, coronal, and sagittal reconstructions producing high quality images. This has increased image interpretation accuracy, helped by the use of intravenous contrast medium, which allows confident differentiation between lymph nodes and blood vessels. CT can accurately identify not only enlarged lymph nodes and categorize these by virtue of their size, shape, and numeracy, but can also demonstrate disease in extra nodal sites, for example the brain, lungs, gastrointestinal tract, kidneys, liver, and spleen. Other cross-sectional imaging modalities complement CT findings in particular anatomical regions and clarify lesions which are indeterminate on CT.

6.2.2.2 Ultrasound

US is useful in assessing indeterminate liver and renal lesions and has a role in imaging splenic lymphoma. The spleen has a high propensity for lymphomatous involvement, particularly in HL. Based on historical series where laparotomy and splenectomy were a routine component of treatment, up to one-third of normal sized spleens contain microscopic HL, whereas only approximately one-third of enlarged spleens were involved. Splenic size alone is therefore not helpful. US can detect splenic lesions down to 3 mm in diameter with higher sensitivity than CT for the detection of splenic lymphoma (63% vs. 37%). The disadvantage of the use of US in lymphoma staging lies in the fact that its performance is best when targeted to specific organs; and it is depth and operator dependent, making assessment of disease less reproducible than CT or MRI, especially in the therapy response setting.

6.2.2.3 Magnetic resonance imaging

With recent advances in MRI technology, whole body MRI is now feasible, with the advantage of no radiation exposure (Figure 6.3). MRI has superior performance to CT in assessing lymph nodes when diffusion-weighted sequences are incorporated within the acquisition protocol, and also in assessing extranodal disease, especially in the assessment of the neural axis, bone marrow, head and neck, and pelvic regions. In bone marrow assessment, MRI enables global assessment of the disease distribution more accurately than single or paired bone marrow aspirates and trephine samples from the iliac crests, identifying bone marrow infiltration in up to 33% of patients who have

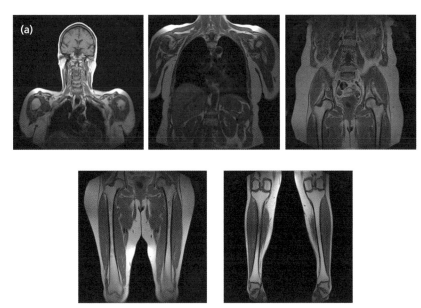

Fig. 6.3a Selected coronal T1-weighted turbo spine echo whole body MRI images showing normal marrow signal intensity.

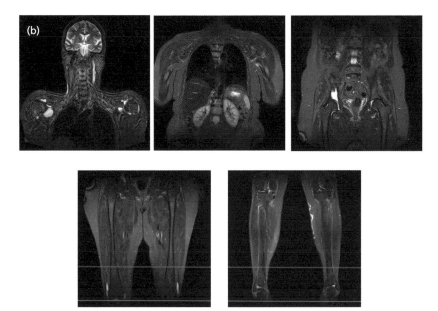

Fig. 6.3b Selected coronal T2-weighted whole body MRI images with STIR fat suppression showing normal marrow signal intensity.

negative iliac crest biopsies. False negatives may occur where there is only scanty infiltration and in indolent lymphomas.

6.2.2.4 Molecular imaging

^{18}F-FDG PET/CT has established itself as an invaluable tool in the management of lymphoma. The principles of ^{18}F-FDG PET/CT are described in Chapter 2. This imaging modality is now advocated as the main modality for staging FDG-avid disease (Table 6.1) in the Lugano Classification 2014.

In the evaluation of lymphoma, the sensitivity of ^{18}F-FDG PET/CT of 85–90% is 15% higher than with CT as PET/CT can identify elevated metabolic activity in normal-sized lymph nodes (Figure 6.4). PET/CT can also detect focal or multi-focal bone marrow involvement where an iliac crest sample is negative (Figure 6.5). Because of this, bone marrow biopsy can be omitted for the routine staging of Hodgkin lymphoma and diffuse large B cell lymphoma (DLBCL). Specificity for CT and PET/CT are equivalent at 70% for lymphomatous involvement. False positive results can result from FDG uptake by granulomatous disorders such as sarcoid and infection (particularly TB), physiological brown fat, muscle, tonsils, and bowel activity. Uptake can also be seen in inflammatory and degenerative arthritis.

^{18}F-FDG PET/CT is less useful in defining involvement with indolent lymphoma as it is not possible differentiate involved nodes from benign, reactive nodes. Nevertheless, FDG PET/CT may have a role in identifying transformation to high-grade disease. Several studies have found PET/CT may identify potential sites of transformation, indicated by elevated metabolic activity, in nodes or organs which can be targeted for biopsy.

Table 6.1 FDG avidity according to different lymphoma subtypes

Lymphoma subtypes	Percentage of FDG avidity
Burkitt lymphoma	100
Mantle cell lymphoma	100
Hodgkin lymphoma	97–100
Diffuse large B cell lymphoma	97–100
Anaplastic large T-cell lymphoma	94–100
Follicular lymphoma	91–100
Natural killer/T cell lymphoma	83–100
Angioimmunoblastic T cell lymphoma	78–100
Peripheral T cell lymphoma	86–98
Mucosa-associated lymphoid tissue (MALT) lymphoma	54–81
Small lymphocytic lymphoma	47–83

Source: data from Barrington SF, Mikhaeel N, Kostakoglu L, et al. 'Role of imaging in the staging and response assessment of lymphoma: consensus of the international conference on malignant lymphomas imaging working group'. *J Clin Oncol* 2014, 32(27), pp.3048–3058.

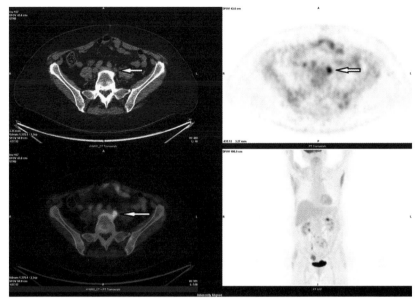

Fig. 6.4 ^{18}F-FDG PET/CT showing areas of increased FDG uptake despite normal left common iliac node on size criteria.

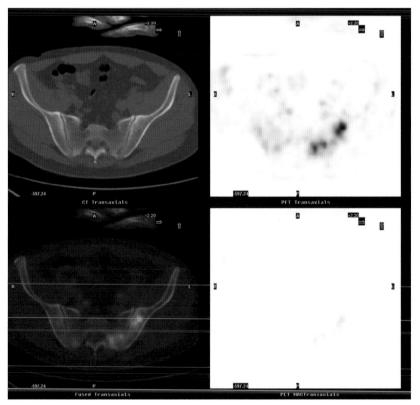

Fig. 6.5 ^{18}F-FDG PET/CT showing bone marrow involvement with lymphoma.

In general, management of both types of lymphoma will depend upon stage, with patients classified into early or advanced disease. Those with early disease, that is stage Ia or IIa, will be treated with short-course chemotherapy and involved node (site) radiotherapy (see below) whilst those with more aggressive disease, that is patients with stage Ib, IIb, III, or IV, will receive more prolonged combination chemotherapy.

A change in stage therefore will only be relevant to treatment if a patient without B symptoms is moved from stage I or II to stage III or IV. With the high sensitivity of ^{18}F-FDG PET/CT in identifying additional sites, that is, stage III or IV disease, this typically does not alter management. Similarly, where additional sites in one anatomical region are identified, the added information from PET/CT will not alter overall management although it might be important in determining radiotherapy volume. In current clinical practice, the baseline PET/CT is compared with an interim imaging (usually done after two cycles of chemotherapy) to assess for an early metabolic response. Evidence suggests that in HL an early response on molecular imaging, in particular PET/CT, predicts outcome and guides further treatment modifications (see below).

6.2.3 Staging

The aim of staging is to identify the full extent of disease prior to treatment, in order to define the best treatment. Currently ^{18}F-FDG PET/CT is routinely recommended for staging all FDG-avid nodal lymphomas. In FDG non-avid histological subtypes such as CLL/small lymphocytic lymphoma, lymphoplasmacytic lymphoma/Walderstrom's macroglobulinaemia, mycosis fungoides, and marginal zone lymphomas, CT scan is used for staging. The Lugano modification of Ann-Arbor staging can be viewed here:[1]

◆ B symptoms: fever (>38.3°C), drenching night sweats, or weight loss >10% body weight over six months. B symptoms only affect HL and therefore this qualifier is only used for HL.

◆ Splenic involvement is defined as diffuse uptake, solitary mass, military lesions or nodules on ^{18}F-FDG PET/CT or splenomegaly is defined as >13 cm in vertical length on CT scan, if FDG non-avid.

6.3 Radiotherapy planning

The role of radiotherapy in the management of lymphoma has changed substantially with the advent of effective combination chemotherapy. It is, however, still the most active single modality in the management of lymphoma, and in HL radiotherapy remains an important component of treatment regimens, particularly in early disease. Similarly, in early stage NHL, radiotherapy remains an important addition to short-course chemotherapy in standard management. There have also been substantial changes in radiotherapy equipment and techniques in the last decade. Routine use of ^{18}F-FDG PET/CT in staging has led to the replacement of involved-field radiotherapy (IFRT: treating the anatomical nodal region involved at diagnosis) with involved-node radiotherapy (INRT: treating a target volume of radiotherapy comprising pre-chemotherapy nodal disease only) (Figure 6.6). However, a pre-requisite

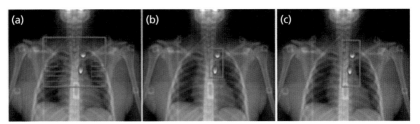

Fig. 6.6 An illustration of evolution of treatment volumes in lymphoma: (a) involved-field radiotherapy; (b) involved-node radiotherapy; and (c) involved-site radiotherapy.

for INRT is imaging with ^{18}F-FDG PET/CT at diagnosis and after chemotherapy in the radiotherapy treatment position and with the same breathing instructions. Since the majority of clinical departments cannot obtain diagnostic PET/CT in radiotherapy treatment position, the current clinical practice is a modification of INRT technique called involved-site radiotherapy (ISRT). The CTV for ISRT comprises the pre-chemotherapy nodal disease with a margin of 15 mm to allow for uncertainties in the contouring. If diagnostic (pre-chemotherapy) PET/CT is not available, IFRT should be considered to avoid any risk of potential recurrences in the anatomical region.

6.3.1 CT

CT based planning is the standard for all lymphoma. CT planning has numerous advantages, including:

♦ More accurate definition of lymph node areas.

♦ More accurate definition of extra nodal sites.

♦ More accurate definition of organs at risk (OAR).

♦ Incorporation of tissue inhomogeneities within the planning algorithm for more accurate dose distributions.

♦ Dose volume histogram analyses for coverage of planning target volume (PTV) and OAR.

Planning CT scan is generally obtained with a slice thickness of 2–3 mm. Intravenous contrast aids identification of the lymph node chains and differentiates nodes from blood vessels. Contrast has no substantial effect upon the dosimetry algorithms for radiotherapy planning. For abdominal and pelvic nodes, oral contrast is useful to delineate intestinal loops. 4D CT imaging may be considered for sites that change with respiration and close to the heart (which may move with respiration and cardiac cycle). Definition of the clinical target volume (CTV) is based on the known lymph node area to be covered using standard published lymph node atlases. OARs should also be outlined in this process, as shown in Figure 6.7.

6.3.2 PET and MRI

^{18}F-FDG PET uptake is required to identify actual sites of involvement with lymphoma distinct from lymph node regions when using the concepts of INRT and ISRT. The CTV

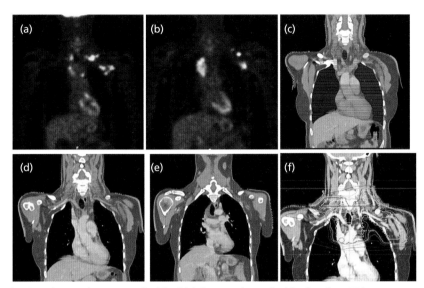

Fig. 6.7 Diagnostic PET scan (a&b) which is co-registered with planning CT images (c–e) in a patient with Hodgkin lymphoma. Coronal planning CT imaging showing OARs (c) and clinical target volume (CTV) for involved-site radiotherapy (d&e). Note: CTV is modified based on post-chemotherapy anatomical changes. (e) Treatment planning using IMRT.

for INRT is defined as the initially involved lymph nodes on the pre-chemotherapy PET/CT, obtained in the treatment position, which is then modified based on post-chemotherapy anatomical changes (Figure 6.7). MRI is useful for radiotherapy planning for lymphomas in the central nervous system, paranasal sinuses, orbit, and musculoskeletal system as MRI provides a greater soft tissue contrast compared to CT.

6.4 **Therapeutic response and follow-up**

As there are various chemotherapy regimens available for treatment, the aim for HL and aggressive NHL is to achieve cure, whereas for low-grade indolent lymphoma, disease control and prolonged survival is often the goal. Imaging plays a pivotal role in selecting treatment regime and assessment of disease response. Contrast enhanced CT is used for indolent lymphoma and PET/CT for FDG-avid lymphoma.

The imaging modality of choice for assessing therapy response will be tailored depending on the distribution of disease at staging. However, if initial staging revealed disease in a region which required another modality for full assessment (e.g. US for testicular, MRI for Waldeyer's ring disease, brain, and bone marrow), then these modalities will also be required for follow-up imaging.

Response can be defined as resolution or reduction in size of the enlarged lymph node or extranodal mass on anatomical imaging and reduced metabolic activity on ^{18}F-FDG PET/CT. A post therapy residual mass will cause uncertainty whether it represents residual active disease or post therapy fibrotic mass. PET/CT assesses

Table 6.2 Deauville five-point scale

Score	FDG uptake based on SUVmax	Interpretation
1	No uptake	Considered to represent complete metabolic response (CMR) at interim and end of treatment
2	≤ Mediastinal blood pool	Considered to represent complete metabolic response (CMR) at interim and end of treatment
3	> Mediastinal blood pool and ≤ liver	Dependent on the timing of assessment, the clinical context and the treatment FDG uptake declines during therapy in chemosensitive disease and residual FDG uptake higher than normal liver uptake is frequently seen at interim in patients who achieve CMR at the end of treatment
4	Moderately > liver at any site	Suggests chemosensitive disease provided uptake has reduced from baseline and is considered to represent partial metabolic response at interim study Represents residual metabolic active disease even if the uptake has reduced from baseline at end of treatment
5	Markedly* > liver at any site and/or new sites of disease	Suggests chemosensitive disease provided uptake has reduced significantly from baseline and is considered to represent partial metabolic response at interim study Represents residual metabolic active disease even if the uptake has reduced from baseline at end of treatment New sites of disease could represent disease progression, biopsy recommended.
X	New areas of uptake unlikely to be related to lymphoma	

SUVmax: maximum standardized uptake value; * SUVmax of the lesion >2x liver uptake

The response evaluation criteria for lymphoma has been published by the International Working Group (RECIL 2017) as shown below:

Source: data from Barrington SF, Mikhaeel N, Kostakoglu L, et al. Role of imaging in the staging and response assessment of lymphoma: consensus of the international conference on malignant lymphomas imaging working group. J. Clin. Oncol 2014, 32 (27), pp. 3048–3058.

the metabolic activity with such mass. An international five-point scoring system (Deauville score) has been developed to give a guidance on residual mass based on its metabolic activity using two reference points of mediastinal blood pool and liver (Table 6.2).

Complete response:

◆ Complete disappearance of all target lesions and all nodes with long axis <10 mm.

- ≥30 decrease in the sum of longest diameters of target lesions with normalization of ^{18}F-FDG-PET/CT (Deauville 1–3).
- Bone marrow is not involved and no new lesion.

Partial response:

- ≥30% decrease in the sum of longest diameters of target lesions with positive ^{18}F-FDG-PET/CT (Deauville score 4–5).
- Bone marrow can be involved, but no new lesion.

Minor response:

- ≥10% decrease but <30% in the sum of longest diameters of target lesions.
- ^{18}F-FDG-PET/CT could be any Deauville score.
- Bone marrow can be involved, but no new lesion.

Stable disease:

- <10% decrease or ≤20% increase in the sum of longest diameters of target lesions.
- ^{18}F-FDG-PET/CT could be any Deauville score.
- Bone marrow can be involved, but no new lesion.

Progressive disease:

- ≥20% increase in the sum of longest diameters of target lesions.
- For small lymph nodes measuring <15 mm post therapy, a minimum absolute increase of 5 mm and the long diameter should exceed 15 mm.
- Appearance of new lesion(s).
- ^{18}F-FDG-PET/CT could be any Deauville score.
- Bone marrow can be involved.

It has been shown that based on the above criteria, a selection of three as opposed to six largest target lesions at baseline for analysis did not jeopardize the final outcome. Target lesions should be lesions from disparate regions of the body, if possible, including mediastinal and retroperitoneal lesions whenever these sites are involved. Where uncertainty remains, then biopsy may be required to give a definitive answer.

6.4.1 Timing of imaging

Conventionally imaging will be timed to identify response during treatment, define the final response, and to monitor disease in follow-up. This will usually mean investigations at the following points:

- During chemotherapy, typically after 2–4 cycles of treatment.
- At completion of chemotherapy.
- At 3–6 months after completion of chemotherapy.

6.4.2 Interim PET/CT

There is emerging data to suggest that an early response on ^{18}F-FDG PET/CT in both HL and aggressive NHL after two cycles of chemotherapy is a strong predictor of subsequent favourable outcome; those patients with negative scans at this point achieving conventional complete remissions and long-term, relapse-free survival times (Figure 6.8a & b), whereas patients with a positive scan at this point are less likely to achieve complete remission and will subsequently progress. The role of an

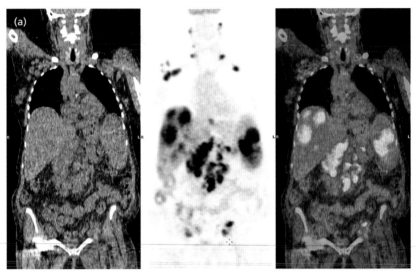

Fig. 6.8a Staging ¹⁸F-FDG PET/CT of a stage IV DLBCL patient.

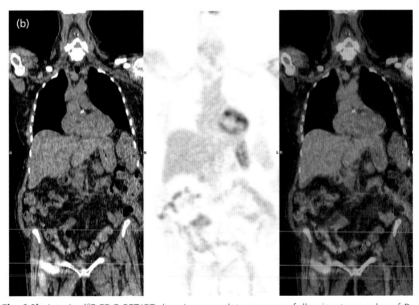

Fig. 6.8b Interim ¹⁸F-FDG PET/CT showing complete response following two cycles of R-CHOP chemotherapy.

interim PET/CT is to identify poor responders at an early stage, hence prevent futile chemotherapy, and prompt to change to more intensive treatment and also to minimize further treatment to those who are in complete remission at this early stage. This interim study should be done just before the third cycle of chemotherapy.

6.4.3 PET/CT at completion of treatment

^{18}F-FDG PET/CT at completion of treatment is an important prognostic indicator. Patients with a negative PET/CT scan at completion of treatment have a short-term progression-free survival of >90%. The predictive value of a positive PET/CT scan at this point, however, is less certain, with a wide range of published figures reflecting the difficulties in interpretation early post-treatment. To avoid these false positive findings, it is recommended that at least six weeks are allowed after completion of all treatment before a definitive completion PET/CT scan is performed. A positive scan in these circumstances has been associated with only a 40% one-year progression-free survival compared to 95% for a contemporary PET/CT negative group. Interpretation of the PET/CT positive scan can be enhanced by reference to a staging PET/CT scan. Criteria for response have been defined by the International Harmonization Project (IHP) as shown in Table 6.3.

In certain situations, ^{18}F-FDG PET/CT can be falsely positive, for example FDG can be taken up in thymic rebound following chemotherapy, in infection, in extramedullary haematopoiesis, and in tissues undergoing inflammatory response to

Table 6.3 International Harmonization Project (IHP) consensus recommendations with inclusion of PET criteria in defining response in lymphoma

The following changes on ^{18}F-FDG PET/CT should be regarded as positive for lymphoma:	
Lymph nodes:	
≥2 cm diameter	Diffuse or focal uptake > mediastinal blood pool structures
<2 cm diameter	Any increase in uptake over background
Lung nodules:	
>1.5 cm diameter	Increase in uptake > mediastinal blood pool structures
<1.5 cm diameter	Cannot be reliably assessed
Hepatic and splenic lesions:	
>1.5 cm	Uptake > or = to normal liver or spleen
<1.5 cm	Uptake > normal liver or spleen
Diffuse splenic disease	Diffuse uptake > normal liver (unless recent cytokine administration)
Bone marrow	Multifocal uptake

Timing of scans after therapy: 6–8 weeks after chemotherapy or chemoimmunotherapy; 8–12 weeks after radiotherapy or chemoradiotherapy.

Source: data from Juweld ME et al. 'Use of positron emission tomography for response assessment of lymphoma: consensus of the Imaging Subcommittee of International Harmonization Project in Lymphoma'. *J Clin Oncol* 2007; Vol. 25, Issue 5, pp.571–8.

radiation reaction. These foci of uptake can be misinterpreted as representing active lymphoma. An initial staging PET/CT image for comparison is valuable in this setting as foci of uptake which were not present on the staging scan are likely to be a consequence of treatment. Biopsy should be considered for any new lesion with high uptake on the interim or completion PET/CT, especially where salvage treatment is considered.

6.4.4 Imaging in follow-up

The role of routine imaging in the follow-up of lymphoma patients is controversial. On the one hand there is increasing concern with regard to the radiation exposure of patients who have a long prognosis, many living their natural lifespan from a relatively young age at treatment, being exposed to unnecessary irradiation. This must be balanced against the ability to detect early relapse enabling further potentially curative treatment. The predictive value of molecular imaging using ^{18}F-FDG PET/CT therefore has considerable importance and interest in this area and the role of additional imaging in patients who are FDG negative at completion of treatment is questionable.

There is no role for routine imaging beyond the initial post-treatment scan at 3–6 months after completion of therapy. Patients, who have residual disease, whether defined by CT criteria or positive disease on ^{18}F-FDG PET/CT scanning, clearly require further monitoring. Where molecular imaging is not available then stable disease on two further CT scans at six-monthly intervals is adequate to justify discontinuation of further routine imaging, and where molecular imaging is available residual disease on a diagnostic CT scan followed by PET/CT which is negative, should also lead to the cessation of further routine imaging. A positive PET/CT scan should, in the absence of other criteria suggesting lymphoma relapse or progression, and be followed by a biopsy of the FDG-positive area.

Finally, the traditional annual chest X-ray no longer has a role in the management of lymphoma patients. The only role for routine radiology following treatment and confirmation of complete remission in lymphoma is in later screening programmes. Currently UK recommendations for female patients having had radiotherapy to chest area involving breast tissue before the age of 36 years are to begin MRI breast screening eight years after completion of treatment. In smokers an increased risk of lung cancer is recognized and studies are underway to identify the optimal means of monitoring such patients to identify early disease for those who persist in their smoking habits.

Further reading

Cheson BD, Fisher RI, Barrington SF, et al. (2014). Recommendations for initial evaluation, staging, and response assessment of Hodgkin and non-Hodgkin lymphoma: the Lugano classification. *Journal of Clinical Oncology,* **32**(27): 3059–3068. doi: 10.1200/JCO.2013.54.8800.

Hoskin PJ, Díez P, Gallop-Evans E, et al. (2016). Recommendations for radiotherapy technique and dose in extra-nodal lymphoma. *Clinical Oncology* (Royal College of Radiology), **28**(1): 62–68.

Juweld ME, Stroobants S, Hoekstra OS, et al. (2007). Use of positron emission tomography for response assessment of lymphoma: consensus of the Imaging Subcommittee of International Harmonization Project in Lymphoma. *Journal of Clinical Oncology*, **25**: 571–578.

Mikhaeel NG, Milgrom SA, Terezakis S, et al. (2019). The optimal use of imaging in radiation therapy for lymphoma: Guidelines from the International Lymphoma Radiation Oncology Group (ILROG). *International Journal of Radiation and Oncology. Biology. Physics*, **104**(3): 501–512.

Specht L, Yahalom J, Illidge T, et al. (2014). Modern radiation therapy for Hodgkin lymphoma: field and dose guidelines from the international lymphoma radiation oncology group (ILROG). *International Journal of Radiation and Oncology. Biology. Physics*, **89**(4): 854–862.

Yahalom J, Illidge T, Specht L, et al. (2015). Modern radiation therapy for extranodal lymphomas: field and dose guidelines from the International Lymphoma Radiation Oncology Group. *International Journal of Radiation and Oncology. Biology. Physics*, **1**, **92**(1): 11–31.

Younes A, Hilden P, Coiffier B, et al. (2017). International Working Group consensus response evaluation criteria in lymphoma (RECIL 2017). *Annals of Oncology*, **28**(7): 1436–1447.

Chapter 7

Oesophageal tumours

Kieran Foley, Carys Morgan, and Tom Crosby

7.1 Clinical background

Oesophageal cancer is the eighth most common cancer in the UK, with >9000 new cases diagnosed per year. The prognosis is poor, with overall five-year survival rates of approximately 15%. The incidence varies widely around the world, ranging from 5 to 10 per 100,000 in developed countries to 100 per 100,000 in endemic areas. Overall, squamous cell carcinoma (SCC) is more common (5.2 per 100,000) than adeno-carcinoma (0.7 per 100,000). SCC is most common in south-east and central Asian countries such as Turkey, Iran, and Northern China (79% of total cases worldwide). Adenocarcinoma is more common in developed countries in northern and western Europe, North America, and Australasia (46% of total cases).

7.2 Diagnosis and staging

7.2.1 Diagnosis

Oesophageal cancer is most commonly diagnosed following upper gastrointestinal (GI) endoscopy. Endoscopy is the first-line investigation and enables direct visualization of the tumour and biopsy for histological diagnosis. The length, location, and degree of obstruction of the visible tumour (measured from the incisors or from the oesophagogastric junction (OGJ)) can be assessed. Contrast studies remain a useful alternative investigation in patients with dysphagia, but far fewer studies are performed now compared to computed tomography (CT) (Figure 7.1). Benign lesions are common and include strictures related to previous surgery, gastro-oesophageal reflux, long-term use of a nasogastric tube, chemical injury, and treatment of oesophageal varices. An advantage of contrast swallow over endoscopy is the detection of motility disorders such as achalasia.

7.2.2 Staging

The accepted standard for staging of oesophageal and OGJ cancers is based on the Union of International Cancer Control (UICC) Tumour Node Metastasis (TNM) staging system, currently in its eighth edition (Table 7.1). Accurate staging is required to determine prognosis and management options, such as curative versus palliative intent and single versus multimodality treatment.

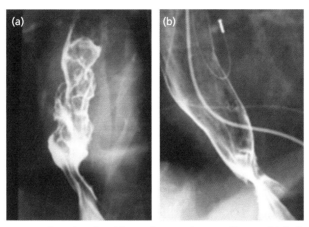

Fig. 7.1 Contrast swallow showing (a) an adenocarcinoma of lower third of oesophagus and (b) a small adenocarcinoma at the oesophagogastric junction.

After a diagnosis of oesophageal cancer, patients are initially staged with CT of the chest and abdomen. This is predominately to assess the primary tumour for potential resectability (loco-regional stage) and to identify distant metastases (commonly liver, lungs, peritoneum, and non-regional lymph nodes). Potentially curable patients who are fit for radical treatment, either with surgery, chemotherapy, radiotherapy, or a combination, should undergo 18-fluorine (^{18}F) fluorodeoxyglucose (FDG) PET/CT followed by endoscopic ultrasound (EUS) for more detailed staging. MRI is occasionally performed in some countries. Invasive EUS-guided fine needle aspiration (EUS-FNA) is also an important diagnostic tool and can help confirm diagnosis and stage, thereby assisting clinical treatment decisions.

7.2.2.1 T stage

There is a strong correlation between the depth of tumour invasion and risk of lymph node metastases in oesophageal cancer. This in turn correlates with risk of distant metastases and a worsening five-year survival. Although CT does not accurately differentiate the anatomical layers of the oesophageal wall to predict T stage, it can identify invasion of adjacent structures such as aorta, vertebral body, pericardium, lungs, and bronchus in patients with locally advanced disease. Fat planes usually separate the oesophagus from adjacent organs. The presence of a visible fat plane can accurately predict absence of invasion into an adjacent organ. However, loss of the fat plane does not necessarily mean that invasion has occurred. The likelihood of irresectability can also be assessed by measuring the extent of tumour surrounding the aorta. If the degree of encasement is >180°, vascular invasion is likely and if >270°, invasion is almost inevitable, both features negating the possibility of surgical resection. However, loss of fat plane between tumour and pericardium is less predictive of invasion, and fat planes can be obscured following radiotherapy.

Table 7.1 TNM eighth edition of oesophageal cancer staging

T primary tumour	
TX	Primary tumour cannot be assessed
T0	No evidence of primary tumour
Tis	Carcinoma *in situ*/high-grade dysplasia
T1	Tumour invades the lamina propria, muscularis mucosae, or submucosa
T1a	Tumour invades the lamina propria or muscularis mucosae
T1b	Tumour invades the submucosa
T2	Tumour invades muscularis propria
T3	Tumour invades adventitia
T4	Tumour invades adjacent structures
T4a	Tumour invades the pleura, pericardium, azygos vein, diaphragm, or peritoneum
T4b	Tumour invades other adjacent structures, such as the aorta, vertebral body, or trachea
N regional lymph nodes	
NX	Lymph node status cannot be assessed
N0	No regional lymph node metastasis
N1	Metastasis in 1–2 regional lymph nodes
N2	Metastasis in 3–6 regional lymph nodes
N3	Metastasis in 7 or more regional lymph nodes
M distant metastasis	
M0	No distant metastasis
M1	Distant metastasis

Reproduced with permission from Sobin LH, Gospodarowicz MK, Wittekind CH. *UICC TNM Classification of Malignant Tumours*. 8th ed. © 2017 Wiley Blackwell.

Transoesophageal EUS combines upper GI endoscopy with ultrasonography (US) using a dedicated US probe. The five layers of the oesophageal wall can be clearly visualized, each with different echogenic appearance. The first layer corresponds to the superficial mucosa, the second layer to the muscularis mucosa, the third layer to the submucosa, the fourth layer to the muscularis propria, and the fifth layer to the adventitia. Therefore, EUS can accurately predict the depth of tumour invasion. Multiple studies using EUS have consistently reported an overall T stage accuracy of >80% compared to surgical pathology, and this improves with increasing T stage to >90% with T3/T4 tumours (Figure 7.2). Meta-analysis of 27 studies demonstrated an accuracy of 89% for EUS T staging. The additional use of EUS staging information can influence the patient's management in approximately 25% of cases. However, there are limitations of EUS. First, distinguishing mucosal (Tis or T1a) from submucosal lesions (T1b) in early tumours is difficult. The primary tumour will be understaged

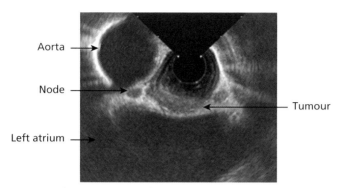

Aorta

Node

Tumour

Left atrium

Fig. 7.2 Endoscopic ultrasound image of a T3N1 tumour.

in 5% and overstaged in 6–11%. Second, it has been reported that around 30% of tumours are non-traversable; however, failure rates as low as 3% have been published using narrow-calibre, blind endoscopes. Third, EUS is operator dependent with a long learning curve of experience and careful audit, as accurate assessment is based on size, shape, margins, and echotexture.

The use of FDG-PET to detect oesophageal tumours is reported to be more sensitive than CT, for both SCC and adenocarcinoma. Combined analysis of seven studies (with a total of 281 patients) using FDG-PET as part of initial staging, showed that the site of primary tumour could be correctly identified in 94%. In the 5% of tumours not identified, small size (<5 mm) was the main reason for false negative results. Also, a small subset of tumours do not take up FDG, irrespective of size. These are usually adenocarcinomas, either mucin-producing, poorly differentiated, or signet-ring subtype. Occasionally, an incidental finding of a small tumour arising within a hiatus hernia or segment of Barrett's oesophagus can be seen on a PET/CT examination performed for a different indication. In patients already known to have oesophageal cancer, FDG-PET does not add any further T stage information compared to CT. False positive FDG-PET uptake in the oesophagus can occur with inflammatory disease, gastro-oesophageal reflux, or radiation-induced oesophagitis, often appearing as diffuse rather than focal uptake, confirming the need for histological diagnosis.

7.2.2.2 N stage

The oesophagus has a rich lymphatic network within the submucosa. Even early T stage tumours are at significant risk of lymph node metastases. This risk ranges from 3–6% for mucosal (T1a) to 21–24% for submucosal (T1b) tumours, 45–75% for intramuscular tumours, and 80–85% for transmural tumours. N stage refers to involvement of regional lymph nodes, defined as those within a peri-oesophageal distribution. Non-regional lymph nodes, including supra-clavicular and coeliac axis nodes, are classified as distant metastases (M1). Accurate identification of lymph node metastases as coeliac axis (M1 disease) rather than left gastric is critical because it can change the patient management from potentially curative to palliative. The presence of lymph node metastases is a major prognostic indicator.

The number, size, and location of lymph nodes relative to the tumour can be demonstrated on CT, with nodes >10 mm in short-axis diameter considered more likely to be involved. However, enlarged nodes are seen in non-malignant processes such as reactive hyperplasia or inflammation. Conversely, involved nodes may not appear enlarged on CT. Therefore, the sensitivity and specificity of CT for detecting involved lymph nodes is poor (31–44%). In general, all modalities are likely to under-stage nodal disease.

EUS provides better assessment of regional nodes. Several studies have compared EUS with CT and FDG-PET. In a study of patients undergoing surgical resection, Flamen et al. reported that EUS was more sensitive than FDG-PET (81% vs. 33%) but less specific (67% vs. 89%). The combined results of CT with EUS did not alter the cumulative specificity over FDG-PET, indicating that nodal detection alone fails to differentiate benign from malignant disease.

One meta-analysis found the sensitivity of CT, EUS, and PET/CT for the detection of regional lymph node metastases was 50%, 80%, and 57%, respectively. The specificity was 83%, 70%, and 85%, respectively, suggesting EUS is better than CT or PET for excluding regional lymph node metastases. The study also found the sensitivity and specificity of diagnosing coeliac lymph node metastases with EUS was 85% and 96%, respectively.

Another meta-analysis of 12 studies (including 490 patients) using FDG-PET to stage regional lymph nodes reported an overall sensitivity of 51% and specificity of 84%. A similar meta-analysis including six studies demonstrated that the pooled sensitivity and specificity of PET/CT was 55% and 76%, respectively. There are two main reasons for the poor sensitivity of PET in detecting involved regional lymph nodes. First, FDG uptake by small volume metastases within involved nodes may be insufficient for detection. Second, despite detectable FDG uptake in involved nodes, the limited spatial resolution of PET cannot differentiate peri-tumoural nodes from the adjacent primary tumour.

The use of EUS-guided fine needle aspiration (EUS-FNA) enables histological confirmation of lymph node involvement within the diagnostic work-up and improves the sensitivity from 85% to >95%.[1] EUS-FNA of gastric and coeliac axis nodes can also be performed to stage non-regional lymph nodes. This procedure has been incorporated into the standard protocol for investigating potential surgical candidates in some centres, particularly when there is uncertainty about involvement of a node that would change management.

7.2.2.3 M stage

The risk of distant metastases increases with the T stage. At presentation, 20–30% of patients with oesophageal cancer have distant metastases. The major additional contribution of FDG-PET in oesophageal cancer is the superior detection of distant metastases that are not identified by CT. Small occult metastases in the liver and bone may be undetectable on CT and common incidental lesions in the thyroid gland, skeletal muscle, and pancreas are often interpreted as benign.

The sensitivity and specificity of CT and PET/CT is 52% and 91%, and 71% and 93%, respectively. Similarly, a meta-analysis showed a pooled sensitivity and specificity of 67% and 97%, respectively. Importantly, PET/CT can change management in up to 38% of patients, with most cases changing because of upstaging. However, in 5% of patients, lesions measuring <1 cm (particularly in the liver or lung) may not be detected by PET/CT. Whole body imaging with PET/CT has also contributed to the detection of synchronous primary tumours, most often in the head and neck, and colon, while false positive findings are seen in inflammatory disorders such as sarcoidosis.

7.3 **Imaging for radiotherapy planning**

The use of radiotherapy in oesophageal cancer can either be for curative or palliative intent. In the curative setting, radiotherapy is often used in combination with chemotherapy (known as chemo-radiotherapy (CRT)) either definitively or as part of a multimodality approach with surgery. This is usually preoperative (neo-adjuvant) or less commonly postoperative (adjuvant).

For radiotherapy planning, a CT is performed with intravenous contrast to improve definition of mediastinal anatomy (Figure 7.3). The planning CT includes the lung apices down to the iliac crest, ensuring full coverage of organs at risk. There is significant movement, particularly in the lower oesophagus and OGJ due to respiratory and cardiac motion, and level of gastric distension. Reproducible stomach filling can be attempted to allow for this movement during treatment and ensure full coverage of disease.

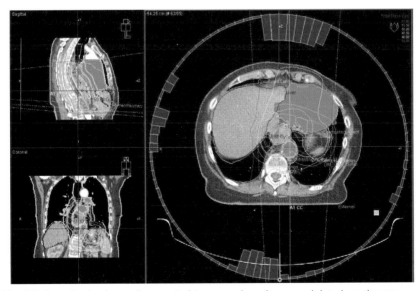

Fig. 7.3 A contrast enhanced computed tomography volume modulated arc therapy (VMAT) radical radiotherapy plan with multi-planar reconstructions and organs at risk outlined.

There is increasing use of four-dimensional CT (4DCT) radiotherapy planning. This technique incorporates organ motion seen particularly during respiration. A 4DCT acquires and reconstructs the data at different time points throughout the respiratory cycle. During the CT, the respiratory cycle is tracked in real-time and divided into 'bins' of respiratory phase. After scanning, the images are sorted into phases, from which several CT datasets (usually 8–10) are reconstructed at the different time points. This process tracks tumour and surrounding organ motion and ensures tumour coverage throughout the respiratory cycle.

Oesophageal tumours are difficult to define on planning CT alone so all diagnostic information including endoscopy, diagnostic CT, EUS, and ^{18}F-FDG PET/CT should be available during gross tumour volume (GTV) delineation. Visible disease on any imaging modality should be included, otherwise the disease extent may be underestimated. Submucosal tumour extension, skip lesions, and involved lymph nodes can be found at significant distances beyond the visible tumour. This is more likely to be detected by EUS than CT. In addition, PET/CT alone may underestimate the length of primary disease and should be used in combination with EUS where possible. As discussed previously, EUS may also define local nodal disease more accurately and should therefore be considered in patients undergoing radical radiotherapy to accurately define disease extent. EUS measurements of the superior and inferior limits of disease need to be related to a reproducible anatomical landmark in the thorax. A suitable reference point is the top of the arch of the aorta or the carina.

7.4 **Therapeutic assessment and follow-up**

Following completion of treatment, the risk of recurrence remains high and usually occurs within the first two years. Recurrent disease is associated with a poor prognosis. The current primary modality to assess treatment response and detect recurrent disease is CT, although the role of ^{18}F-FDG PET/CT to detect disease recurrence is emerging. A limitation of CT is the difficulty in reliably differentiating post-treatment changes from recurrent or residual disease. In patients receiving neo-adjuvant treatment, an early response detectable on PET/CT may predict for long-term outcome but this is not currently standard of care. Post-treatment CT can be difficult to interpret and additional endoscopic assessment is recommended in those patients where surgical salvage is a potential option.

7.4.1 **Assessing response to therapy**

The treatment options for oesophageal cancer include surgical and non-surgical approaches. The addition of neo-adjuvant CRT prior to resection improves survival when compared with surgery alone. Patients who respond well to neo-adjuvant CRT and achieve a pathological complete response (pCR) may not benefit from surgical resection. Reported pCR rates range from 8% to 56% (mean 24%) following preoperative CRT and resection. As patients are unlikely to benefit from surgical resection, the ability to predict pCR would contribute significantly to the patient's management and reduce treatment morbidity.

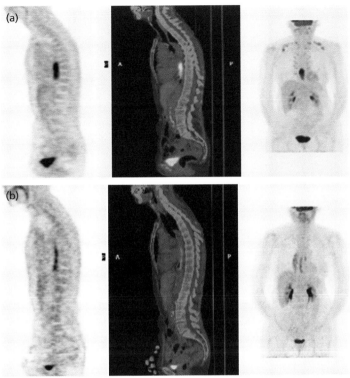

Fig. 7.4 A 70-year-old woman with a T3 N0 M0 squamous cell carcinoma of the lower oesophagus. Pre-treatment ^{18}F-FDG PET, fused PET/CT, and MIP images (a) show a tumour with an SUV_{max} of 14.9. FDG uptake in brown fat in the supraclavicular fossae is a normal variant. Images four months later (b) following neoadjuvant CRT show a 50% reduction in tumour SUV_{max}. Note FDG-uptake in the right adjacent lung margin due to radiotherapy.

Currently, a combination of modalities is relied upon to assess response. CT is relatively inaccurate for determining tumour and lymph node response, with studies showing little correlation between reduction in tumour size and pathological response. Although EUS is a good tool for preoperative staging, its utility is limited for assessing response, as it cannot differentiate residual tumour from post-treatment fibrosis. Metabolic imaging with ^{18}F-FDG PET can be used to assess response to therapy (Figure 7.4). A baseline scan is required to compare with subsequent scans and the degree of FDG uptake within the tumour objectively measured using the maximum standard uptake value (SUV_{max}). Studies have shown that a reduction in SUV_{max} at 14 days after commencement of pre-operative chemotherapy or CRT correlates with good histological tumour regression and improved survival. However, one study assessing FDG uptake after seven days failed to demonstrate this correlation, possibly due to the short interval allowing insufficient metabolic response to occur.

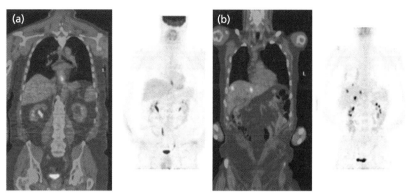

Fig. 7.5 (a) A 63-year-old man with T3 N0 M0 adenocarcinoma of the lower oesophagus on baseline fused ^{18}F-FDG PET/CT and PET images. (b) Following a complete response to neoadjuvant CRT and subsequent surgery, new liver metastases indicate distant disease recurrence.

Ongoing studies are also assessing how this information from early ^{18}F-FDG PET/CT can potentially be used to change or intensify treatment in non-responders. The MUNICON studies assessed use of FDG-PET to assess response to preoperative chemotherapy, In the initial trial, 'metabolic responders' were associated with improved outcomes. The MUNICON II trial looked at the addition of radiation to the treatment regime in metabolic 'non-responders'. The results of these studies confirmed that early PET-CT can differentiate patients with better outcomes but radiation did not improve survival in non-responders in this trial. Further studies in this area are ongoing.

7.4.2 Follow-up

The role of regular CT imaging in the follow-up of asymptomatic patients who have completed curative treatment is unproven as recurrent disease is rarely salvaged successfully. ^{18}F-FDG PET/CT may detect recurrent loco-regional or distant metastatic disease (Figure 7.5). However, like CT, this is not used routinely in the follow-up of asymptomatic patients. False positive findings at the anastomotic site or in adjacent mediastinal lymph nodes can occur due to inflammation.

7.5 Summary

- A combination of imaging modalities is required to improve oesophageal cancer staging accuracy.
- Lymph node metastases are an important prognostic indicator but diagnostic accuracy remains relatively poor.
- Diagnostic CT should be used to identify patients with unresectable primary tumours or distant metastases before proceeding to ^{18}F-FDG PET/CT and EUS.

- ◆ ¹⁸F-FDG PET/CT is an important modality in oesophageal cancer staging by increasing the sensitivity of distant metastasis detection and changing patient management.
- ◆ The use of PET/CT to assess early treatment response and potentially guide treatment is an area of interest and active research.

Further reading

Flamen P, Lerut A, Van Cutsem E, et al. (2000). Utility of positron emission tomography for the staging of patients with potentially operable oesophageal carcinoma. *Journal of Clinical Oncology*, **18**: 3202–3210.

Foley KG, Christian A, Fielding P, Lewis WG, Roberts SA (2017). Accuracy of contemporary oesophageal cancer lymph node staging with radiological-pathological correlation. *Clinical Radiology*, **72**(8): e691–e697.

Kayani B, Zacharakis E, Ahmed K, Hanna GB (2011). Lymph node metastases and prognosis in oesophageal carcinoma-a systematic review. *European Journal of Surgical Oncology*, **37**(9): 747–753.

Lordick F, Ott K, Krause BJ, et al. (2007). PET to assess early metabolic response and to guide treatment of adenocarcinoma of the oesophagogastric junction: the MUNICON phase II trial. *Lancet Oncology*, **8**: 797–805.

Monjazeb AM, Riedlinger G, Aklilu M, et al. (2010). Outcomes of patients with esophageal cancer staged with 18F-fluorodeoxyglucose positron emission tomography (FDG-PET): can postchemoradiotherapy FDG-PET predict the utility of resection? *Journal of Clinical Oncology*, **28**: 4714–4721.

Ott K, Wolfgang A, Lordick F, et al. (2006). Metabolic imaging predicts response, survival, and recurrence in adenocarcinomas of the esophogastric junction. *Journal of Clinical Oncology*, **24**: 4692–4698.

Puli SR, Reddy JB, Bechtold ML, et al. (2008). Staging accuracy of esophageal cancer by endoscopic ultrasound: a meta-analysis and systematic review. *World Journal of Gastroenterology*, **14**: 1479–1490.

Sobin LH, Gospodarowicz MK, Wittekind CH (2017). *UICC TNM Classification of Malignant Tumours* (eighth edn). Chichester: Wiley Blackwell.

van Hagen P, Hulshof MCCM, van Lanschot JJB, et al. (2012). Preoperative chemoradiotherapy for esophageal or junctional cancer. *New England Journal of Medicine*, **366**: 2074–2084.

Reference

1. van Vliet EP, Heijenbrok-Kal MH, Hunink MG, Kuipers EJ, Siersema PD (2008). Staging investigations for oesophageal cancer: a meta-analysis. *British Journal of Cancer*, **98**(3): 547–557.

Chapter 8

Gastric tumours

Nicholas Carroll and Elizabeth C. Smyth

8.1 Clinical background

Gastric adenocarcinoma is the world's fifth most common cancer and the third most common cause of cancer death. There is a particularly high incidence in Asia and South America. The incidence of adenocarcinomas of the gastric cardia has rapidly increased over the past 20 years, whilst the incidence of distal stomach cancers has decreased. Adenocarcinomas of the lower oesophagus have also increased at the same rate. It is often difficult to distinguish the origin of tumours at the oesophagogastric junction (OGJ). Tumours within 5 cm of the oesophagogastric junction and those in the proximal gastric cardia can be grouped together as "junctional tumours". These are subclassified in to Siewert type 1, centred in the distal oesophagus. Siewert type 2, centred on the junction itself and Siewert Type 3, those centred in the gastric cardia, the latter staged as gastric tumours.[1]

8.2 Diagnosis and staging

8.2.1 Diagnosis

Endoscopy is the modality of choice for diagnosing gastric tumours, allowing for exact localization and biopsy for histology.[2] In the diagnosis of scirrhous carcinoma, which diffusely infiltrates the stomach wall (linitis plastica) the endoscopic appearance may be normal as the infiltration is submucosal and a lack of stomach distension on endoscopic insufflation or imaging studies may be the only indication of disease. More specific tailored computed tomography (CT) protocols (see section 8.2.2) allow for higher detection rates. Endoscopic ultrasound (EUS) may be used to perform submucosal biopsies if the endoscopic guided mucosal biopsies are inconclusive.

8.2.2 Staging

CT is the cornerstone of staging of gastric tumours. EUS, diagnostic laparoscopy, and occasionally ^{18}F-fluorodeoxyglucose positron emission tomography/computed tomography (FDG PET/CT) are useful modalities, particularly as problem-solving tools. As described, EUS can be used to perform submucosal biopsies to confirm a cancer diagnosis, but may also be utilized to distinguish subtle infiltration and involvement of adjacent organs such as the pancreas or liver, indicating T4 disease. EUS can also accurately define lymph node involvement and be used to biopsy lymph nodes outside a normal operative field to exclude in effect what would be metastatic disease. Although CT is adequate for visualization of most liver metastases MRI is more sensitive for detection of subtle liver lesions.[2,3] Staging of gastric cancers is based on the TNM (tumour, node, metastasis) classification.[4]

8.2.2.1 T stage

In order to improve the sensitivity and specificity of cancer detection and staging, the stomach should be distended with water, or other low Hounsfield unit fluid, prior to CT image acquisition. This is helpful in distinguishing subtle thickening or mass lesions arising from the gastric wall from the pseudo-thickening which can result from an undistended stomach. Appearances of gastric cancers on CT can range from focal wall thickening with or without ulceration (Figure 8.1), to a soft tissue mass, to diffuse wall thickening in linitis plastica. Following injection of intravenous contrast medium tumours can show variable degrees of contrast enhancement. Lower attenuation lesions may correspond with fibrosis or mucinous tumours. It can be helpful to study the stomach using multiplanar reconstructions (MPRs). Curved MPRs are useful to distinguish tumours abutting adjacent organs from invading adjacent organs (Figure 8.2).[5] The overall accuracy of CT in staging gastric cancer ranges from 77% to 89%.[6] Studies using these specific tailored scanning and reconstruction techniques with multidetector CT and 'virtual gastroscopy', show increasing accuracy in T staging, and sensitivity for detecting the early gastric cancers (EGCs). Using these state-of-the-art techniques, CT can detect gastric cancer (in mixed series of advanced gastric cancers (AGCs) and EGCs) with 94–98% accuracy and T stage correctly in 84–89%.

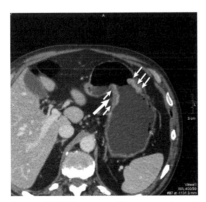

Fig. 8.1 Axial contrast-enhanced CT demonstrating circumferential mural thickening caused by a lesser curve adenocarcinoma. The gastric wall is intact (small arrows).
A vessel in the gastrohepatic ligament simulates infiltrative disease (large arrow), which can be a pitfall.

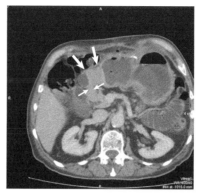

Fig. 8.2 Axial contrast-enhanced CT demonstrating an annular antral tumour (large arrows) extending into the pancreatic head. A T4 poorly differentiated adenocarcinoma was confirmed at palliative surgery.

MRI has similar accuracy to CT but is limited in routine practice by artefacts and the complexity and time taken to perform the examination.

EUS is probably the best method of predicting the pathological T stage of EGCs, with published overall accuracy rates of 65–92%. As in the oesophagus, the normal layers of the stomach wall can be clearly visualized on EUS. Most tumours appear hypoechoic with irregular margins, disrupting these layers. EUS is particularly sensitive for early stage tumours confined to the mucosa and submucosa (T1 and T2). However, it is operator dependent with a learning curve, hence its availability is often confined to regional centres. Where there is coexisting inflammation, the extent of disease can be overestimated.

8.2.2.2 N stage

Although current N staging depends on the number of positive lymph nodes rather than the previously described nodal stations, the latter is important as prognosis is also dependent on extent of lymphadenectomy. Involvement of the hepatoduodenal nodes, retropancreatic, mesenteric, para-aortic, or more distant nodes are considered as metastatic disease being outside the most widely performed operative field. CT is the modality of choice for lymph node staging. It can detect the more distant lymph nodes (compartments 3 and 4) that may influence the surgeon to either perform an extended lymphadenectomy or not to offer curative resection at all. The overall accuracy of lymph node staging by CT is, at best, around 80%. The main limitation of using CT to assess lymph node size and shape as a means of predicting tumour involvement is that this is unreliable, often over- as well as under-staging the disease.

EUS is a useful adjunct for confirming lymph node involvement but limited to nodes within the limited imaging field. EUS has been reported as having diagnostic accuracy of 70–90%. In a comparative series of 63 patients, similar accuracies were reported between EUS (79%) and CT (75%). There may be a role for FDG PET/CT in the staging of gastric cancer in detecting involved but normal sized nodes and distant metastases.[7]

8.2.2.3 Distant metastases

CT is the modality of choice. Liver metastases are present in approximately 25% of newly diagnosed patients with AGC. Other sites including lung, bone, and adrenal metastases are less common but can be also detected with CT. Subtle peritoneal deposits are the most commonly missed form of metastasis using cross-sectional imaging and will require laparoscopy for diagnosis. The presence of ascites may, however, indicate peritoneal disease. In a female patient, it is important to include the pelvis as ovarian drop metastases, otherwise known as 'Krukenberg tumours', may be found. If there are no metastases on imaging, staging laparoscopy is indicated and this can influence the clinical management in up to 20% of cases. FDG PET/CT may be useful in non-diffuse cancers to exclude suspected occult metastatic disease.[7]

8.3 **Treatment**

The standard treatment in non-Asian patients with gastric cancers which are T2 or greater is perioperative chemotherapy followed by surgery. In Asia, primary surgery is more often followed by adjuvant chemotherapy. For junctional adenocarcinoma, there is a survival benefit for preoperative chemoradiotherapy (CRT) or perioperative chemotherapy.[8,9]

Following curative resection, many patients remain at high risk of locoregional recurrence. The US Intergroup 0116 Trial showed that the use of postoperative CRT (45 Gy in 25 fractions with synchronous 5-fluorouracil (5FU) and folinic acid) improved overall survival when compared with surgery alone in patients who had curative resection (R0). This approach has decreased in use since perioperative chemotherapy has been more widely adopted.[10]

8.3.1 **Role of radiotherapy and imaging for treatment planning**

Following good quality surgery, the role of postoperative CRT remains uncertain. If the decision is to treat the patient with postoperative CRT (e.g. if circumferential resection margin positive tumours), preparation should include ensuring that the patient has sufficiently recovered from surgery, has an adequate nutritional intake (with or without support), and has optimal renal function. Both glomerular filtration rate (GFR) as well as differential renal function—DMSA (dimercaptosuccinic acid) or MAG3 (mercaptoacetyl triglycine)—should be assessed, as the radiation dose to one kidney will often exceed tolerance and it is important to ensure that the function of the other kidney is adequate.

The planning CT scan should be in the supine position with the arms raised, starting from above liver to below kidneys to allow generation of dose volume histograms (DVH) for organs at risk. Addition of intravenous contrast and dilute gastrograffin to opacify the bowel is helpful to define the various anatomical structures. The oncologist needs to be familiar with the original site and extent of tumour, using information from preoperative CT, endoscopy, surgical notes, histology report, and, importantly, multidisciplinary team discussion. Intensity modulated radiotherapy (IMRT) or image guided radiotherapy (IGRT) should be used for optimal sparing of normal tissue.

In the palliative setting, short courses of radiotherapy (30 Gy in 10 fractions or 20 Gy 5 fractions) to the stomach using parallel opposed anterior and posterior fields simulated with barium contrast can help to control bleeding or pain. In addition, single dose radiotherapy to painful bony metastases can be effective in controlling symptoms and improving quality of life.

8.4 **Therapeutic assessment and follow-up**

Disease recurrence is common within the first two years of surgery and is associated with a poor prognosis. The benefit of postoperative imaging to identify asymptomatic recurrent disease remains unproven. When there is clinical suspicion of recurrence, CT is the imaging modality of choice. It is also used to assess response to further therapy using standard reporting criteria (Response Evaluation in Solid Tumors—RECIST).[11] The ability of FDG PET/CT to detect abnormal metabolic function has an emerging role, as CT cannot reliably differentiate post-treatment changes from recurrent or residual active disease. In the setting of neoadjuvant treatment FDG PET/CT may have a role in predicting response early in the course of therapy.

8.5 **Summary**

- ◆ CT remains the main modality for staging and determining resectability, but more comprehensive information is provided by a multimodality approach (CT, EUS, laparoscopy, and PET).
- ◆ The role for routine imaging following curative treatment remains unproven.

References

1. **Siewert RJ, Feith M, Werner M, et al.** (2000). Adenocarcinoma of the esophagogastric junction: results of surgical therapy based on anatomical/topographic classification in 1002 consecutive patients. *Annals of Surgery*, **232**: 353–361.

2. **Smyth EC, Verheij M, Allum W, et al.** (2016). Gastric cancer: ESMO Clinical Practice Guidelines for diagnosis, treatment and follow-up. *Annals of Oncology*, **27**(suppl 5): v38–v49.

3. **Miller FH, Kochan ML, Talamonti MS, et al.** (2007). Gastric cancer: Radiologic staging. *Radiologic Clinics of North America*, **35**: 331–348.

4. **Kwee RM, Kwee TC.** (2007). Imaging in local staging of gastric cancer: a systematic review. *Journal of Clinical Oncology*, **25**: 2107–2116.

5. **Smyth E, Schöder H, Strong VE, et al.** (2012). Prospective evaluation of the utility of 2-deoxy-2-[(18) F]fluoro-D-glucose positron emission tomography and computed tomography in staging locally advanced gastric cancer. *Cancer*, **118**(22): 5481–5488.

6. **Al-Batran SE, Homann N, Pauligk C, et al.** (2019). Perioperative chemotherapy with fluorouracil plus leucovorin, oxaliplatin, and docetaxel versus fluorouracil or capecitabine plus cisplatin and epirubicin for locally advanced, resectable gastric or gastro-oesophageal junction adenocarcinoma (FLOT4): a randomised, phase 2/3 trial. *Lancet*, **393**(10184): 1948–1957.

7. **van Hagen P, Hulshof MC, van Lanschot JJ, et al.** (2012). Preoperative chemoradiotherapy for esophageal or junctional cancer. *New England Journal of Medicine*, **366**(22): 2074–2084.

8. **Noh SH, Park SR, Yang HK, et al.** (2014). Adjuvant capecitabine plus oxaliplatin for gastric cancer after D2 gastrectomy (CLASSIC): 5-year follow-up of an open-label, randomised phase 3 trial. *Lancet Oncology*, **15**(12): 1389–1396.

9. **Suzuki C, Jacobsson H, Hatschek T, et al.** (2008). Radiologic measurements of tumor response to treatment: practical approaches and limitations. *Radiographics*, **28**: 329–344.

10. **Sobin LH, Gospodarowicz MK, Wittekind CH (2017).** *UICC TNM Classification of Malignant Tumours* (eighth edn). Oxford: Wiley Blackwell.

11. **Kim JH, Eun HW, Goo DE, et al.** (2006). Imaging of various gastric lesions with 2D MPR and CT gastrography performed with multidetector CT. *Radiographics*, **26**: 1101–1116, discussion 1117–1118.

Chapter 9

Hepatic and biliary tumours

Marika Reinius, Edmund Godfrey, and Bristi Basu

9.1 Introduction

Hepatobiliary tumours account for the largest increase in cancer-specific mortality worldwide. They are broadly categorized by cell type and site of origin: hepatocytes (hepatocellular carcinoma (HCC)), bile duct (cholangiocarcinoma (CCA)), mixed HCC-CCA, and gallbladder carcinoma.

9.1.1 Differential diagnosis

Imaging facilitates differentiation between benign and primary malignant lesions of the hepatobiliary system (Tables 9.1 and 9.2). The liver is the most common site of metastasis from tumours that drain initially via the portal circulation and in around 25% of cases of colorectal cancers, is a unique site of metastasis. However, other primary solid tumours, for example breast and lung cancers frequently disseminate here.

9.2 Diagnosis and staging

9.2.1 Hepatocellular carcinoma

9.2.1.1 Background and anatomy

The liver is divided into right and left anatomical lobes by the falciform ligament. Functionally, it is subdivided into eight segments, each supplied by a distinct branch of the portal triad. Part of the anatomical right lobe is thus functionally left-sided and referred to as the left medial section (segment IV), due to its supply by the branches of the left hepatic artery and portal vein. The dual vascular supply to the liver (75% portal vein, 25% hepatic artery) has important implications for intravenous contrast examinations and vascular intervention.

HCC represents 85–90% of all primary hepatic malignancies. Morphologies include solitary, multifocal, or diffusely infiltrating patterns. Local spread occurs via bile ducts and branches of the hepatic and portal veins, the latter acting as conduits for intrahepatic metastases. Extrahepatic spread occurs late, commonly to local lymph nodes, lungs, bone, and adrenal glands. HCC usually develops on the background of a cirrhotic liver, which can have typical morphological features such as atrophy, diffuse heterogeneity from fibrosis, or nodularity from regenerative nodules, in addition to

Table 9.1 Typical imaging characteristics of benign lesions

Pathology	Typical imaging characteristics	Comment
Simple cyst	CT/MRI: thin-walled, well-defined, fluid-containing lesions. No internal septae or enhancement with contrast enhancement. US: anechoic with posterior acoustic enhancement.	Commonest lesion.
Haemangioma	Well-defined, lobulated lesions. Peripheral, nodular, discontinuous enhancement with progressive centripetal filling post-contrast. Small lesions can show flash filling. Large lesions may have a scar. Enhancement follows vascular density at all phases.	Second commonest lesion, more frequent in females, often multiple.
Focal nodular hyperplasia	Hyper-enhancing, iso to mild T2 hyper-intensity. May have a T2 hyperintense central scar. Often does retain liver specific contrast agent.	Nineteen times more common than adenoma. Associated with elevated circulating oestrogen levels. More common in women of childbearing age.
Hepatic adenoma	Hyper-enhancing, mild T2 hyper-intensity, does not retain liver specific contrast agent. May contain fat.	More common in women of childbearing age.
Focal fat infiltration	No deviation of intrahepatic vessels or bile ducts. Diagnosed on 'in and out of phase' MR sequences. Often in typical locations within the liver, for example adjacent to the falciform ligament.	
Hepatic abscess	Variable appearance, often with mixed fluid/soft tissue attenuation. Can be difficult to distinguish from other lesions without aspiration/biopsy.	

evidence of associated portal hypertension such as splenomegaly, oesophageal varices, and ascites.

Early disease is typically identified on surveillance ultrasound (US) in the context of known cirrhosis (Figure 9.1), and frequency of imaging may depend on size or growth and vascular pattern of nodules. Advanced disease is more common in emergency or symptomatic presentations.

9.2.1.2 Non-invasive diagnosis

Contrast-enhanced multiphasic computed tomography (CT) or magnetic resonance imaging (MRI) are gold standard first-line investigations in the diagnosis of primary liver cancers (Figure 9.2). The Liver Imaging-Reporting and Data System (LI-RADS) is widely adopted for the diagnosis of primary liver cancer in high-risk patients based on imaging alone. The 'LR-M' category comprises definitely or probably malignant

Table 9.2 Typical imaging characteristics of metastatic lesions

US	CT/MRI	Comment
Typically hypoechoic, ill-defined, irregular, rounded lesions +/- hypoechoic ring. US may help discriminate between small metastases versus simple cysts.	CT: often ill-defined, low-attenuation in portal phase. Sometimes ring enhancement (early phase) with washout (delayed phases). Hypervascular metastases (e.g. neuroendocrine, renal, sarcoma, melanoma, occasionally colon/breast cancers): arterial enhancement followed by rapid washout, isodense/hypodense to surrounding liver on portal phase (can be invisible on portal phase). MRI: typically low to intermediate signal (T1W), moderately high signal (T2W). Enhancement characteristics as above. Restrict diffusion. Do not retain liver specific contrast agents.	Cystic metastases less common (ovary, colon, stomach), but cystic change in larger solid lesion or following chemotherapy not uncommon. Transcoelomic spread from ovarian cancer commonly cystic and found on peritoneal surface of liver.

observations which are not specifically HCC, including atypical HCC, CCA, and mixed HCC-CCA where a confirmatory biopsy is needed. Features of LR-M lesions include a targetoid mass or infiltrative appearance, marked diffusion restriction, necrosis, or severe ischaemia. LI-RADS has been validated for high-risk (e.g. cirrhotic) patients only. The diagnostic hallmark of HCC on multiphasic CT/MRI consists of initial arterial phase hyperenhancement, followed by washout during portal venous or delayed phases. This phenomenon relies on the differential vascular supply of HCCs (hepatic artery) and surrounding benign liver (portal vein). In the context of existing cirrhosis, radiological hallmarks of HCC in nodules measuring 1 cm or greater indicate a high pre-test probability of HCC. This allows for radiological diagnosis in the absence of confirmatory biopsy, as risk of seeding and decompensation during the process is a concern for potentially curable disease. CT/MRI also have the ability to differentiate between thrombosis and malignant invasion of the portal vein, where the latter constitutes a key negative prognostic factor. Hepatobiliary-specific contrast agents, for example gadoxetate or gadobutrol, can be used in MR protocols to improve detection and characterization of lesions, such as focal nodular hyperplasia. Anatomic structure and function of the biliary tree can be delineated by evaluating biliary excretion of these agents.

9.2.1.3 Other imaging modalities

On US, HCC often appears hypoechoic, but appearances vary from hyperechoic to mixed. Contrast-enhanced US should not be used first line for radiological diagnosis of HCC, as it cannot distinguish between intrahepatic CCA (iCCA) and HCC.

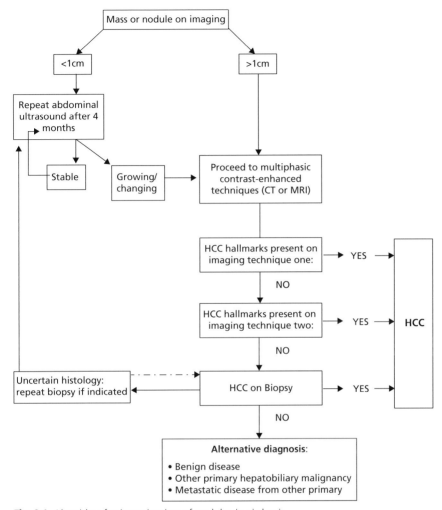

Fig. 9.1 Algorithm for investigation of nodules in cirrhosis.
Adapted with permission from EASL Clinical Practice Guidelines, 'Management of hepatocellular carcinoma'. *J Hepatol.* Vol. 69, Issue 1, pp.182–236. Copyright © 2018 Elsevier.

Contrast enhanced US may, however, facilitate diagnosis of HCC where CT/MRI are contraindicated or inconclusive.

Positron emission tomography CT (PET/CT) is not used to diagnose HCC, as high false-negative rates have been observed, particularly in early/well-differentiated HCC. A role of PET-CT may include assessment of avidity as a marker of poor prognosis during patient selection for surgery.

9.2.1.4 Invasive diagnosis

Biopsy, almost always guided by US, is required for tumours arising in non-cirrhotic livers, although histological confirmation, if safe and feasible, is

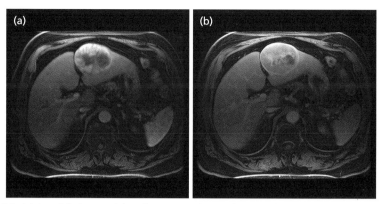

Fig. 9.2 (a) Arterial phase axial T1 fat saturated MR. There is a hyperenhancing mass in the left lateral section of the liver. (b) Delayed phase axial T1 fat saturated MR. The mass demonstrates washout (the signal is now lower than the adjacent liver parenchyma) and a capsular enhancement pattern (the hyperintense ring surrounding the lesion). In the presence of cirrhosis and arterial phase hyperenhancement, these features are diagnostic of hepatocellular carcinoma.

increasingly being required for all HCC patients to access systemic therapies in the advanced disease setting. This can facilitate differentiation of HCC from other hepatobiliary primaries, benign nodules, and metastatic disease from other sites. Immunohistochemical tests can provide further diagnostic certainty, particularly for poorly differentiated or mixed morphology tumours. Background tissue can also be taken to confirm presence of fibrosis or cirrhosis if this may influence surgical or ablative decisions.

9.2.1.5 Staging

A multitude of HCC staging systems exist; however, the Barcelona Clinic Liver Cancer (BCLC) system is currently the most widely validated and implemented system. It integrates staging and treatment by stratifying patients into five groups (0, A–D), according to tumour size and multiplicity, vascular invasion, extrahepatic spread, liver function, and performance status (Table 9.3).

9.2.2 Cholangiocarcinoma

9.2.2.1 Background and anatomy

CCA represents 15–20% of primary hepatobiliary cancers. Macroscopic patterns include mass-forming, periductal-infiltrating, and intraductal-papillary morphologies. Divisions of the biliary tree inform subclassification of CCA into distal (dCCA), perihilar (pCCA), and iCCA. pCCA can be further classified anatomically into five types according to the Bismuth-Corlette system to inform surgical planning (Figure 9.3).

iCCA (10–20%) often present non-specifically or incidentally, with a propensity for early intrahepatic metastasis. Extrahepatic CCA present with obstructive

Table 9.3 HCC staging and management based on the modified BCLC system

Prognostic BCLC stage group	Tumour characteristics	Liver function	ECOG PS	Treatment	Treatment intent
0 Very early stage	Solitary nodule <2 cm	Preserved (i.e. Child-Pugh A and no ascites)	0	◆ Surgical resection, or ◆ Ablative therapy (RFA).	Curative
A Early stage	Solitary nodule >2 cm	Preserved	0	◆ If optimal surgical candidate, surgical resection. ◆ If resection not possible, transplant if suitable candidate. ◆ If candidate for neither, ablative therapy.	Curative
	2–3 nodules =<3 cm	Preserved	0	◆ Transplant if suitable candidate. ◆ If not, ablative therapy.	Curative
B Intermediate stage	Multinodular, unresectable	Preserved	0	◆ TA(C)E.	Palliative
C Advanced stage	Portal invasion/ extrahepatic spread	Preserved	1–2	◆ Systemic therapy (current first line: sorafenib/lenvatinib, regorafenib second line).	Palliative
D Terminal stage	HCC, non-transplantable	End-stage liver failure	3–4	◆ Best supportive care.	Palliative

Source: data from EASL Clinical Practice Guidelines, 'Management of hepatocellular carcinoma'. *J Hepatol.* Vol. 69, Issue 1, pp.182–236. Elsevier 2018.

complications, including jaundice and cholangitis, and are classified into pCCA (50–60%) and dCCA (20–30%). The latter require distinction from pancreatic, ampullary, or duodenal tumours, which is sometimes challenging.

9.2.2.2 Intrahepatic cholangiocarcinoma

Radiological diagnosis of iCCA requires differentiation from HCC. The role of US is limited in this regard. Contrast-enhanced CT and MRI are the imaging modalities of choice, where CT is ideal for vascular assessment to determine resectability. Unlike HCC, iCCA typically demonstrate peripheral or rim enhancement on arterial phase, with subsequent central delayed phase enhancement. Biopsy is indicated if iCCA is suspected, as imaging appearances alone are not sufficient to make the diagnosis (there is an overlap with the appearances of metastases to the liver, Figure 9.4).

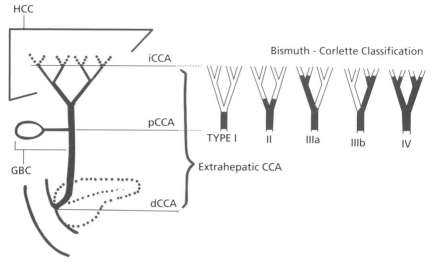

Fig. 9.3 Schematic of hepatobiliary anatomy. Tumours proximal to secondary branches of the right and left hepatic ducts constitute iCCA. pCCA are located at the right or left hepatic ducts or common bile duct cranial to the level of the cystic duct. dCCA are located inferior to this and cranial to the Ampulla of Vater.

9.2.2.3 Distal and perihilar cholangiocarcinoma

CT can accurately demonstrate vascular invasion and any anatomical anomalies, whilst MRCP is superior for assessing biliary involvement. The main differential diagnosis for extrahepatic CCA includes benign strictures and IgG4 cholangiopathy.

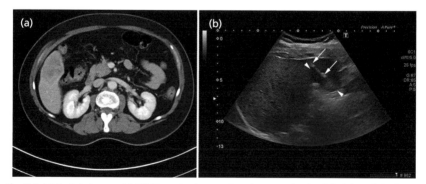

Fig. 9.4 (a) Portal phase axial CT. There is a hypoenhancing mass in the right lobe of the liver. The lesion does not demonstrate any specific features, but appears malignant. The differential diagnosis for this lesion includes an intrahepatic cholangiocarcinoma and a metastasis.
(b) Oblique US. To confirm the nature of the lesion seen in 9.4A, a US guided biopsy has been carried out. The needle (arrows) is visible as a hyperechoic line, and the lesion (arrowheads) as a hypoechoic region. The biopsy confirmed intrahepatic cholangiocarcinoma.

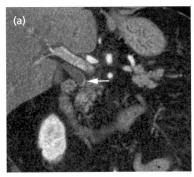 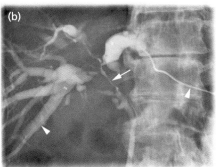

Fig. 9.5 (a) Arterial phase coronal CT. Inferior common duct cholangiocarcinoma, demonstrated as a hyperenhancing, shouldered stricture in the inferior common duct. Diagnosis is typically confirmed using EUS-FNA. (b) Frontal fluoroscopic image. In this patient with perihilar cholangiocarcinoma, the tumour is visible as a stricture in the common hepatic duct (arrow). The tumour also involves the left hepatic duct and the confluence of the right anterior and right posterior hepatic ducts, in keeping with a Bismuth-Corlette type 3a lesion. External drains (arrowheads) are present in the right and left ductal systems, enabling the contrast medium to be injected to produce the image.

For pCCA (Figure 9.5), obtaining tissue in resectable cases is often impossible prior to resection. There is some concern regarding seeding, hence the use of endoscopic US fine needle aspiration (EUS FNA) in this context varies between centres. Endoscopic retrograde cholangiopancreatography (ERCP) brushings have a low sensitivity but are highly specific for both pCCA and dCCA. If ERCP brushings are negative, EUS FNA is used to make a preoperative diagnosis in dCCA. PTC (percutaneous transhepatic cholangiography) guided biopsy is, like ERCP brushings, specific but not sensitive. Both approaches may also allow for stent insertion.

9.2.2.4 Staging

The majority of required staging information can be obtained from a multiphasic liver/pancreas protocol CT with MRCP. Contrast enhanced liver MRI is also helpful to assess disease extent. PET-CT may have some value in assessing metastatic disease in select cases, but is not currently used routinely. iCCA, pCCA, and dCCA are staged according to separate criteria. Whilst the respective TNM AJCC/UICC systems are most widely applied, alternative systems are under development to better reflect prognostic outcomes.

9.2.3 Gallbladder carcinoma

This is uncommon and often associated with cholelithiasis. US typically shows a mass within or extending from the gallbladder or variable wall thickness. If resectable, tissue is not obtained prior to surgery.

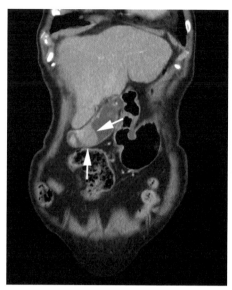

Fig. 9.6 Portal phase coronal CT. Gall bladder cancer (arrows) is seen as a mass arising from the gall bladder.

The sensitivity of contrast-enhanced CT reportedly approaches 90%, and demonstrates a gallbladder mass or discontinuous gallbladder wall thickening (Figure 9.6). CT can also demonstrate direct hepatic spread, biliary tract dilatation, or vascular involvement, and is key to staging and identification of candidates for curative resection. MRI can further aid differentiation of malignant lesions from benign pathologies, including xanthogranulomatous cholecystitis.

9.2.4 Mixed hepatocellular cholangiocarcinoma

Biphenotypic tumours (Figure 9.7) are a rare and poorly characterized entity, thought currently to represent less than 1% of primary hepatobiliary cancer diagnoses. Clinically, age of diagnosis and male preponderance reflect those of HCC, whereas poor survival figures resemble those of iCCA. Published data to date is sparse and insufficient to conclude on any definitive radiological hallmarks for mixed hepatocellular cholangiocarcinoma (HCC-CCA).

9.3 Therapeutic assessment and follow-up

9.3.1 Overview

CT is the main radiological modality, with MRI or PET being used as problem-solving tools. Defined imaging protocols may be necessary to assess response to specific surgical or interventional management. For instance, a pre- and post-contrast CT is performed to assess for viable residual or recurrent disease following radiofrequency ablation (RFA) or transarterial (chemo)embolization (TA(C)E).

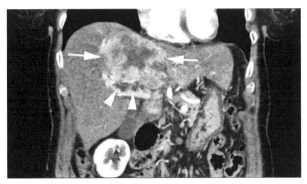

Fig. 9.7 Arterial phase coronal CT. Biphenotypic tumours share imaging features with both hepatocellular carcinoma and intrahepatic cholangiocarcinoma. In this case, arterial hyperenhancement is present (arrows), as well as tumour thrombus in the right portal vein (arrowheads).

9.3.2 Ablative techniques

Percutaneous ablative therapies act by causing coagulative tumour necrosis, using thermal techniques (including RFA, microwave ablation, laser ablation, and cryoablation) or chemical injection of ethanol (PEI) or acetic acid. RFA is a standard first-line treatment option in stage BCLC 0 or A HCC when deemed unsuitable for surgery, with the same overall survival outcomes compared to surgical resection in lesions measuring less than 2 cm. US or CT are used for image guidance (Figure 9.8), and image fusion may improve procedure accuracy, particularly for ill-defined lesions on US.

9.3.3 Transarterial (chemo)embolization

(TA(C)E is an established standard of care in BCLC stage B (asymptomatic large or multinodular) HCC, with an established overall survival advantage in HCC. Altered

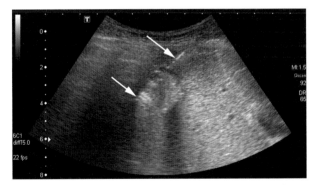

Fig. 9.8 Oblique US. US can be used to guide radiofrequency ablation for the treatment of HCC. The needle is visible as an echogenic line (arrows) and the ablation zone as an echogenic region surrounding it.

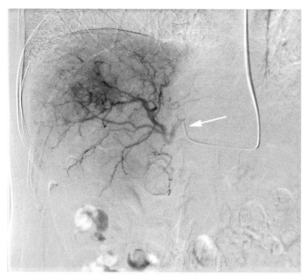

Fig. 9.9 Arterial phase frontal fluoroscopic image. HCC can be treated using transarterial embolization. In this case a catheter has been inserted into the hepatic artery to allow the injection of embolic material.

portal venous circulation, deteriorating performance status, hepatic decompensation, biliary stenting, biliary-enteric anastomoses, and segmental portal vein invasion are known factors associated with poor outcomes. With good patient selection, median survival figures are in the region of 40–50 months.

Embolization of the tumour feeding artery (Figure 9.9) uses embolizing agents such as polyvinyl alcohol or gelfoam, and may involve, in addition, direct delivery of an anthracycline or platinum-based cytotoxic agent followed by occlusion of the tumour vascular supply to cause tumour ischaemia and infarction. Drug eluting beads can also be used in the procedure. Treatment response is assessed with contrast-enhanced CT or MRI at four weeks post-treatment and the change in viable tumour bulk is evaluated (see section 9.3.6).

9.3.4 Selective internal radiation therapy

SIRT, also referred to as transarterial radioembolization (TARE), is image-guided brachytherapy using beta-radiation from Yttrium-90 microspheres and subsequent ischaemia through arterial embolization to mediate a cytotoxic effect. Planning angiography is undertaken pre-treatment, including prophylactic embolization of non-target arteries and identification of any anatomical variants. SPECT scanning with the radiotracer 99mTc-macroaggregated albumin (MAA) is performed to ensure safe levels of hepatopulmonary shunting prior to SIRT (Figure 9.10).

Although SIRT has been used for solitary HCC lesions too large for, refractory to, or anatomically unlikely to respond to TA(C)E, with objective response rates between

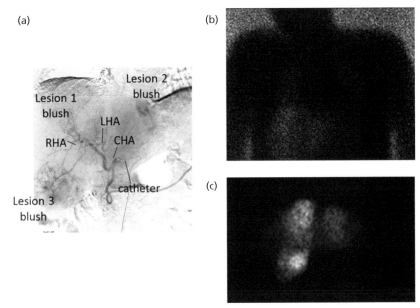

Fig. 9.10 (a) During SIRT work-up the presence of collateral shunts from hepatic vessels (common hepatic artery (CHA), left hepatic artery (LHA), right hepatic artery (RHA)) which can affect distribution of radioactive microspheres is established by angiography. Angiography here shows three lesions by the presence of focal contrast accumulation as a 'tumour blush'. (b) 99 mTc MAA, which is a similar size to the treatment microspheres, is injected, and distribution assessed here using a SPECT scan to calculate lung shunts by evaluating uptake in liver and lung versus liver alone. Radiation exposure is considered too high if lung shunt value is over 10%. (c) SPECT scan of liver shows good distribution of activity in both lobes with uptake around the tumour and no extra-hepatic uptake.

35–50%, published evidence of overall survival advantage, particularly in BCLC C disease, is lacking to date.

9.3.5 Radiotherapy

Clinical trials are exploring the safety and efficacy of external beam radiotherapy techniques including IMRT (intensity-modulated radiotherapy) and SBRT (stereotactic body radiation therapy) for hepatobiliary cancers, for instance in resected CCA or unresectable iCCA. However, the role of radiotherapy for these tumours is yet to be established, and is largely performed within a research setting at present.

9.3.6 Systemic therapies

For advanced cholangiocarcinomas and gallbladder cancers, gemcitabine and cisplatin have been established as a standard of care treatment. For efficacy of cytotoxic treatment in solid cancers, tumour response by Response Evaluation Criteria in Solid Tumors (RECIST) criteria is frequently used as a surrogate for survival outcomes.

However, use of anatomic tumour response parameters, such as change in sum of maximal diameters of lesions, can be ambiguous when evaluating the loco-regional therapies of the molecularly targeted agents (MTAs) or anti-angiogenic therapies used in management of advanced HCC. These now include the multi-targeted tyrosine kinase inhibitors sorafenib (VEGFR, PDGFR, Raf family), lenvatinib (VEGFR1-3, FGFR1-4) in the first-line treatment setting, and in the second-line setting regorafenib (VEGFR2, TIE2, FGFR1), cabozantinib (VEGFR, AXL, MET), and the anti-angiogenic monoclonal antibody against VEGFR2, ramucirumab.

RECIST criteria have, therefore, been amended to encompass the notion of viable tumoural tissue showing uptake in the arterial phase of contrast-enhanced imaging techniques, the modified RECIST (mRECIST). Reports suggesting activity from the immune checkpoint PD-1 inhibitors, nivolumab and pembrolizumab as monotherapy or in combination with MTAs in advanced HCC means that immune-related response criteria may also become incorporated into the response assessments for this tumour in the future.

9.4 **Summary**

+ Dynamic contrast-enhanced CT and MRI form the basis of radiological diagnosis and surgical planning.

+ HCC often arises in the background of abnormal cirrhotic liver and demonstrates typical features, which have previously permitted diagnosis in the absence of histological confirmation on non-invasive criteria.

+ It may not be possible to acquire tissue from pCCA or gallbladder cancer prior to resection—alternative diagnoses are excluded and then confirmation of malignancy is only possible after surgical removal.

+ Modified RECIST criteria have been developed to address the concept of viable tumour following treatment of HCC with loco-regional therapies or MTAs within response assessments, although these require validation.

Further reading

Blechacz B (2017). Cholangiocarcinoma: current knowledge and new developments. *Gut Liver*, **11**(1): 13–26.

Chernyak V, Fowler KJ, Kamaya A, et al. (2018). Liver Imaging Reporting and Data System (LI-RADS) version 2018: imaging of hepatocellular carcinoma in at-risk patients. *Radiology*, **289**, 816–830.

Chow PKH, Gandhi M, Tan SB, et al. (2018). SIRveNIB: selective internal radiation therapy versus sorafenib in Asia-Pacific patients with hepatocellular carcinoma. *Journal of Clinical Oncology*, **36**(19): 1913–1921.

European Association for the Study of the Liver (2018). EASL Clinical Practice Guidelines: management of hepatocellular carcinoma. *Journal of Hepatology*, **69**(1): 182–236.

Forner A, Reig M, Bruix J (2018). Hepatocellular carcinoma. *Lancet*, **391**(10127): 1301–1314.

Hennedige TP, Neo WT, Venkatesh SK (2014). Imaging of malignancies of the biliary tract—an update. *Cancer Imaging*, **14**: 14.

Lencioni R, Petruzzi P, Crocetti L (2013). Chemoembolization of hepatocellular carcinoma. *Seminars in Interventional Radiology*, **30**(1): 3–11.

McEvoy SH, McCarthy CJ, Lavelle LP, et al. (2013). Hepatocellular carcinoma: illustrated guide to systematic radiologic diagnosis and staging according to guidelines of the American Association for the Study of Liver Diseases. *Radiographics*, **33**(6): 1653–1168.

Roberts LR, Sirlin CB, Zaiem F, et al. (2018). Imaging for the diagnosis of hepatocellular carcinoma: a systematic review and meta-analysis. *Hepatology*, **67**(1): 401–421.

Wang EA, Broadwell SR, Bellavia RJ, Stein JP (2017). Selective internal radiation therapy with SIR-Spheres in hepatocellular carcinoma and cholangiocarcinoma. *Journal of Gastrointestinal Oncology*, **8**(2): 266–278.

Chapter 10

Pancreatic tumours

David Bowden and Thankamma Ajithkumar

10.1 Introduction

Approximately 9400 new cases of pancreatic cancer are diagnosed in the UK and 367,000 new cases globally every year. The peak incidence is in the 65–75-year age group, with 60% of patients being older than 65 years of age. Approximately 10–15% patients present with early stage disease amenable to curative surgery, 30–40% with locally advanced inoperable disease, and the remainder with metastatic disease. The overall five-year survival is less than 5%.

Common symptoms at presentation are painless jaundice, epigastric pain radiating to the back, and unexplained weight loss. Radical resection (typically with a pancreatico-duodenectomy: Whipple's procedure) with a negative margin (R0) is the only curative treatment but is associated with a 1–5% mortality and 20% morbidity; however, R0 resection is only feasible in 40–60% patients with localized disease. After R0 resection the median survival is 24 months, which falls to 18 months with a margin-positive resection. Accurate imaging is important in optimal therapeutic decision making, especially in order to identify tumours in which an R0 resection is potentially achievable.

10.2 Diagnosis and staging

10.2.1 Diagnosis

10.2.1.1 Transabdominal ultrasound

Transabdominal ultrasound (TAUS) is often the initial examination in patients with painless jaundice. It can detect biliary and/or pancreatic duct dilatation (double duct sign), larger tumours >2 cm, and liver metastases. Image quality is, however, significantly affected by multiple factors, including operator expertise, patient body habitus, and the presence of overlying bowel gas. As a result, sensitivity may be as low as 75%, making it an unsuitable imaging modality for the surveillance of individuals at high risk of malignancy.[1]

10.2.1.2 Computed tomography

Triple-phase computed tomography (CT) is the investigation of choice for diagnosis and staging. A typical scanning protocol will use 1000 mL oral water as negative

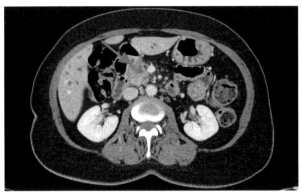

Fig. 10.1 Axial contrast-enhanced CT image showing a hypoenhancing mass arising within the head of the pancreas (arrow). Note dilatation of the intrahepatic ducts secondary to biliary obstruction (dilated ducts near the asterisk).

intraluminal contrast with 100–150 mL intravenous iodinated contrast injected at 4 mL/s via a power injector. Thin (1–2 mm) slices are obtained in both a pancreatic parenchymal phase (approximately 40 s or using bolus tracking) and a later portal venous phase (70 s). The main aim is to maximize the attenuation difference between the tumour and normal pancreas. Approximately 90% of tumours will be hypo-enhancing relative to normal pancreatic parenchyma (Figure 10.1). The late arterial pancreatic phase also allows more accurate detection of vascular involvement. An early arterial phase (at approximately 20 s) can subsequently be acquired if additional surgical planning of vascular anatomy is required, thereby facilitating the generation of multiplanar and 3D (volume rendered) images with post-processing tools. Accuracy of CT in detecting pancreatic adenocarcinoma is 85–100%.

A well-recognized sign of an obstructing pancreatic tumour is the classical 'double duct' sign in which both the common bile and pancreatic ducts are obstructed with resultant upstream dilatation. In cases where the primary lesion cannot be seen, more subtle secondary signs are useful (Table 10.1). If the primary lesion cannot be identified

Table 10.1 Secondary signs of a pancreatic tumour

Sign	Remark
Pancreatic duct cut-off	Subtle sign
Upstream pancreatic atrophy	Subtle sign
Vascular occlusion	Look for development of collateral vessels
Loss of normal pancreatic margins	Use gastroduodenal artery as a landmark
Double duct sign	Always abnormal but can also be seen in chronic pancreatitis as a result of benign strictures

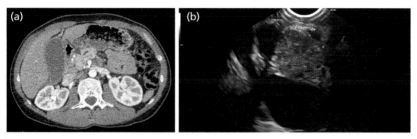

Fig. 10.2 Axial CT image (a) showing dilatation of the pancreatic duct with an abrupt cut-off of a dilated pancreatic duct (arrow), but no visible tumour; EUS (b) clearly demonstrates an obstructing tumour, marked with calipers.

with CT, in the presence of these secondary signs, further evaluation with endoscopic ultrasound (EUS) or magnetic resonance imaging (MRI) is indicated (Figure 10.2).

10.2.1.3 Endoscopic ultrasound

A pancreatic cancer will typically appear as an irregular hypoechoic mass relative to the normal pancreatic tissue. Its accuracy rates for diagnosing tumours are higher than multidetector CT (MDCT) (97%), particularly for tumours <2 cm in size. A normal EUS can reliably exclude a tumour with a negative predictive value approaching 100%. In a majority of patients EUS-guided fine needle biopsy is the method of choice for histological diagnosis and carries a lower risk of peritoneal seeding compared to other percutaneous approaches. EUS-guided coeliac axis nerve block can be also be useful in the palliative setting.

10.2.1.4 Magnetic resonance imaging

MRI, in particular the use of magnetic resonance cholangiopancreatography (MRCP), has an established role for evaluating biliary tree pathology, but is less commonly used to diagnose pancreatic cancer. However, it may be useful where secondary signs are present but the primary lesion is not seen at CT. The 'duct penetration sign', in which a dilated pancreatic duct is seen to traverse a stricture or possible mass without complete obstruction, can be useful to differentiate between chronic pancreatitis and adenocarcinoma. Studies have demonstrated diagnostic accuracies of 76–89%. Unenhanced fat-saturated T1-weighted imaging is also of particular use in the evaluation of pancreatic parenchyma, given its innate hyperintensity as a result of abundant endoplasmic reticulum, high manganese, and protein content. Tumours typically are therefore visible as a focus of hypo-intensity relative to background parenchyma.

10.2.1.5 Endoscopic retrograde cholangiopancreatography

Endoscopic retrograde cholangiopancreatography (ERCP) is often performed to palliate obstruction to the biliary tract by stenting. However, the presence of stents in the common bile duct and any post-procedural inflammation can hinder interpretation of subsequent staging imaging and ideally these should be performed prior to ERCP.

10.2.1.6 F-fluorodeoxyglucose positron emission tomography/CT

F-fluorodeoxyglucose positron emission tomography/CT ([18]FDG PET/CT) in routine staging of pancreatic cancer has not been defined. However, it may be considered for patients with equivocal para-aortic nodal or other disease, but otherwise resectable disease.

10.2.2 Staging

This is performed to assess for potential resectability of the primary tumour (locoregional stage) and to identify distant metastases (commonly peritoneum, liver, and lungs). The accepted standard for staging of pancreatic cancers is based on the TNM (tumour, node, metastasis) staging system.[2]

10.3 Therapeutic staging classification

Localized pancreatic cancers are classified into resectable, borderline resectable, and locally advanced disease.[3] Patients with resectable disease proceed with primary surgery followed by adjuvant chemotherapy, whereas those with borderline-resectable and locally advanced tumours are considered for neoadjuvant treatment, usually with combination chemotherapy (Figure 10.3). Patients who continue to be inoperable after neoadjuvant chemotherapy may be considered for radical chemo-radiotherapy.

There are a number of criteria for classification of localized tumours (e.g. MD Anderson, NCCN, etc.). The 2017 International consensus on criteria for classification of localized tumours are given in Table 10.2

The accuracy of MDCT in staging and resectability ranges from 85% to 95%, with an accuracy up to 90% for the exclusion of unresectable disease. Since pancreatic cancer tends to spread early via the lymphatics, it is important to try to recognize subtle involvement of the peripancreatic tissue, as well as early peritoneal or perineural spread.

Distant metastases in pancreatic cancer commonly occur in the liver, peritoneum, and lungs. Liver metastases generally appear as low attenuation, ill-defined lesions on CT and are typically solid on US. The presence of ascites is often a sign of peritoneal

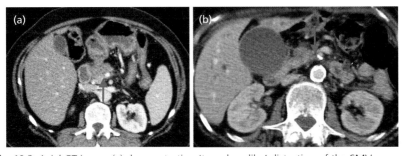

Fig. 10.3 Axial CT image (a) demonstrating 'tear-drop-like' distortion of the SMV secondary to encasement by an adjacent tumour within the pancreatic head. Axial CT image (b) in a separate patient shows subtle early involvement of the SMA (with calcified wall) by tumour extension from an uncinate process mass.

Table 10.2 International consensus on classification of localized tumours

Criteria	Resectable	Borderline		Locally advanced
		Borderline-PV	Borderline-A (arterial)	
Venous involvement: superior mesenteric vein (SMV)/portal vein (PV)	No tumour contact or unilateral narrowing	Tumour contact 180° or greater or bilateral narrowing/ occlusion, not exceeding the inferior border of the duodenum	—	Bilateral narrowing/ occlusion, exceeding the inferior border of the duodenum
Arterial involvement: superior mesenteric artery (SMA), coeliac axis (CA), common hepatic artery (CHA)	No tumour contact	No tumour contact/invasion	SMA, CA: tumour contact of less than 180° without showing deformity/stenosis CHA: tumour contact without showing tumour contact of the PHA and/or CA	SMA, CA: tumour contact/invasion of 180° or more degree CHA: tumour contact/invasion showing tumour contact/invasion of the proper hepatic artery and/or CA

Source: data from Isaji S, et al. 'International consensus on definition and criteria of borderline resectable pancreatic ductal adenocarcinoma 2017'. *Pancreatology.* Jan 2018, Vol. 18, Issue 1, pp. 2–11.

spread. Small tumour deposits on the peritoneum and liver surface will be subtle on imaging and require a high index of suspicion, although modern thin-section CT has improved sensitivity for their detection. If imaging findings continue to be non-specific, staging laparoscopy is useful prior to definitive resection.

10.4 Mucinous neoplasms of the pancreas

With the widespread use of CT and MRI in modern imaging, incidental cystic lesions within the pancreas are being detected with relative frequency. These are classified as mucinous cystic neoplasms (MCNs) and intraductal papillary mucinous neoplasm (IPMNs).[5,6] Other benign cystic lesions include serous cystadenomas, pseudocysts, and epithelial cysts.

MCNs predominate in the body and tail of the pancreas occurring at a median age of 40–50 years, almost exclusively in women. They have an ovarian-type stroma secreting mucin and do not communicate with the pancreatic duct. The classic appearance of an MCN is of a unilocular or multilocular cystic lesion, each cyst >2 cm in diameter, perhaps containing a solid or papillary nodule or exhibiting punctuate mural calcification. Serous cystadenomas, on the other hand, are usually located around the head, contain smaller cysts, and have an extremely low (but not non-existent) malignant potential.

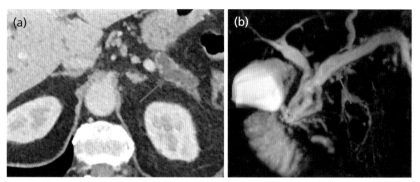

Fig. 10.4 Contrast-enhanced axial CT (a) shows marked pancreatic duct dilatation secondary to an intraductal papillary mucinous tumour (arrow). Coronal MRCP image (b) demonstrates diffuse dilatation of the entire main pancreatic duct (arrow).
Images courtesy of Dr. Ed Godfrey, Cambridge University Hospitals NHS Foundation Trust, Cambridge, UK.

IPMNs are slow- growing tumours, subdivided into main duct and side branch duct types. Side-branch duct type is most commonly found in the pancreatic head, neck, and uncinate process, often appearing as a cystic lesion on imaging. Main duct type IPMN has the higher risk of developing malignancy (50% at five years) compared with side branch duct type (15% at years). Imaging appearances can often be very similar to those seen in chronic pancreatitis or other cystic lesions. Features suggestive of IPMN include location in the head and uncinate process, communication with the main pancreatic duct, presence of solid components within the lesion, and bulging of the duodenal papilla due to mucin secretion (Figure 10.4). A study demonstrated accuracies for the diagnosis of IPMN of 76% for MDCT and 80% for MRCP.

Differentiation of MCN from the other cystic lesions is often not easy on CT, MRI, or US appearances alone. EUS, however, is able to aid in this differentiation by enabling EUS fine needle aspiration, and obtaining fluid from these cystic lesions. This can be analysed for cytological malignancy, amylase content, and carcinoembryonic antigen (CEA) levels. Using this approach, a study demonstrated 100% sensitivity and 89% specificity for differentiating benign from malignant lesions.

10.5 Imaging for radiotherapy planning

While external beam radiotherapy can be used in pancreatic cancer as a curative or palliative treatment, randomized trials have reported conflicting results regarding its benefit. In the postoperative setting, a meta-analysis and the RTOG 9704 trial did not show any benefit with adjuvant chemo-radiotherapy.

In patients with borderline tumour, ongoing studies are evaluating the role of conventional radiotherapy or stereotactic ablative body radiotherapy (SABR) in improving overall resection and margin-negative resection rates. In patients with locally advanced unresectable tumours, the LAP-07 study did not show any difference in median survival between chemotherapy and chemo-radiotherapy (16.5 vs. 15.2 months, p = 0.83) after four months of chemotherapy.

However, most guidelines recommend consideration for radical chemo-radiotherapy if there is at least stable localized disease after 3–4 months of chemotherapy.[7,8] Alternatively, patients could be enrolled into clinical trials. Radical fractionated radiotherapy is often combined with synchronous fluoropyrimidine-based chemotherapy, such as oral capecitabine (chemoradiotherapy or CRT) as a radiosensitizer. A meta-analysis suggests that SABR (35–50 Gy in five fractions) is equally effective in locally advanced pancreatic cancer.[9]

Treating pancreatic cancers with radiotherapy is technically challenging. Target volume delineation is particularly challenging as there are uncertainties in defining the extent of tumour, especially identifying tumour spread along the splanchnic plexus and identifying lymph node involvement. For 3D radiotherapy planning, CT imaging with ≤3 mm slice thickness during free breathing is obtained with the patient appropriately immobilized (supine position with arms above head).

For 4D planning, exhale breath-hold, contrast-enhanced, 3D-CT scan (CE-3DCT) using a pancreatic protocol followed by a 4D-CT is used. Intravenous contrast with or without opacification of the bowel will help to delineate the anatomy, particularly to distinguish bowel loops and vasculature from tumour and lymph nodes. Critical structures including the duodenum, liver, spinal cord, and both kidneys are outlined. The tumour and visible lymph nodes of >1 cm in short axis (gross tumour volume—GTV) are then identified and outlined, often with the help of a cross-sectional radiologist. The CTV margin is generally 5 mm.

For 3D planning, a 15 mm margin is added to CTV in superior-inferior directions and 10 mm circumferentially to obtain the PTV margin. This is to allow for microscopic spread of the tumour beyond CT resolution, organ movement, and daily variation of patient positioning. The PTV margin for 4D planning is typically 3–5 mm. Taking into account the predefined dose constraints to the critical structures, a 3–4-field coplanar conformal or IMRT/VMAT plan is made and used to deliver radiotherapy (Figure 10.5). Conventional fractionated radiotherapy is given to a dose of 50.4 Gy in 28 fractions delivering five fractions daily with concurrent chemotherapy (usually capecitabine).

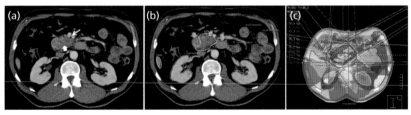

Fig. 10.5 Contrast-enhancing planning CT scan (a) shows an ill-defined hypodense lesion in the head of the pancreas (thick arrow) which is involving superior mesenteric vessels (thin arrow). The lesion is located in the C-loop of the duodenum (b) and treated with IMRT (c) for optimal sparing of the duodenum and bowel.

Palliative radiotherapy is given for pain relief or bleeding into the duodenum. Localization of the tumour should be performed using CT and treated with a 2–3 cm margin using parallel opposed anterior and posterior fields, 3D conformal radiotherapy using a 3–4-field plan or IMRT/VMAT. Painful bone and soft tissue metastatic disease can respond well to short courses of palliative radiotherapy.

10.6 Therapeutic assessment and follow-up

Follow-up of patients after surgical resection usually involves clinical assessment with or without tumour marker (CA19-9 and CEA) measurements. Further evaluation (usually with CT) is indicated if there is clinical suspicion of recurrent disease. Common sites of relapse include local and lymph node recurrence, peritoneal, liver, and lung metastases. The use of FDG PET/CT scanning may be useful to distinguish recurrent disease from postoperative changes.

For selected patients who have completed definitive CRT for locally advanced unresectable pancreatic cancer, a reassessment CT may be performed at 4–8 weeks to document treatment response and to exclude metastatic disease. Curative resection may be considered in a small proportion of these patients as salvage for treatment failure.

10.6 Summary

- Ductal adenocarcinoma is the most common malignant pancreatic tumour and >80% are unresectable at diagnosis.
- CT is performed for staging and to determine resectability.
- EUS is useful for detecting small cancers not visible on CT and for obtaining histological confirmation of malignancy.
- There is no role for routine surveillance following curative treatment.

References

1. **Ashida R, Tanaka S, Yamanaka H, et al.** (2018). The role of transabdominal ultrasound in the diagnosis of early stage pancreatic cancer: review and single-center experience. *Diagnostics* (Basel), **9**(1): ii: E2. doi: 10.3390/diagnostics9010002.
2. **Sobin LH, Gospodarowicz MK, Wittekind CH (2017).** *UICC TNM Classification of Malignant Tumours* (eighth edn). Oxford: Wiley Blackwell, p.93.
3. **Ducreux M, Cuhna AS, Caramella C, et al.** (2015). ESMO Guidelines Committee. Cancer of the pancreas: ESMO Clinical Practice Guidelines for diagnosis, treatment and follow-up. *Annals of Oncology*, **26**(5): v56–68.
4. **Isaji S, Mizuno S, Windsor JA, et al.** (2018). International consensus on definition and criteria of borderline resectable pancreatic ductal adenocarcinoma 2017. *Pancreatology*, **18**(1): 2–11.
5. **Lim J, Allen PJ** (2019). The diagnosis and management of intraductal papillary mucinous neoplasms of the pancreas: has progress been made? *Updates in Surgery*, **71**(2): 209–216.
6. **Chandwani R, Allen PJ** (2016). Cystic neoplasms of the pancreas. *Annual Reviews in Medicine*, **67**: 45–57.

7. **O'Reilly D, Fou L, Hasler E, et al.** (2018). Diagnosis and management of pancreatic cancer in adults: a summary of guidelines from the UK National Institute for Health and Care Excellence. *Pancreatology*, **18**(8): 962–970.

8. **Balaban EP, Mangu PB, Yee NS** (2017). Locally advanced unresectable pancreatic cancer: American Society of Clinical Oncology Clinical Practice Guideline Summary. *Journal of Oncology and Practicals*, **13**(4): 265–269.

9. **Petrelli F, Comito T, Ghidini A, Torri V, Scorsetti M, Barni S** (2017). Stereotactic body radiation therapy for locally advanced pancreatic cancer: a systematic review and pooled analysis of 19 trials. *International Journal of Radiation Oncology. Biology. Physics*, **97**(2): 313–322.

Chapter 11

Gastrointestinal stromal tumours

Haesun Choi

11.1 Introduction

Gastrointestinal stromal tumour (GIST) accounts for only 0.2% of all gastrointestinal (GI) neoplasm but is the most common tumour of non-epithelial origin in the GI tract. The term *gastrointestinal stromal tumour* was first used by Mazur and Clark[1] to describe an unusual type of non-epithelial GI tumour that lacked the traditional features of smooth muscle or Schwann cells. GISTs are now thought to derive from a precursor of the interstitial cells of Cajal, which are normally present in the myenteric plexus, and are clearly distinct from other mesenchymal tumours, such as leiomyomas and leiomyosarcomas.

The true incidence rate of GISTs in all population is not known. The reported population-based incidence rates vary from 6.5 to 14.5 per million. Assuming the annual incidence rate of 10 per million, approximately 3000 cases might be diagnosed in the USA a year. The median age at diagnosis is 66–69 years.

11.2 Clinical presentation

GISTs can occur anywhere along the GI tract and is associated with a broad range of clinical presentations. In adult GISTs, the stomach (60%) and small intestine (30%) are the most common primary sites and the duodenum the third (5%). Oesophageal and colorectal GISTs are rare. On rare occasions GISTs occurs in the mesentery, omentum, or retroperitoneum. Extragastrointestinal (soft tissue) stromal tumours are histologically and immunophenotypically similar to their gastrointestinal counterpart, but have an aggressive course similar to small intestinal rather than gastric stromal tumours.

The tumours are often large at the time of initial presentation but bowel obstruction is rare due to its exophytic nature of growth. In a population-based study, the median tumour size of GISTs that were detected based on symptoms, incidental findings, or during an autopsy were 8.9, 2.7, and 3.4 cm, respectively. Small GISTs (smaller than 2 cm) usually do not produce symptoms and are detected incidentally during abdominal exploration, endoscopy, or radiologic imaging. Symptoms are often non-specific, including, early satiety, vague abdominal pain or dyspepsia, and palpable mass. It is not infrequent for the patient to present at the emergency room with an acute abdomen (GI bleeding, perforation, intraperitoneal bleeding due to tumour rupture, and, rarely, gastrointestinal obstruction). Nearly 50% of patients present with metastasis. Most common sites of metastasis are liver and peritoneal cavity. Unlike GI adenocarcinomas, lymph node metastasis is extremely uncommon. Less frequently, the metastasis can be found in the lungs, pleura, and soft tissue.

11.3 Diagnosis

11.3.1 Imaging studies

Imaging is important not only for diagnosing and staging the tumours, but also for monitoring the tumours during and following treatments. Computed tomography (CT) is currently the modality of choice for these purposes, although other imaging techniques, such as fluorine-18-fluorodeoxyglucose (FDG) positron emission tomography (PET), magnetic resonance (MR) imaging, and ultrasonography, can also be used.[2] Further detail is discussed in a separate section in this chapter.

11.3.2 Pathology

The tumours are highly vascular, submucosal in location (Figure 11.1), and grow out away from the originating bowel lumen but may form polypoid masses. Mucosal ulceration is not uncommon in large tumours that are often associated with GI bleeding. Most GISTs present as a single, well-circumscribed nodule.

A core biopsy is recommended for an adequate tissue sampling, although obtaining adequate tumour tissue material for definitive diagnosis before surgical resection can be challenging because these tumours tend to be soft and friable with a risk of rupture. A biopsy may not be necessary if the tumour is suspected and is easily resectable without preoperative therapy on CT.

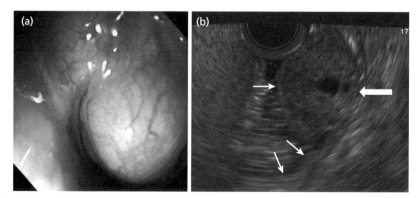

Fig. 11.1 Typical submucosal presentation of GIST seen on endoscopy and endoscopic ultrasound. (a) Typical appearances of a submucosal bilobulated GIST of the stomach. Note the intact mucosa. Endoscopic biopsies were expectedly, unremarkable.
(b) Endoscopic US appearances of a typical GIST. A 2.5 cm, heterogeneous GIST arises from the first submucosal layer (large arrow), and contains an anechoic space suggesting central necrosis. Note the normal intact mucosa (small arrows).

11.3.3 Prognostic features

Based on previously published series of GISTs, the two most important prognostic features of a primary tumour are the size and mitotic index. Smaller studies indicate that anatomic location affects the risk of disease recurrence and progression. Small intestinal GISTs are more aggressive than gastric GISTs of equal size, and this should be factored into the risk assessment of a primary tumour. Based on the summary in Table 11.1[3] GISTs that are 2 cm or less in size can be regarded as essentially benign, but lesions larger than 2 cm have a risk of recurrence.

11.4 **Treatment**

The optimal management of GIST requires a multidisciplinary approach. The remarkable efficacy of imatinib mesylate (Gleevec; Norvatis, Basel, Switzerland), a tyrosine kinase inhibitor, has revolutionized the management approach for GIST. Imatinib mesylate, a phenylaminopyrimidine derivative, is a small molecule that is known to inhibit the specific kinase action of Abl and the chimeric BCR-Abl fusion protein. Approximately 4% of patients with GIST are intolerant of imatinib. Furthermore, 50% of patients will eventually develop resistance to imatinib at a median of 24 months, commonly (70%) the result of secondary mutations in specific *KIT* loci. New second-line targeted agents are now also available for those with imatinib-resistant GISTs.[4]

Table 11.1 Risk stratification of primary GIST by mitotic index, size, and site

Tumour parameters		Risk of progressive disease * (%)			
Mitotic index	**Size**	**Gastric**	**Duodenum**	**Jejunum/ileum**	**Rectum**
≤5 per 50 hpf	≤2 cm	None (0%)	None (0%)	None (0%)	None (0%)
≤5 per 50 hpf	>2 ≤ 5 cm	Very low (1.9%)	Low (4.3%)	Low (8.3%)	Low (8.5%)
≤5 per 50 hpf	>5 ≤ 10 cm	Low (3.6%)	Moderate (24%)	(Insuff. data)	(Insuff. data)
≤5 per 50 hpf	>10 cm	Moderate (10%)	High (52%)	High (34%)	High (57%)
>5 per 50 hpf	≤2 cm	None+	High+	(Insuff. data)	High (54%)
>5 per 50 hpf	>2 ≤5 cm	Moderate (16%)	High (73%)	High (50%)	High (52%)
>5 per 50 hpf	>5 ≤10 cm	High (55%)	High (85%)	(Insuff. data)	(Insuff. data)
>5 per 50 hpf	>10 cm	High (90%)	High (90%)	High (86%)	High (71%)

GIST—gastrointestinal stromal tumour, hpf—high power field, insuff—insufficient.

*Defined as metastatsis or tumour-related death.

+Denotes small numbers of cases.

Reproduced with permission from Demetri GD et al. 'NCCN Task Force report: management of patients with gastrointestinal stromal tumor (GIST)--update of the NCCN clinical practice guidelines'. J Natl Compr Canc Netw. Vol. 5, Suppl 2, pp. S1–29. Copyright © 2007 National Comprehensive Cancer Network.

The tumours less than 2 cm found incidentally can be monitored using endoscopy or a cross-sectional imaging. In patients with the localized, potentially resectable tumours without significant risk of comorbidity, surgical resection is the choice. For those with comorbidity, the US national comprehensive cancer network (NCCN) guideline recommends neoadjuvant imatinib along with appropriate imaging work-up prior to and during the course of treatment until surgical resection is feasible (usually in 3–6 months). For those unresectable, recurrent, or metastatic GISTs, imatinib is the initial treatment of choice. The imatinib is also recommended in post-surgical patients with a high risk of recurrence, such as resection with margin positive.[5]

For those undergoing systemic treatment, image assessment is critical to evaluate the tumour response (see later) to explore further treatment options without delay when needed. Those who develop resistance to imatinib may be overcome by increasing the imatinib dose from 400 to 800 mg/day, typically in those tumours with mutations in *KIT* exon 9.[6] While focal resistance may be controlled transiently, by surgical removal of the resistant lesion, there is a general consensus that multifocal imatinib resistance should be treated with an alternative targeted agent, such as sunitinib malate (SUTENT®, Pfizer Inc., CA, USA). Sunitinib is an oral multitargeted RTK inhibitor of KIT, PDGFR-α and -β, VEGF receptors (VEGFR-1, -2, and -3), FMS-like tyrosine kinase 3, colony-stimulating factor 1 receptor, and glial cell line-derived neurotrophic factor receptor (rearranged during transfection). Sunitinib is effective in imatinib-refractory patients, including those with the *KIT* exon 9 mutation, at the standard daily dose of 50 mg/day (schedule 4/2).

11.5 Imaging

11.5.1 Computed tomographic imaging

In patients with biopsy-proven GISTs, computed (CT) is the imaging modality of choice at initial presentation, for staging, and for monitoring the disease during its course. When a submucosal tumour is found incidentally during endoscopy (Figure 11.1), the extraluminal extent of disease should be evaluated with CT.

Typically, CT images of the abdomen and pelvis are acquired prior to and following bolus administration (usually 3–5 cc/sec of injection rate) of an iodinated intravenous contrast agent and oral and rectal contrast agents. For contrast-enhanced CT, arterial- and portal-venous-phase images (obtained using a biphasic or triphasic technique) are required to optimize the detection and characterization of the hepatic metastasis or hypervascular masses, such as GISTs.

The CT features of GISTs can vary depending on the size, location, and aggressiveness of tumour. They are typically highly vascular enhancing masses, submucosal in location, growing away from the original bowel lumen. The tumours can be heterogeneous and predominantly hypodense when they become necrotic, haemorrhagic, or myxoid degenerating. The primary GIST can occasionally present with an ulceration and a fistula to the originating bowel lumen. Air or oral contrast agent may be seen within the fistularized mass on the CT images. At the time of presentation, the mass

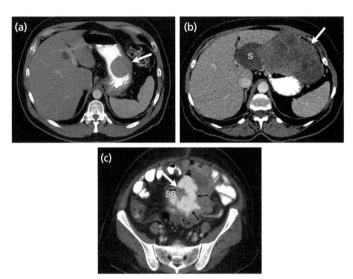

Fig. 11.2 (a) Polypoid gastric GIST (arrow), (b) exophytic gastric GIST (arrow), (c) exophytic small bowel GIST (arrow) with a fistulous tract. Note the contrast (small arrows) within the tumour cavity. S: stomach; SB: small bowel.

is often large and may be difficult to identify its origin. Despite the large size, clinical evidence of GI obstruction is uncommon (Figure 11.2).

Most common metastasis are to the liver and peritoneal cavity which can be readily identified on CT. Metastasis in the pleura, lungs, or soft tissues, such as abdominal wall, can occur less frequently. Lymph node metastases are rare. These metastatic lesions have CT features similar to those of the primary tumours: they may be (depending on the tumour size) homogeneously to heterogeneously enhancing soft-tissue masses, often with tumour vessels visible.

11.5.2 Positron emission tomography

The primary role for positron emission tomography (PET) in the initial evaluation of biopsy-proven GISTs is in staging (Figure 11.3). Baseline FDG-PET is recommended in patients in whom FDG-PET will be used to monitor therapy or who require a very short follow-up (2–3 weeks), such as those with marginally resectable GIST.[3]

In general, for tumours less than 1 cm in size, FDG-PET may not be reliable in identifying metabolically active lesions.[2] In GIST, it has been reported that the overall sensitivity of FDG-PET is approximately 80% in detection at initial presentation; patients with negative uptake on pretreatment FDG-PET had tumours ranging from 1.0 to 4.7 cm. Similarly, Hersh et al. found negative results on pretreatment FDG-PET in four of eight patients. These four patients had homogeneous tumours on CT images, with a mean diameter of 6 cm (range 3–8 cm).[7]

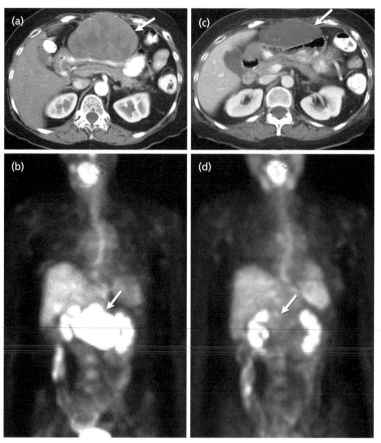

Fig. 11.3 Responding gastrointestinal stromal tumour in a 59-year-old woman with recurrent gastric GIST in the omentum. (a, b) Pretreatment contrast-enhanced CT scan (a) shows a large, enhancing omental mass (arrow) abutting the anterior surface of the stomach corresponding to the mass (arrow) with markedly increased glucose update shown on pre-treatment FDG-PET (B). (c, d) Contrast-enhanced CT scan (c) obtained two months after treatment showed that the mass (arrow) has decreased in size and become homogeneous, with a marked decrease in CT density corresponding to the mass (arrow) with no appreciable glucose uptake shown on FDG-PET (d) obtained at the same time.

11.5.3 Ultrasound

Endoscopic ultrasonography (EUS) may be used in evaluating small (<2 cm) GISTs that are incidentally found during endoscopy. The high-frequency probe (12–30 MHz) used in EUS can delineate each layer of bowel wall and, therefore, may reliably locate tumour origin within or outside of the wall. EUS also can evaluate the tumour vascularity when used in conjunction with Doppler ultrasonography. EUS is most useful in the oesophagus, stomach, duodenum, and anorectum. EUS is, however, not a routine imaging modality because of its limited penetration and field of view, and CT should always be performed to accurately estimate the extent of disease.

Although transabdominal ultrasonography may be used to evaluate hepatic metastasis, this technique is inappropriate for evaluating the peritoneal cavity or large tumours in staging or monitoring the disease following treatment.

11.5.4 Magnetic resonance imaging

Well-performed magnetic resonance imaging (MRI) is superior to contrast-enhanced CT in evaluating hepatic metastasis and rectal GIST with superior soft-tissue contrast and direct multiplanar acquisition capability. However, MRI is not the primary imaging modality of choice in evaluating GIST patients because of its limited sensitivity in detecting peritoneal tumours.

On MR images, GISTs are generally well defined; the solid portions of the masses are typically of low to intermediate signal intensity on T1-weighted images and high signal intensity on T2-weighted images. As in CT, the tumours enhance after administration of an intravenous contrast agent.[8] Intravenous contrast helps to delineate viable solid components and non-enhanced necrotic areas. Internal haemorrhage may have signal intensity varying from high to low on both T1- and T2-weighted images, depending on the time from the haemorrhage.

11.6 Response evaluation and surveillance

11.6.1 Response evaluation

In patients who have undergone surgical resection of GISTs, CT scan every 3–6 months is performed for surveillance of metastatic or recurrent disease. In patients with unresectable advanced disease or metastasis, CT is recommended within three months of the start of systemic treatment.[5]

Responding GISTs are characterized by a dramatic change in the pattern of enhancement on contrast-enhanced CT images, from heterogeneous hyperattenuation to homogeneous hypoattenuation, accompanying the resolution of enhancing tumour nodules and a decrease in tumour vessels, regardless of whether the tumour size decreases (Figures 11.3, 11.4). These changes can be observed within one or two months and may be seen as early as one week after treatment (unpublished data).

Traditional size-based response evaluation criteria, such as the Response Evaluation Criteria in Solid Tumours (RECIST) or World Health Organization criteria, underestimate the response of the GIST treated with targeted agents. The median time to evidence of tumour shrinkage on CT is about 3–4 months, although it sometimes may take 6–12 months or longer. More importantly, responding GISTs sometimes increase in size because of intratumoural haemorrhage, necrosis, or myxoid degeneration (Figure 11.4).[9] In these cases, observation of changes in tumour density (indicating a decrease in density) and in the enhancement pattern (indicating a decrease in tumour vasculature) aid to reaching the correct conclusion. New CT response evaluation criteria have been advocated.[10–12] A 10% decrease in the sum of the uni-dimensional tumour size or a 15% decrease in tumour density, as determined by the CT attenuation

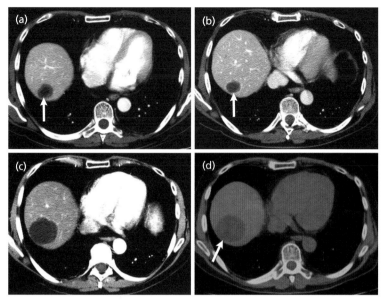

Fig. 11.4 Responding hepatic metastasis with pseudoprogression in a 56-year-old male with duodenal GIST. (a) Pre-treatment contrast-enhanced CT showed an enhancing hepatic metastasis (arrow) in segment seven with the tumour density measured 40 HU. Note the peripheral enhancing component (small arrows). (b) Contrast-enhanced CT image obtained at two months after treatment demonstrated a minimal decrease in size of the hepatic metastases (arrow) but with a significant decrease in CT density (27 HU). The peripheral enhancement is no longer evident. This is typical of responding GIST. Contrast-enhanced CT image (c) obtained seven months after treatment showed a homogenously hypoattenuating tumour with a continuous decrease in tumour density (18 HU). Notice the significant increase in tumour size with no appreciable glucose uptake on FDG-PET image (d). The enlarging homogenous tumour with a continuous decrease in tumour density should not be confused with a progressing tumour.

coefficient in Hounsfield units, at the first follow-up (two months) following treatment can best separate the good responders and poor responders and response at this time is an excellent predictor of progression-free survival.[10,11] The same authors proposed modified CT response criteria (Table 11.1) using both tumour density and uni-dimensional measurement of tumour size, of which reproducibility was confirmed in an extended group of patients. Similar results are reported using the sum of products of bi-dimensional measurement (BDM)[12] with a 8.25% decrease in tumour size at one month following treatment best identifying the group of patients in whom treatment failed. It was concluded that stability or any decrease in the sum of products of bi-dimensional measurement at one month following treatment was a strong indicator of time-to-treatment failure in 52 patients. Perfusion CT and PET/CT in GIST patients before and after treatment with imatinib mesylate at three, five, or seven days found that PET responders (>30% decrease in SUV) had decreases in both blood flow and blood volume to tumours, while non-responders had an increase in blood flow and less increase in blood volume.[13] Use of perfusion CT requires special post-processing software, careful monitoring of data acquisition, and data analysis for reducibility.

11.6.2 Surveillance

Contrast-enhanced CT plays an important role in surveillance and the early detection of tumour recurrence or progression that might signal the clonal emergence of resistance to ongoing targeted treatment.

Recurrence or disease progression is traditionally diagnosed by finding an increase in tumour size or the development of new lesions at the site of previous disease or distant metastasis. However, as mentioned previously, increased tumour size alone, without a change in tumour enhancement or tumour vessels, may not accurately represent the disease progression. Development of an intratumoural enhancing nodule is often the earliest sign of disease progression. This is observed within a treated hypodense tumour without a change in tumour size (Figure 11.5). Thorough analysis of each treated lesion is required to identify these new intratumoural nodules. If tumour recurrence or disease progression is suspected, short-term follow-up (e.g. one month) using well-designed, contrast-enhanced CT imaging may be performed for confirmative diagnosis. Whenever the CT findings are inconclusive or inconsistent with clinical findings, FDG-PET is indicated.

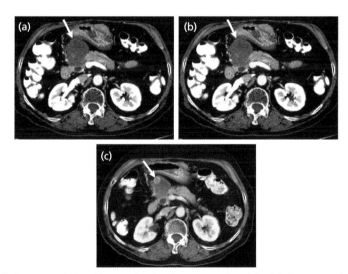

Fig. 11.5 Recurrent GIST with an enlarging intratumoral nodule. (a) Contrast-enhanced CT obtained at nine months after treatment showed a typical responding GIST (arrow). (pretreatment CT is not shown here). (b, c) Note a tiny enhancing nodule (arrows) developed within the treated tumour at ten months after treatment (b), with an increase in size 11 months later (c).

11.7 **Conclusion**

GIST is a mesenchymal tumour of the GI tract. It often used to be misdiagnosed as leiomyomas and leiomyosarcomas without optimal therapeutic options until KIT receptor protein was identified in the tumour cells. Correct diagnosis is critical to take advantage of the early targeted agents, KIT tyrosine kinase receptor inhibitor, such as imatinib, with dramatic improvement of the survival. Its unique immunohistochemical profile and mutational analysis of the kinase genes *KIT* and platelet-derived growth factor receptor alpha (*PDGFRA)* help to make a correct diagnosis. Understanding the unique imaging features has become important not only at the time of initial presentation but also during the time of response evaluation to the targeted agents.

References

1. **Mazur MT, Clark HB** (1983). Gastric stromal tumours. Reappraisal of histogenesis. *American Journal Surgeical Pathology*, **7**(6): 507–519.

2. **Choi H, Charnsangavej C, de Castro Faria S, et al.** (2004). CT evaluation of the response of gastrointestinal stromal tumours after imatinib mesylate treatment: a quantitative analysis correlated with FDG PET findings. *American Journal of Roentgenology*, **183**(6): 1619–1628.

3. **Demetri GD, Benjamin RS, Blanke CD, et al.** (2007). NCCN Task Force report: management of patients with gastrointestinal stromal tumour (GIST)—update of the NCCN clinical practice guidelines. *Journal of National Comprehensive Cancer Network*, **5**(2): S1–29; quiz S30.

4. **Demetri GD, van Oosterom AT, Garrett CR, et al.** (2006). Efficacy and safety of sunitinib in patients with advanced gastrointestinal stromal tumour after failure of imatinib: a randomised controlled trial. *Lancet*, **368**(9544): 1329–1338.

5. **Network NCC (2018).** *NCCN Guidelines Version 1.2018 Gastrointestinal Stromal Tumours (GIST)*. Fort Washington, PA: NCCN.

6. **Debiec-Rychter M, Sciot R, Le Cesne A, et al.** (2006). KIT mutations and dose selection for imatinib in patients with advanced gastrointestinal stromal tumours. *European Journal of Cancer*, **42**(8): 1093–1103.

7. **Hersh MR, Choi J, Garrett C, Clark R** (2005). Imaging gastrointestinal stromal tumours. *Cancer Control*, **12**(2): 111–115.

8. **Levy AD, Remotti HE, Thompson WM, Sobin LH, Miettinen M** (2003). Gastrointestinal stromal tumours: radiologic features with pathologic correlation. *Radiographics*, **23**(2): 283–304, 456; quiz 532.

9. **Hong X, Choi H, Loyer EM, Benjamin RS, Trent JC, Charnsangavej C** (2006). Gastrointestinal stromal tumour: role of CT in diagnosis and in response evaluation and surveillance after treatment with imatinib. *Radiographics*, **26**(2): 481–495.

10. **Benjamin RS, Choi H, Macapinlac HA, et al.** (2007). We should desist using RECIST, at least in GIST. *Journal of Clinical Oncology*, **25**(13): 1760–1764.

11. **Choi H, Charnsangavej C, Faria SC, et al.** (2007). Correlation of computed tomography and positron emission tomography in patients with metastatic gastrointestinal stromal tumour treated at a single institution with imatinib mesylate: proposal of new computed tomography response criteria. *Journal of Clinical Oncology*, **25**(13): 1753–1759.

12. **Holdsworth CH, Manola J, Badawi RD, et al.** (2004). Use of computerized tomography (CT) as an early prognostic indicator of response to imatinib mesylate (IM) in patients with gastrointestinal stromal tumours (GIST). *Journal of Clinical Oncology*, **22**(14): 197s.

13. **McAuliffe JC, Hunt KK, Lazar AJ, et al.** (2009). A randomized, phase II study of preoperative plus postoperative imatinib in GIST: evidence of rapid radiographic response and temporal induction of tumour cell apoptosis. *Annals of Surgical Oncology*, **16**(4): 910–919.

Chapter 12

Rectal cancer

Vivek Misra and Rohit Kochhar

12.1 Clinical background

Colorectal cancer is the fourth most common cancer in the UK. Of the approximately 40,000 new cases annually, a quarter to a third are located in the rectum. Rectal cancer is more common in men and the highest rate is in the 85–89 years age group for both males and females. Adenocarcinomas account for over 90% of tumours, the remainder consist of squamous carcinomas, carcinoid, lymphoma, melanoma, and gastrointestinal stromal tumours. Presentation includes rectal bleeding, change in bowel habit, frequency of defaecation, tenesmus, rectal fullness, and pelvic pain. With the introduction of bowel screening in the UK for people between the ages of 50 and 74 years, asymptomatic patients are increasingly diagnosed. Distant spread most commonly occurs to the liver, lung, and peritoneum. Metastases are less commonly seen in the bones, brain, and other areas.

Advances in surgical technique and more accurate radiotherapy planning and delivery have improved rectal cancer outcome. Anterior resection combined with total mesorectal excision (TME) has become the standard surgical procedure, facilitating the radial clearance of the primary tumour, mesorectal tissue, and associated vascular, lymphatic, and perineural deposits, thus improving local recurrence rates. Abdominoperineal resection is now reserved for low rectal tumours when sphincter integrity cannot be preserved.

In the UK, preoperative radiotherapy (RT) or chemoradiotherapy (CRT) prior to surgery is recommended to reduce the risk of local relapse or to downstage inoperable disease. Recent non-randomized evidence suggests that a non-operative approach for patients with a complete clinical response following neo-adjuvant CRT may be safe, with reduced long-term morbidity and preservation of sphincter function.[1] This approach is currently the subject of randomized controlled trials. In patients otherwise unfit for neoadjuvant CRT and with localized rectal cancers, radiotherapy alone may provide meaningful downstaging of the disease and allow surgery in a significant proportion of patients.

Accurate staging is essential to ensure the correct therapeutic approach is undertaken. Imaging plays a pivotal role in defining which patients may benefit from radical surgery, selecting the most relevant surgical procedure, and identifying patients in whom a postoperative margin (R0) resection is not possible with surgery alone, and for whom preoperative RT or CRT may be appropriate.

12.2 **Diagnosis and staging**

12.2.1 Diagnosis

Rectal cancer is most commonly diagnosed by lower gastrointestinal endoscopy (fibreoptic colonoscopy) and biopsy, although imaging is an alternative where computed tomography (CT) colonography has superseded barium enema for diagnosis.[2] The capability of CT to reconstruct images into dynamic navigable 3D views of the colon simulating fibreoptic colonoscopy has popularized the technique. A systematic review has suggested that CT colonography has high average sensitivity and specificity for large and medium colorectal polyps (>10 mm and 6–10 mm respectively), and excellent sensitivity for cancer in the symptomatic population, with >96% of cancers detected.

12.2.2 Staging

A clear understanding of the anatomy (Figure 12.1) and pathway of spread is important for accurate staging. A commonly used definition for rectal cancer is an

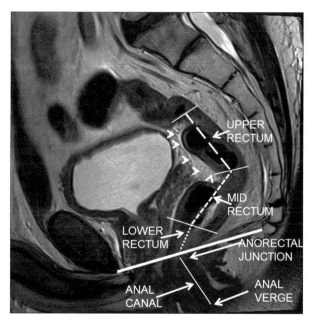

Fig. 12.1 Sagittal T2-weighted MR image demonstrating the divisions of the rectum extending from S3 to the level of the levator plate. The anorectal junction is identified by the pubococcygeal line (solid bold line) extending from inferior tip of symphysis to the last coccygeal joint. The lower rectum (round dotted line) extends from the anorectal junction to 6 cm from the anal verge. The mid rectum (short dash line) extends to 10 cm from the verge and the upper rectum (long dash line) extends to S3. Anteriorly, the peritonealized surface of the upper rectum can be identified (arrowheads).

adenocarcinoma with a distal margin ≤15 cm from the anal verge, as measured by rigid sigmoidoscopy. 'Low' rectal cancers are those with the lower edge, at or below the origin of the levators at the pelvic side-wall on magnetic resonance imaging (MRI), which usually corresponds to within 6 cm of the anal verge. Once a tumour has penetrated through the muscularis propria, growth can extend deep into perirectal fat. Below the supporting structures of the anus, tumour can extend into the ischiorectal fossa, a potential space around the anal canal and sphincter. Hence, there is a high risk of locoregional failure for low tumours. Lymphatic drainage to regional nodes is dependent on site. Mid-upper rectal tumours drain to perirectal nodes and along the superior rectal vessels to the inferior mesenteric vessels. Low-mid rectal tumours drain to perirectal nodes and along mid-rectal vessels to the internal iliac vessels. Most involved perirectal nodes within the mesorectum lie either at the level of, or within 5 cm proximal to, the primary tumour. Lateral pelvic lymph nodes (external iliac and obturator nodes) may be involved in 10–25% of patients with rectal cancer. As lateral pelvic and internal iliac nodes are not removed with a standard TME, there is risk of local recurrence at these sites with surgery alone. Venous drainage of the upper rectum is via the superior rectal vein to the inferior mesenteric vein and portal system, while drainage of the mid and lower rectum is to the iliac veins and inferior vena cava, thus metastases can develop either in the liver or lungs, depending on tumour site.

Accurate staging is essential for defining the most appropriate treatment strategy. The accepted standard for staging cancer is based on the Union for International Cancer Control (UICC) Tumour Node Metastasis (TNM) staging, currently in its eighth edition (Table 12.1), although Dukes' classification also remains in use (Table 12.2). Staging should also address synchronous colonic cancers. Additional information beyond TNM staging which is vital for treatment decisions is: (1) the relationship of the tumour to the potential circumferential resection margin (CRM) indicating the likelihood of a clear R0; (2) the presence of extramural venous invasion (EMVI), a prognostic feature; and (3) the relationship of the tumour to the anal sphincter complex which defines whether sphincter-sparing surgery is possible for low rectal cancer, as well as the need for preoperative RT.

MRI is the modality of choice for locoregional staging (Figure 12.2). T-staging accuracies ranging from 71% to 91% have been reported, although differentiation between T2 and early T3 tumours remains challenging due to desmoplasis and microscopic disease. MRI has also been validated prospectively (MERCURY) with an accuracy of 87% and specificity of 92% in predicting a clear CRM (>1 mm).[3] Patients with tumours that extend to within a small distance of the mesorectal fascia (e.g. 1 mm), that lie outside the mesorectum, or that extend inferiorly to the anorectal junction should be offered adjuvant RT. The distance of tumour to the CRM is also a prognostic factor for overall five-year survival.

Extramural venous invasion (EMVI) is defined by the presence of tumour cells beyond the muscularis propria in endothelium-lined vessels. It is an important and independent risk factor for local and distant recurrence as well as reduced survival requiring treatment intensification.[4] On MRI intermediate signal intensity tumour is seen invading or expanding a vessel. The invaded vessel has similar signal intensity to the tumour (Figure 12.2). EMVI is recorded as positive or negative and a note is made as to whether the involved vessels lie close to the mesorectal fascia.

Table 12.1 TNM staging, eighth edition

T primary tumour

TX	Primary tumour cannot be assessed
T0	No evidence of primary tumour
Tis	Carcinoma *in situ*: invasion of lamina propria[a]
T1	Tumour invades submucosa
T2	Tumour invades muscularis propria
T3	Tumour invades subserosa or into non-peritonealized pericolic or perirectal tissues
T4	Tumour directly invades other organs or structures[b,c,d] and/or perforates visceral peritoneum
T4a	Tumour perforates visceral peritoneum
T4b	Tumour directly invades other organs or structures

Notes

[a] Tis includes cancer cells confined within the mucosal lamina propria (intramucosal) with no extension through the muscularis mucosae into the submucosa.

[b] Invades through to visceral peritoneum to involve the surface.

[c] Direct invasion in T4b includes invasion of other organs or segments of the colorectum by way of the serosa, as confirmed on microscopic examination, or for tumours in a retroperiotoneal or subperiotoneal location, direct invasion of other organs or structures by virtue of extension beyond the muscularis propria.

[d] Tumour that is adherent to other organs or structures, macroscopically, is classified cT4b. However, if no other tumour is present in the adhesion, microscopically, the classification should be pT1-3, depending on the anatomical depth of wall invasion.

N regional lymph nodes

NX	Regional lymph nodes cannot be assessed
N0	No regional lymph node metastasis
N1	Metastasis in 1–3 regional lymph nodes
N1a	Metastasis in 1 regional lymph node
N1b	Metastasis in 2–3 regional lymph nodes
N1c	Tumour deposit(s), that is, satellites*, in the subserosa, or in non-peritonealized peicolic or perirectal soft tissue *without* regional lymph node metastasis
N2	Metastasis in 4 or more regional lymph nodes
N2a	Metastasis in 4–6 regional lymph nodes
N2b	Metastasis in 7 or more regional lymph nodes

Note

* Tumour deposits (satellites) are discrete macroscopic or microscopic nodules of cancer in the pericolorectal adipose tissue's lymph drainage area of a primary carcinoma that are discontinuous from the primary and without histological evidence of residual lymph node or identifiable vascular or neural structures. If a vessel wall is identifiable on H&E, elastic or other stains, it should be classified as venous invasion (V1/2) or lymphatic invasion (L1). Similarly, if neural structures are identifiable, the lesion should be classified as perineural invasion (Pn1). The presence of tumour deposits does not change the primary tumour T category, but changes the node status (N) to pN1c if all regional lymph nodes are negative on pathological examination.

(continued)

Table 12.1 Continued

M distant metastasis	
M0	No distant metastasis
M1	Distant metastasis
M1a	Metastasis confined to one organ (liver, lung, ovary, non-regional lymph node(s)) without peritoneal metastases
M1b	Metastasis in more than one organ
M1c	Metastasis to the peritoneum with or without other organ involvement

Reproduced with permission from Sobin LH, Gospodarowicz MK, Wittekind CH. *UICC TNM Classification of Malignant Tumours*. 8th ed. © 2017 Wiley Blackwell.

Table 12.2 Duke's classification

A	Tumour confined to bowel wall
B	Tumour penetrates bowel wall
C	Regional lymph nodes involved
D	Distant metastases

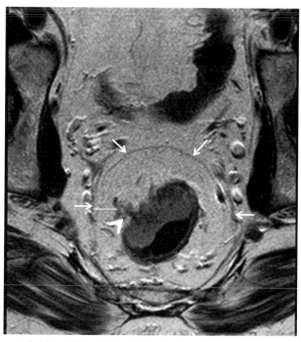

Fig. 12.2 Transaxial oblique T2-weighted MRI showing a T3c rectal cancer with contiguous extramural vascular invasion extending 8mm beyond the hypointense muscularis propria into the mesorectal fat (bold arrow head). The CRM (short arrows) is not threatened as the distance to the CRM (thin straight line) is >1mm.

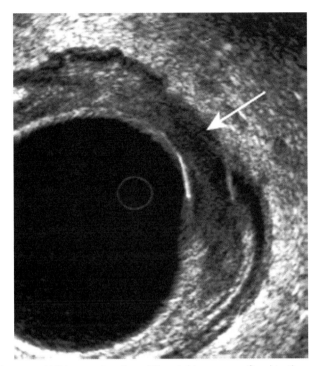

Fig. 12.3 Transrectal US image showing a T2 rectal tumour confined to the muscularis propria (arrow).

Transrectal ultrasound (TRUS) is preferred for small early tumours (T1N0 or T2N0; <3 cm; within 8 cm of anal verge) to assess if local excision is appropriate. Infiltration of the rectal wall layers by tumour is well demonstrated (Figure 12.3). However, T2 tumours may be overstaged due to peritumoural inflammation and the technique is inferior to MRI for depiction of the potential surgical CRM due to its limited field of view. A meta-analysis examining the accuracy of TRUS, MRI, and CT for local staging has suggested that TRUS has better diagnostic accuracy for perirectal tissue invasion than CT or MRI with sensitivities of 90% vs. 79% and 82%, but comparable accuracy for invasion of adjacent organs (sensitivities of 70–74%).[5]

[18]F-fluorodeoxyglucose (^{18}F-FDG) positron emission tomography (PET)/CT is not recommended for initial distant staging. However, it is recommended when CT is equivocal or when synchronous metastases are potentially suitable for resection.[6] Studies on rectal cancer have shown nearly a 30% change in tumour stage or treatment plan on ^{18}F-FDG PET/CT, more frequent for low rectal cancers.[7]

Reliable detection of nodal involvement still remains a challenge for imaging. The majority of histologically involved lymph nodes are <5 mm and will not raise suspicion on size criteria alone. Furthermore, many involved nodes are <3 mm and may not be seen on imaging. Accuracies with a variation of 62–83% have been reported for TRUS while accuracies with a variation of 39–95% have been reported for MRI. The use of morphological appearances on high resolution MRI based on the nodal outline

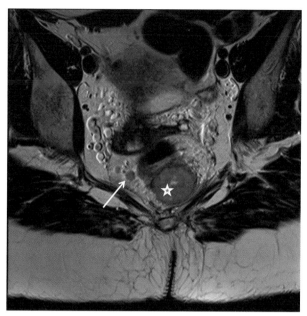

Fig. 12.4 T2-weighted coronal oblique image shows an 8 mm mesorectal node (arrow) at 9 o'clock showing an irregular outline and heterogeneous signal, similar to the tumour (star).

and signal intensity are more reliable than size. Nodes are judged suspicious if they have irregular borders, mixed signal intensity, or both (Figure 12.4). FDG PET/CT has also not been shown to be superior to conventional imaging for nodal staging, with sensitivity of only 29%.

About 20% of patients will be diagnosed with metastases at initial presentation, the liver, lungs, and peritoneum being the most common sites. CT is the most commonly used imaging modality for distant staging. However, ^{18}F-FDG PET/CT is more sensitive than CT (Figure 12.5) and may identify occult disease missed on conventional CT. Several studies have shown the impact of ^{18}F-FDG PET/CT on the management of this subgroup, avoiding futile surgery.

A meta-analysis of CT, MRI, and ^{18}F-FDG PET staging performance reported per-patient sensitivities of 64.7%, 75.8%, and 94.6% respectively.[8] ^{18}F-FDG PET/CT is routinely recommended for restaging patients with recurrence being considered for radical surgery and/or metastatectomy. Additionally, hepatic MRI with diffusion and contrast enhancement should be performed for patients planned for resection of hepatic metastases.

Recurrent disease occurs in one-third of patients, usually within three years of curative surgery; patients with rectal cancer are at a higher risk (11.3%) of local recurrence compared with patients with colon cancer (6.1%). Although pelvic MRI has high accuracy for detecting local recurrence, ^{18}F-FDG PET/CT is now recommended for patients with rising tumour markers and/or clinical suspicion of recurrence with normal or equivocal findings on other imaging.

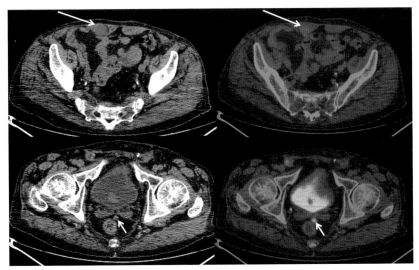

Fig. 12.5 Right rectus abdominis metastasis (long arrow) and a mesorectal deposit (short arrow) are easily identified on the axial ^{18}F-FDG PET/CT images as increased uptake compared to the conventional CT.

12.3 **Imaging for radiotherapy**

Preoperative RT may be delivered as: (1) short-course RT only; (2) long-course RT with concurrent chemotherapy. A preoperative approach reduces the risk of tumour seeding, increases the likelihood of an R0 resection, has less acute toxicity and enhanced radiosensitivity due to better oxygenated cells, and is favoured in the UK. Postoperative treatment is rarely used and has been shown to be inferior in a large RCT.

Short-course radiotherapy (SCRT) is 25 Gy in five daily fractions and long-course radiotherapy is commonly 45 Gy in 25 daily fractions or 50.4 Gy in 28 daily fractions. This is typically given with concurrent fluoropyrimidine chemotherapy (LCCRT).

12.3.1 **Treatment planning**

Individualized CT-based volume definition is superior to the previously used field-based planning technique. The individualized planning CT is performed from the superior aspect of L5 to 2 cm beyond the anal margin, which may be defined by an anal marker placed prior to the CT scan. Images ≤3 mm slice thickness are acquired. Oral dilute gastrograffin or barium contrast to opacify the bowel, and intravenous contrast to highlight vessels, and delayed imaging for ureteric opacification is recommended. Patients may be scanned supine or prone. A full bladder and the use of special immobilization devices such as the 'belly board' can reduce the volume of small-bowel in the pelvis, thus reducing both acute- and long-term toxicity.

The radiotherapy volume should encompass the gross tumour in terms of primary and discontinuous spread, the lymph nodes that are suspected of being involved, and

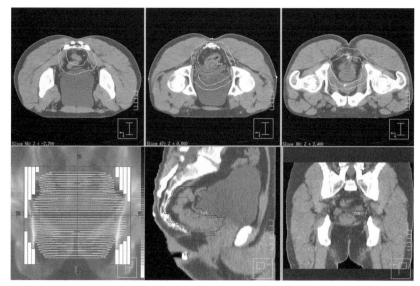

Fig. 12.6 Planning CT demonstrating definition of GTV, CTV expanded, CTV2, and PTV for a mid-rectal cancer from its superior to inferior aspect.

potential areas of microscopic spread. The gross tumour volume (GTV) includes the visible tumour and involved lymph nodes, which is then expanded by 1 cm in all directions to create the clinical target volume (CTV). The final planning target volume (PTV) is then obtained by expanding the CTV in all directions, typically, by 1 cm. The PTV allows for inter-fraction organ displacement and set-up errors.

The volumes and expansions used currently are based on data from previous and current phase III trials, patterns of spread, and local failure. However, different philosophies towards defining the treatment volumes remain. The main thrust of research and development in this field is towards achieving smaller treatment volumes by more accurate imaging for treatment planning along with image-guided radiotherapy (IGRT) to minimize the volume of irradiated normal tissues whilst still accurately treating the target volume. The ultimate aim is to increase the therapeutic ratio.

12.4 **Therapeutic assessment and follow-up**

12.4.1 Therapeutic assessment

A number of radiation-induced tissue changes including oedema, inflammation, necrosis, and fibrosis may make post-neoadjuvant therapy assessment challenging. However, MRI is most commonly performed. Response to neoadjuvant therapy may be assessed by an MRI tumour regression grade (TRG, Table 12.3)),[4] akin to pathology, where MRI signal intensity changes of the whole tumour are evaluated, including extramural disease and areas of vascular invasion, whether contiguous or

Table 12.3 MRI tumour regression grading

Grade	Description
Grade 1	Complete radiological response (linear scar only), no evidence of treated tumour
Grade 2	Good response (dense hypointense fibrosis, no obvious tumour signal) signifying no tumour or minimal residual disease
Grade 3	Moderate response (>50% fibrosis or mucin and visible intermediate signal intensity) signifying residual tumour
Grade 4	Minimal response (mostly tumour, minimal fibrosis/mucinous degeneration)
Grade 5	No response in the primary tumour or frank tumour progression

Source: data from 1) Patel UB, et al. 'MRI after treatment of locally advanced rectal cancer: how to report tumor response-The MERCURY Experience'. *American Journal of Roentgenology* (2012), Vol. 199, Issue 4, pp.W486–W9, and 2) Mandard AM, et al. 'Pathologic assessment of tumor regression after preoperative chemoradiotherapy of esophageal carcinoma'. *Cancer* (1994), Vol. 73, Issue 11, pp.2680–2686.

not (Figure 12.7). Tumour regression grading is a better predictor of outcome after treatment than T stage.[9]

Currently, MRI is recommended 8–10 weeks after the completion of treatment. However, the optimum timing is not established, and this remains a clinical decision. Some clinicians prefer to scan 12 weeks post treatment. This is based on studies which demonstrate that the volume-halving time for rectal cancers is 14 days. Thus, the time for an average tumour to regress to <0.1 cm³ is about 15 weeks post CRT. However, there is no evidence that such a delayed assessment and subsequent surgery improves cancer-specific or overall survival and there are concerns about an increase in resection margin positivity with a delayed approach.[10]

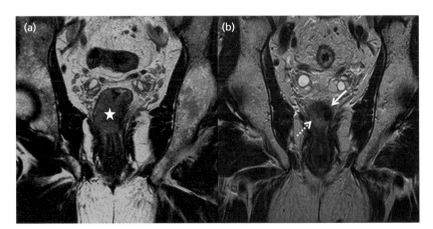

Fig. 12.7 T2-weighted coronal MR images. There is a low rectal tumour seen with intermediate signal (* in (a)). Follow up three months post CRT shows moderate response with both low signal fibrosis (sold arrow in (b) and intermediate signal residual tumour (dotted arrow in (b) scored as mrTRG 3.

Identification of a complete response is best done with a combination of digital rectal examination (DRE), endoscopy, and MRI (for nodal regression). Typically a flat white scar is seen on endoscopy, with only signs of fibrosis and complete nodal regression on MRI.[11] The value of additional ^{18}F-FDG PET/CT is still unclear and not routinely recommended.

12.4.2 Surveillance

There has been debate over the best approach for surveillance. An American Society of Clinical Oncology expert panel concluded that periodic clinical evaluation with carcinoembryonic antigen (CEA) and colonoscopy were justifiable, but other testing added little benefit. Randomized trials of more intensive versus less intensive strategies have been difficult to conduct. Older trials, mainly from the 1990s, have included colon and rectal cancers, early to advanced stage, less well-defined indications for adjuvant therapy, and differing frequency and type of screening for intensive and less intensive groups. Results from these studies have suggested that the number of recurrences is similar for either group, but are detected earlier with more intensive surveillance. More recent trials and a recently published meta-analysis[12] suggest an improvement in overall survival with more intense follow-up regimes and an improvement in cancer specific survival in patients who have more tests as compared to those who have fewer tests. However, these studies included colon and rectal cancer patients and are heterogeneous and used very different follow-up schedules, tests, and duration of follow-up.

In patients who have an initial complete response and remain on active surveillance, this should focus on early detection and treatment of regrowth. Although a uniform protocol has not yet been established, expert opinion favours intensive surveillance with DRE, flexible endoscopy, and MRI including diffusion in the first two years,[13] and decreasing intensity in subsequent years.[14] In practice, three- or six-monthly CEA tests and yearly body CT scans are commonly performed for surveillance for at least three years in the UK, but clearly further clarification is needed.

12.5 Summary

- MRI is the modality of choice for locoregional staging and assessment of potential resectability.
- CT is performed for staging metastatic disease; however, ^{18}F-FDG PET/CT is more sensitive and may play a greater role in the future, particularly if surgical excision of oligometastatic disease is being considered.
- RT planning using CT has limitations that CT/MRI fusion, ^{18}F-FDG PET/CT, or MRI planning may overcome, but these techniques require further validation.
- MRI is the preferred modality for assessing neoadjuvant therapy, typically at 8–10 weeks following completion.
- Debate continues as to the optimum method for surveillance. Yearly body CT is advocated currently.

References

1. **Renehan A**, **Malcomson L**, **Emsley R, et al.** (2016). Watch-and-wait approach versus surgical resection after chemoradiotherapy for patients with rectal cancer (the OnCoRe project). *Lancet*, **17**(2): 174–183.

2. **Cunningham C**, **Leong K**, **Clark S, et al.** (2017). Association of Coloproctology of Great Britain & Ireland (ACPGBI): Guidelines for the Management of Cancer of the Colon, Rectum and Anus (2017)—Diagnosis, Investigations and Screening. *Colorectal Disease*, **19**(Suppl. 1): 9–17.

3. **Mercury Study Group** (2006). Diagnostic accuracy of preoperative magnetic resonance imaging in predicting curative resection of rectal cancer: prospective observational study. *British Medical Journal*, **333**: 779–784.

4. **Patel UB**, **Blomqvist LK**, **Taylor F, et al.** (2012). MRI after treatment of locally advanced rectal cancer: how to report tumor response—the MERCURY experience. *American Journal of Roentgenology*, **199**(4): W486–W489.

5. **Bipat S**, **Glas AS**, **Slors FJM, et al.** (2004). Rectal cancer: local staging and assessment of lymph node involvement with endoluminal US, CT and MR imaging-a meta-analysis. *Radiology*, **232**: 773–783.

6. **Evidence-based indications for the use of PET-CT in the United Kingdom** (2016). London: The Royal College of Radiologists. https://www.rcr.ac.uk/publication/evidence-based-indications-use-pet-ct-united-kingdom-2016 (accessed 11 January 2021).

7. **Petersen RK**, **Hess S**, **Alavi A**, **Hoilund-Carlsen PF** (2014). Clinical impact of FDG-PET/CT on colorectal cancer staging and treatment strategy. *American Journal of Nuclear Medicine Molecular Imaging*, **4**(5): 471–482.

8. **Bipat S**, **van Leeuwen MS**, **Comans EF, et al.** (2005). Colorectal liver metastases: CT, MR imaging, and PET for diagnosis—meta-analysis. *Radiology*, **237**(1): 123–131.

9. **Taylor FG**, **Swift RI**, **Blomqvist L**, **Brown G** (2008). A systematic approach to the interpretation of preoperative staging MRI for rectal cancer. *American Journal of Roentgenology*, **191**: 1827–1835.

10. **Sclafani F** and **Chau I** (2016). Timing of therapies in the multidisciplinary treatment of locally advanced rectal cancer: available evidence and implications for routine practice. *Seminars in Radiation Oncology*, **26**(3): 176–185.

11. **Maas M**, **Lambregts DM**, **Nelemans PJ, et al.** (2015). Assessment of clinical complete response after chemoradiation for rectal cancer with digital rectal examination, endoscopy, and MRI: selection for organ-saving treatment. *Annals of Surgical Oncology*, **22**: 3873–3880.

12. **Jeffery M**, **Hickey BE**, **Hider PN**, **See AM** (2016). Follow-up strategies for patients treated for non-metastatic colorectal cancer. *Cochrane Database Systematic Reviews*, **11**(11): CD002200.

13. **Lambregts DM**, **Lahaye MJ**, **Heijnen LA, et al.** (2016). MRI and diffusion-weighted MRI to diagnose a local tumour regrowth during long-term follow-up of rectal cancer patients treated with organ preservation after chemoradiotherapy. *European Radiology*, **26**: 2118–2125.

14. **Van der Valk MJM**, **Hilling DE**, **Bastiaannet E, et al., and the IWWD Consortium** (2018). Long-term outcomes of clinical complete responders after neoadjuvant treatment for rectal cancer in the International Watch & Wait Database (IWWD): an international multicentre registry study. *Lancet*, **391**: 2537–2545.

Chapter 13

Anal cancer

Rebecca Muirhead and Vicky Goh

13.1 **Clinical background**

Anal cancer is rare, with 1500 new presentations annually in the UK, but its incidence is increasing both nationally and internationally. They occur at the anal verge (25%) or within the anal canal tumours (75%). Squamous cell carcinomas make up 97% of anal cancers, with other rarer types including adenocarcinomas, neuroendocrine tumours, undifferentiated carcinomas, melanomas, gastrointestinal stromal tumours, verrucous carcinomas, and lymphomas.

Peak incidence is in the sixth decade of life. The pathogenesis is multifactorial. However, the predominant risk factor is exposure to the human papilloma virus, primarily HPV-16 and HPV-18. It is positive in 90% of anal squamous cell carcinoma (ASCC). The impact of the implementation of HPV vaccination may reduce incidence. However, the full impact of this will not become apparent for decades. Additional risk factors include other sexually transmitted viruses, smoking, multiple sexual partners, anal intercourse, chronic inflammation, and immunosuppression, including HIV. Patients with anal cancer are more likely to have had a previous malignancy and more likely to develop a further malignancy (e.g. cervix, vulva, or vagina). Small early cancers may cause few symptoms, and are sometimes diagnosed serendipitously with the removal of anal tags. More advanced lesions present as non-healing ulcers, with perineal pain, sensation of a mass, rectal bleeding, itching, discharge, and faecal incontinence. Tumours may be diagnosed concomitantly with a benign anal condition such as haemorrhoids, anal fissure, or fistula.

Anal cancer is predominantly a locoregional disease, metastasizing first to the local lymph nodes such as mesorectal, internal iliac, pre-sacral, obturator, external iliac, or inguinal. Only 10% of patients present with metastatic disease. A small cohort of early anal cancers, particularly at the anal verge, can undergo a local excision, maintaining their sphincter with curative intent. If these patients have disease within 1 mm of the margin they undergo adjuvant chemoradiotherapy. For the majority of those with localized disease, the standard curative treatment is definitive chemoradiation (CRT) with concomitant mitomycin and either 5-fluorouracil or capecitabine. The three-year disease free survival (DFS) following this treatment is 73%.[1] For those with metastatic disease the standard treatment is systemic therapy with palliative intent, the median survival is approximately 12 months.

13.2 **Diagnosis and staging**

Diagnosis is made typically by clinical examination, proctoscopy, and biopsy. Direct proctoscopy is often difficult in more advanced lesions because of pain; patients then undergo examination under anaesthetic (EUA) and biopsy. Digital rectal examination (DRE), magnetic resonance imaging (MRI), and computed tomography (CT) are required for full staging. DRE allows clinical measurement of tumour size, site, and distance from anal verge. MRI pelvis offers information on size, infiltration of adjacent organs, whether there is extension above the dentate line and below the anal margin, and nodal status. Figure 13.1 demonstrates anal cancer on T2 weighted MRI. CT of the thorax and abdomen offers further information on involved nodes as well as assessing whether or not there is metastatic disease.

Although not standard, diagnostic imaging in anal cancer, 18-F fluorodeoxyglucose positron emission tomography/CT (FDG PET/CT), is highly sensitive and increasingly used for patients in selected cases. A recent systematic review reported the sensitivity for PET was 99%, while only 67% for CT. In inguinal lymph nodes the sensitivity was 93% and specificity 76%. There is a cohort of patients who are upstaged or downstaged by FDG PET/CT (5.1–37.5% and 8.2–26.7% respectively).[2] However, Mistrangelo et al. compared findings on PET/CT with pathological conformation on SNB and reported that PET/CT demonstrated a high number of false positive results.[3] Therefore, positive results on PET/CT should be discussed in multidisciplinary

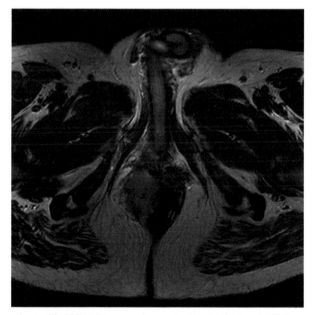

Fig. 13.1 A patient with T2W MRI scans demonstrating high signal ASCC.

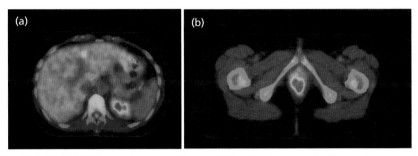

Fig. 13.2 FDG PET/CT scan demonstrating an FDG avid primary and a liver metastasis not picked up on routine CT scan.

setting in order to decide whether an FDG avid lymph node is involved, not involved, or requires further investigation such as an FNA, to facilitate a treatment decision. Figure 13.2 demonstrates the FDG avid primary and one of multiple liver metastases not detected by CT scan.

Investigation is ongoing regarding the use of molecular metabolic imaging as a predictive factor of outcome. A number of studies have suggested that baseline levels of FDG avidity can predict for presence of lymph node metastasis, locoregional failure, and disease-free survival following treatment.[4] Two small studies have suggested that the FDG derived metabolically active volume on diagnostic images correlate with areas of local recurrence, although this may be due to larger tumours being more metabolically active and large tumours are proven to do worse.[5,6] A further study highlighted that heterogeneity analysis performed on a baseline MRI can predict for outcome.[7] All these potential predictive imaging markers require further investigation in larger cohorts.

Staging is based on the TNM (tumour, node, metastasis) classification.[8] This classification is based on clinical factors such as tumour size (assessed by clinical examination and imaging studies) and the site rather than number of local nodes. This is applicable to all carcinomas arising from the canal apart from melanoma.

13.3 Imaging for radiotherapy

13.3.1 Radiation treatment

Radiation is now delivered routinely using intensity modulated radiotherapy (IMRT). In comparison to conformal treatment, IMRT reduces the grade 3 non-haematological toxicity of treatment from 49% to 40% and the number of patients requiring interruptions in their treatment, or discontinuing early due to toxicity.[9] A simultaneous integrated boost (SIB) technique is used to deliver a radical dose to the primary tumour as well as a prophylactic dose to lymph nodes at risk of micrometastatic disease at the same time. Early primary tumours (T1,2 N0) receive 50.4 Gy in 28 fractions; more locally advanced (T3,4 or node positive) receive 53.2 Gy; the prophylactic nodes receive 40 Gy.

13.3.2 Treatment planning process

Patients undergo a single planning CT scan in the supine position, with immobilization for popliteal fossa and feet. Patients are scanned with a comfortably full bladder. If there is infiltration of the buttocks they are placed on a pyrex sheet to enable build-up of dose. If there is infiltration of the skin around involved inguinal nodes, bolus is placed on the affected skin. Intravenous contrast is routinely delivered to enable easier delineation of vessels and GTV. An anal marker is often placed at the anal verge or on the excision scar or surrounding the disease if it is infiltrating the buttocks and difficult to define on CT.

13.3.3 Target volume definition

Co-registration of the diagnostic MRI and PET with the planning scan may improve accuracy of target volume delineation. However, differences in set-up during image acquisitions and poor registration could lead to potential inaccuracies which should be considered. Other imaging formats are being investigated for target volume delineation, for example DW MRI has been demonstrated to improve inter-observer agreement in assigning T stage and aid delineation of gross tumour volume[10] and the potential of an FDG derived biological GTV has been highlighted due to the reproducibility of the biological boost over a course of CRT.[11] These need further investigation in larger cohorts.

The primary tumour GTV (*GTV_A*) includes all areas of macroscopic primary tumour visible on contrast enhanced planning CT; length and distance from anal verge on DRE, EUA, or proctoscopy, and the MRI. The volume is limited to the gross tumour and does not include the whole lumen.

The nodal GTV (*GTV_N*) should be determined using the planning CT, inguinal node examination, MRI, and FDG PET/CT. All macroscopically involved nodes should be encompassed.

The GTV_A is then enlarged by 1 cm (for early tumours) and 1.5 cm (for locally advanced tumours) in order to encompass microscopic disease to create the CTV_A. These margins are based on pathological data from skin squamous cell cancers, suggesting larger tumours have larger distance of microscopic infiltration from the primary tumour. The CTV_A is then enlarged by a further 1 cm to create the PTV_A which is the target for the high dose boost.

The GTV_N is enlarged by 0.5 cm to encompass microscopic disease within CTV_N and finally an additional 0.5 cm to allow for set-up errors to create PTV_N. The PTV_N receives 50.4 Gy unless the nodes are >3 cm, in which case they receive 53.2 Gy.

The elective nodes (CTV_E) are the nodes that are at risk of microscopic disease. These are the mesorectal, internal iliac, external iliac, pre-sacral, obturator, and inguinal lymph nodes. A UK national guidance is available to aid with delineation.[12] The CTV_E is enlarged by 0.5 cm to create the PTV_E which receives 40 Gy in 28 fractions. Figure 13.3 demonstrates a radiotherapy plan with all the appropriate volumes delineated.

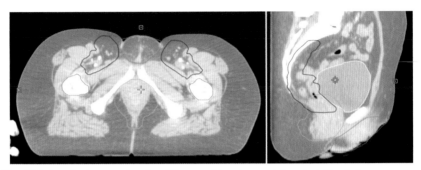

Fig. 13.3 A radiotherapy planning CT scan with volumes delineated. Genitalia: green; bladder: yellow, PTV_E: navy blue; PTV_A: pink.

For, IMRT, the OARs such as the femoral heads, genitalia, urinary bladder, and the small bowel should be delineated.

13.3.4 Treatment modality

Photons (6 MV) are delivered with fixed coplanar beams or arc delivery (VMAT) (Figure 13.4). Prescription point is 100% to the median dose in PTV in keeping with ICRU 83.

13.3.5 Verification images

During treatment, cone-beam CT (CBCT) images are acquired on days 1–5 and then weekly for online assessment of target and organs at risk (OAR) coverage and adjustments in patient position are made, if necessary, to improve coverage. Figure 13.5 shows a fused CBCT and planning scan to verify positioning. On all other days, paired orthogonal kV images are used for online assessment comparing the position of the

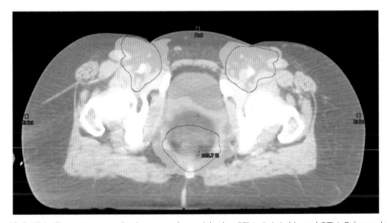

Fig. 13.4 This illustrates a radiotherapy plan with the PTV_A (pink) and PTV_E (navy blue) and dose illustrated in colour-wash.

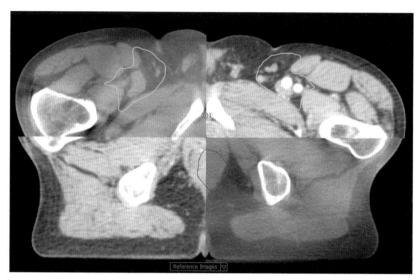

Fig. 13.5 Planning CT scan and CBCT fused to facilitate patient set up with CTV_E (green) and GTV (red) volume from the planning scan highlighted.

patient on that day relative to to the digitally reconstructed radiographs (DRRs) created from the planning scan; adjustments are made as appropriate. Figure 13.6 demonstrates paired orthogonal kV image fused with DRR from planning scan.

13.4 **Therapeutic assessment and follow-up**

There are two small studies highlighting the potential for interim imaging to act as early predictors of outcome. Muirhead et al. demonstrated that the change between DW MRI scans at baseline and after 8–10 fractions correlated with outcome.[13] In another study, the total lesion glycolysis on a FDG PET/CT after 30 Gy correlated with freedom from local progression.[5]

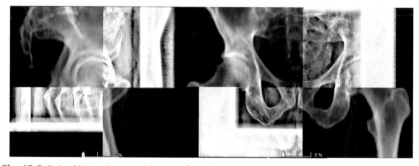

Fig. 13.6 Paired kV orthogonal images fused with DRR created from the planning scan to facilitate patient set-up.

Approximately 10% of patients do not respond to chemoradiotherapy (CRT), and are usually treated with salvage abdominoperineal resection (APR). The rate of APR in patients with an incomplete response to CRT is only 40%.[14] Hence it is important to assess patients closely following treatment to ensure an ongoing response. A DRE exam is performed at six weeks following completion of CRT to ensure the ASCC is reducing in size. An MRI at this stage is of limited benefit.[15] If the tumour increases in size at any point following completion of CRT of the primary tumour, an early APR should be pursued as these patients can rapidly become inoperable. The optimal time to assess response following CRT is 26 weeks following treatment,[16] which is used as the time point for definitive CR assessment in trials.

Surveillance is typically performed by clinical examination three-monthly, MRI at three and six months and CT of the thorax, abdomen, and pelvis annually to exclude macroscopic metastasis. It is known that 75% of anal relapses occur at the site of the primary tumour, and DRE picks these up before any imaging; hence the high frequency of clinical follow-up. If a local recurrence can be identified early those with local recurrence can still undergo curative salvage APR if localized. Of those with local relapse, 80% undergo APR with a two-year DFS of 70%.[14]

FDG PET/CT on completion of treatment has demonstrated correlation with one or more of: local control rate, progression-free survival, cancer-specific survival, or overall survival.[17] This holds potential for reducing the intensive clinical follow-up that occurs in these patients but must be tested in a prospective study prior to clinical use.

13.5 **Summary**

◆ MRI is the preferred modality for local staging due to its superior contrast resolution. CT is the standard modality for assessing metastatic disease. However, FDG PET/CT is increasingly being used routinely to contribute valuable information on nodal and metastatic staging.

◆ Co-registration of staging MRI and PET with the planning CT can allow more accurate contouring.

◆ Following treatment, clinical evaluation and MRI is performed to assess therapeutic response; the use of FDG PET/CT to predict response is investigational.

◆ CT of the thorax, abdomen, and pelvis is performed for metastatic surveillance annually.

References

1. **James RD, Glynne-Jones R, Meadows HM, et al.** (2013). Mitomycin or cisplatin chemoradiation with or without maintenance chemotherapy for treatment of squamous-cell carcinoma of the anus (ACT II): a randomised, phase 3, open-label, 2×2 factorial trial. *Lancet Oncology*, **14**(6): 516–524.

2. **Mahmud A, Poon R, Jonker D** (2017). PET imaging in anal canal cancer: a systematic review and meta-analysis. *British Journal of Radiology*, **90**: 20170370.

3. **Mistrangelo M, Pelosi E, Bello M, et al.** (2010). Comparison of positron emission tomography scanning and sentinel node biopsy in the detection of inguinal no.de metastases in patients with anal cancer. *International Journal of Radiation Oncology Biology. Physics*, **77**(1): 73–78.

4. **Rusten E, Rekstad B, Undseth C, et al.** (2019). Anal cancer chemoradiotherapy outcome prediction using 18F-fluorodeoxyglucose positron emission tomography and clinicopathological factors. *British Journal of Radiology*, **92**: 20181006.

5. **Hong JC, Cui Y, Patel BN, et al.** (2018). Association of Interim FDG-PET imaging during chemoradiation for squamous anal canal carcinoma with recurrence. *International Journal of Radiation Oncology. Biology. Physics*, **102**(4): 1046–1051.

6. **Mohammadkhani Shali S, Schmitt V, Behrendt FF, et al.** (2016). Metabolic tumour volume of anal carcinoma on (18)FDG PET/CT before combined radiochemotherapy is the only independant determinant of recurrence free survival. *European Journal of Radiology*, **85**(8): 1390–1394.

7. **Owczarczyk K, Prezzi D, Cascino M, et al.** (2019). MRI heterogeneity analysis for prediction of recurrence and disease free survival in anal cancer. *Radiotherapy & Oncology*, **134**: 119–126.

8. **Sobin LH, Gospodarowicz MK, Wittekind CH** (2017). *UICC TNM Classification of Malignant Tumours* (eighth edn). Oxford: Wiley Blackwell.

9. **Muirhead R, Drinkwater K, O'Cathail SM, et al.** (2017). Initial results from the Royal College of Radiologists' UK National Audit of Anal Cancer Radiotherapy 2015. *Clinical Oncology* (Royal College of Radiology), **29**(3): 188–197.

10. **Prezzi D, Mandegaran R, Gourtsoyianni S, et al.** (2018). The impact of MRI sequence on tumour staging and gross tumour volume delineation in squamous cell carcinoma of the anal canal. *European Radiology*, **28**(4): 1512–1519.

11. **Sabbagh A, Jacobs C, Cooke R, et al.** (2019). Is there a role for an 18F-fluorodeoxyglucose-derived biological boost in squamous cell anal cancer? *Clinical Oncology* (Royal College of Radiologists), **31**(2): 72–80.

12. **Muirhead R, Adams RA, Gilbert DC, et al.** (2014). Anal cancer: developing an intensity-modulated radiotherapy solution for ACT2 fractionation. *Clinical Oncology* (Royal College of Radiologists), **26**(11): 720–721.

13. **Muirhead R, Bulte D, Cook R, et al.** (2019). A prospective study of diffusion-weighted magnetic resonance imaging for predicting outcome following chemoradiotherapy, in squamous cell carcinomas of the anus. *Annals of Oncology*, **30**(Supp 5): V204.

14. **Shakir R, Adams R, Cooper R, et al.** (2020). Patterns and predictors of relapse following radical chemoradiotherapy delivered using intensity modulated radiotherapy with a simultaneous integrated boost in anal squamous cell carcinoma. *International Journal of Radiation Oncology. Biology.* **106**(2): 329–339.

15. **Goh V, Gollub FK, Liaw J, et al.** (2010). Magnetic resonance imaging assessment of squamous cell carcinoma of the anal canal before and after chemoradiation: can MRI predict for eventual clinical outcome? *International Journal of Radiation Oncology. Biology. Physics*, **78**(3): 715–721.

16. **Glynne-Jones R, Sebag-Montefiore D, Meadows HM, et al.** (2017). Best time to assess complete clinical response after chemoradiotherapy in squamous cell carcinoma of the anus (ACT II): a post-hoc analysis of randomised controlled phase 3 trial. *Lancet Oncology*, **18**(3): 347–356.

17. **Cardenas ML, Spencer CR, Markovina S, et al.** (2017). Quantitative FDG-PET/CT predicts local recurrence and survival for squamous cell carcinoma of the anus. *Advances in Radiation Oncology*, **2**(3): 281–287.

Chapter 14

Urological cancers

Ananya Choudhury and Peter Hoskin

14.1 **Prostate cancer**

14.1.1 **Clinical background**

Prostate cancer is the most common cancer in males and is the second leading cause of cancer deaths in the Western world. In 2015, there were over 47,000 new cases diagnosed, with over 11,000 deaths and a ten-year survival of 84%. For patients with organ-confined prostate cancer, management options include observation, active surveillance, radical prostatectomy, or radiotherapy (external beam or brachytherapy). For patients with locally advanced or metastatic disease treatment, options include a combination of hormone therapy, radiotherapy, or chemotherapy.

14.1.2 **Diagnosis and staging**

14.1.2.1 Diagnosis

Prostate cancer is usually diagnosed by multiparametric magnetic resonance imaging (mpMRI) and trans-rectal ultrasound (TRUS) guided needle biopsy. As standard, 12 cores are taken, although the diagnostic yield increases when more cores are taken. If more biopsies are required for diagnostic purposes or for more targeted approaches, transperineal template biopsies are acquired, also using TRUS guidance. Although prostate cancer classically appears hypoechoic in comparison to the surrounding peripheral zone, its ultrasonic appearance is variable. For this reason, TRUS is not used to detect or direct biopsies to malignant lesions but to target the gland for systematic sampling. Recent studies have confirmed the superiority of MRI for prostate cancer, with mpMRI now the standard of care for diagnosis and targeting of biopsies.[1] The PI-RADS (Prostate Imaging Reporting and Data System) reporting scheme is used to standardize evaluation of prostate MRI as shown in Table 14.1. The score is made up of parameters from T2-weighted, diffusion-weighted (DWI), and dynamic-contrast enhanced MRI (DCE-MRI). The scale is based a score of 1–5 for T2-weighted and DWI, and on a score of yes or no for DCE-MRI. A composite likelihood score is given for each lesion, with 1 being most likely benign and 5 being highly likely to be a clinically significant cancer.

14.1.2.2 Staging

Prostate cancer may be staged clinically with digital rectal examination (DRE), but more accurate estimates of tumour burden will be obtained using imaging. The

Table 14.1 PI-RADS (prostate imaging reporting and data system) score

PI-RADS 1	Very low (clinically significant cancer is highly unlikely to be present)
PI-RADS 2	Low (clinically significant cancer is unlikely to be present)
PI-RADS 3	Intermediate (the presence of clinically significant cancer is equivocal)
PI-RADS 4	High (clinically significant cancer is likely to be present)
PI-RADS 5	Very high (clinically significant cancer is highly likely to be present)

Reproduced with permission from American College of Radiology, 'Prostate Imaging—Reporting and Data System (PI-RADS) 2019, Version 2.1'. Copyright © American College of Radiology.

tumour, node, metastasis (TNM) staging classification is shown in Table 14.2. TRUS is not used for staging as its accuracy is no better than DRE and there is significant inter-operator variability. Computed tomography (CT) does not allow reliable tumour visualization but gross disease extension or enlarged adenopathy may be seen.

T stage mpMRI is the imaging modality of choice for local staging, including T1-weighted, T2-weighted, DCE and DWI sequences. Intraprostatic lesions and zonal anatomy are best demonstrated on T2-weighted images (Figure 14.1). Approximately 70% of prostate cancers arise in the PZ, 30% in the central gland.

Prostate cancers are typically of low-signal intensity within the PZ on T2-weighted images (Figure 14.1). However, low-signal intensity lesions in the PZ can also be caused by prostatitis, scarring, and post-biopsy haemorrhage. MRI is performed ideally before biopsy. The PROMIS study[1] has shown that pre-biopsy multi-parametric MRI can reduce the over-diagnosis of clinically insignificant prostate cancer while improving that of clinically significant cancer.

If biopsy has taken place, it is recommended to delay the MRI for a minimum of 3-4 weeks after biopsy[2] to allow post-biopsy trauma to settle. In terms of staging accuracy, the reported sensitivity and specificity of MRI in detecting extracapsular spread is highly variable.[3,4] The sensitivity and specificity of MRI in detecting seminal vesicle invasion (Figure 14.2) is also variable, ranging from 85–97% and 21–63% respectively.[5]

Functional MRI sequences, such as DCE-MRI, DWI, and MR spectroscopy (MRS) have been described in the assessment of prostate cancer. DWI and DCE-MRI have become part of routine staging in recent years. DWI measures Brownian motion of water, reflecting the cellularity of tissue. Diffusion of water is reduced in prostate cancer compared to normal tissue and is measured using the apparent diffusion co-efficient (ADC). The values can be mapped by voxel, with an area of malignant tissue showing a 20–40% lower ADC measurement compared to normal tissue reflecting higher cell density.

DCE-MRI provides a means of assessing tissue perfusion and permeability by imaging the passage of intravenous gadolinium through the tissues. In prostate cancer, MR spectra from protons in choline and citrate can be assessed. High levels of citrate and intermediate levels of choline are observed within the normal PZ. However, prostate cancer cells have a reduced capacity for citrate production and increased

Table 14.2 TNM classification for prostate cancer

T primary tumour

TX	Primary tumour cannot be assessed
T0	No evidence of primary tumour
T1	Clinically inapparent tumour that is not palpable
T1a	Tumour incidental histological finding in 5% or less of tissue resected
T1b	Tumour incidental histological finding in more than 5% of tissue resected
T1c	Tumour identified by needle biopsy (e.g. because of elevated PSA)
T2	Tumour that is palpable and confined within prostate
T2a	Tumour involves one half of one lobe or less
T2b	Tumour involves more than half of one lobe, but not both lobes
T2c	Tumour involves both lobes
T3	Tumour extends through the prostatic capsule*
T3a	Extraprostatic extension (unilateral or bilateral) including microscopic bladder neck involvement
T3b	Tumour invades seminal vesicle(s)
T4	Tumour is fixed or invades adjacent structures other than seminal vesicles: external sphincter, rectum, levator muscles, and/or pelvic wall

Note

*Invasion into the prostate apex or into (but not beyond) the prostatic capsule is not classified as T3, but as T2.

N regional lymph nodes

NX	Regional lymph nodes cannot be assessed
N0	No regional lymph node metastasis
N1	Regional lymph node metastasis

Note

Metastasis no larger than 0.2 cm can be designated pNmi.

M distant metastasis

M0	No distant metastasis
M1	Distant metastasis
M1a	Non-regional lymph node(s)
M1b	Bone(s)
M1c	Other site(s)

Note

When more than one site of metastasis is present, the most advanced category is used. (p)M1c is the most advanced category.

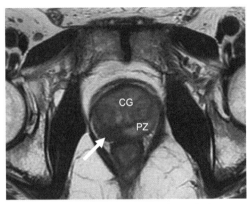

Fig. 14.1 Prostate cancer. Axial T2-weighted images through the prostate showing the zonal anatomy: central gland (CG) and peripheral zone (PZ). Prostate cancer is seen as the low signal area (arrow) in the right PZ.

cell turnover results in higher choline levels. Although MRS was initially reported as promising an increase in diagnostic yield, it is rarely used in routine practice.

Most prostate imaging is undertaken using a 1.5 T magnet; however, 3 T imaging provides an opportunity for better spatial, contrast, or temporal resolution with smaller voxel sizes.

There will be a small group of patients for whom MR is contraindicated, usually because of implanted devices such as a pacemaker. In these patients, computed tomography (CT) will usually be undertaken, but will show only gross changes in gland pathology although it remains a useful tool for lymph node staging (see below).

N stage CT and MRI are the principal imaging modalities used in the detection of lymph node spread (Figure 14.2). The routine use of mpMRI means that as well as staging the primary tumour, the regional lymph nodes will be assessed. The detection of lymph node metastases by CT or MR is based on size (Table 14.2). Hyperplastic or

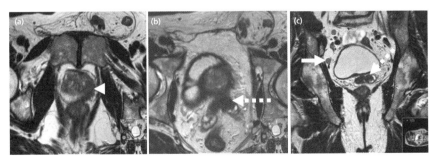

Fig. 14.2 T2-weighted MR images (a) and (b) axially through the prostate, and (c) coronally through the seminal vesicles shows prostate cancer with extraprostatic spread (arrowhead), seminal vesicle invasion (dashed arrow) (stage T3b), and nodal disease (arrow).

reactive nodes with no tumour involvement will give rise to false positive results. The sensitivity and specificity of CT in the detection of node metastases has a range of 25–78% and 77–98% respectively.[6] The sensitivity and specificity of MRI in the detection of lymph node metastases has a range of 30–100% and 94–100% respectively.[7,8]

Lymph node-specific contrast agents, ultra-small particles of iron oxide (USPIO), have been evaluated in the detection of node involvement with malignancy. The USPIO are taken up by macrophages in the reticuloendothelial system, causing loss of signal on T2- and T2*-weighted sequences in normal nodes. A portion of the nodes infiltrated with metastatic disease do not take up the USPIO and hence remain of high signal intensity. A systematic review has shown that sensitivity and specificity of USPIO with MRI is higher than that of MRI alone.[9] However, the limited availability of USPIO has meant that its application has been mainly in the Netherlands where it is licensed for production.

While positron emission tomography/CT (PET/CT) has limited value currently in local tumour staging (due to uptake in benign prostatic hyperplasia and prostatitis), it has a role in nodal staging in high-risk prostate cancer. To date, the most commonly used PET tracer has been choline (11-C or 18F-choline) with pooled sensitivity and specificity of 60% and over 90%, respectively, with uptake in both enlarged and normal sized involved lymph nodes. More recently, new tracers have been introduced. 18F-fluciclovine, a synthetic amino acid analogue, has been licensed for suspected prostate cancer recurrence with sensitivity and specificity >85%; increased fluciclovine uptake into prostate cancer cells is due to upregulated amino acid transporters, including ASCT2 and LAT1. Also, 68-Ga and 18F-labelled tracers targeting prostate-specific membrane antigen (PSMA) are promising, with superiority compared to CT[10] as over 90% of prostate cancers overexpress PSMA, a transmembrane glycoprotein. Sensitivity has been shown to be 60–70% with specificity of over 95%. At present there is limited data on its routine use and no evidence that PSMA PET/CT at staging impacts on survival. Nevertheless, it is expected that PSMA PET will replace other tracers as the first choice in the future (Figure 14.3).

M stage Distant metastasis in prostate cancer is most commonly to the bone, with the axial skeleton involved in 85% of patients dying from prostate cancer. Bone scintigraphy with technetium 99m diphosphonate is the main imaging modality used in staging to screen for metastatic bone disease (Figure 14.4).[11] Bone metastases demonstrate increased uptake of tracer; however, plain film correlation may be needed to exclude other causes of increased tracer uptake, such as degenerative disease or Paget's disease since the technetium uptake in fact represents osteoblastic activity. The use of whole body MRI (Figure 14.5) has been increasing, with recent international guidelines published recommending its use for patients where there is some uncertainty regarding the presence of bone metastases as its sensitivity is higher than either choline PET/CT or bone scintigraphy. However, whole body MRI may be less sensitive than either 68Ga-PSMA-PET/CT or NaF-PET/CT. Other sites of metastatic disease are extremely rare and occur late.

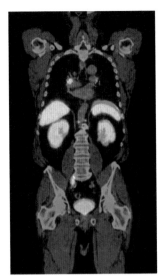

Fig. 14.3 Coronal PSMA PET/CT image in a patient with biochemical relapse after radical prostatectomy shows recurrence with increased uptake in right common iliac and hilar nodes.

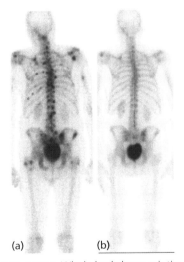

(a)   (b)

Fig. 14.4 Metastatic prostate cancer. Whole body bone scintigraphy (a) showing multiple bone metastases. (b) Following treatment with hormone therapy there has been resolution of the metastatic disease.

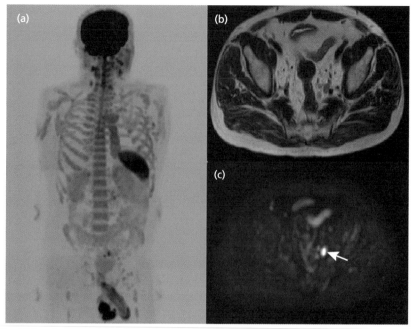

Fig. 14.5 Whole body MRI with inverted grey-scale high-b-value DWI image (a), corresponding T2-weighted (b) and high b-value DWI (c) image showing left mesorectal and internal iliac nodal disease (white arrow) from prostate cancer.

14.1.3 Imaging for radiotherapy planning

14.1.3.1 External beam radiotherapy

Cross-sectional imaging plays a central role in the definition of target volumes, treatment planning, and verification of treatment.

Modern external beam radiotherapy (EBRT) relies on CT for treatment planning. However, it is clear that MRI can offer advantages for radiotherapy treatment planning (RTP). In prostate planning studies of co-registered CT-MRI, investigators have reported better definition of prostate boundaries and substantially smaller treatment volumes by up to 40%.[12] MRI can substantially reduce uncertainty in target volume definition compared to CT, especially at the prostatic base and apex. The smaller but more appropriate treatment volumes may also enhance the therapeutic ratio when dose escalation schemes are employed.

In order to use MRI information for RTP, several important issues need to be addressed. These include defining and correcting for MR image distortions, overcoming the lack of electron density information in MR images which are needed for dose computation, as well as other potential limitations such as patient claustrophobia, and other contraindications (e.g. *in situ* pacemakers). Sources of MR image distortion include system-related and object-induced (i.e. patient dependent) effects. These

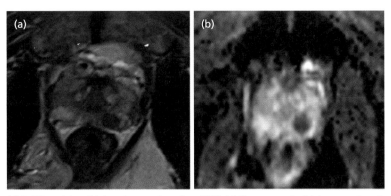

Fig. 14.6 T2-weighted (a) and corresponding DWI ADC parametric (b) images showing a restricted, left peripheral zone, dominant intraprostatic lesion.

effects are important as accurate geometric imaging data is needed for RTP and they can now be assessed, quantified, and minimized through the use of correction algorithms. After distortion correction, MR images can either be assigned bulk attenuation factors for the relevant volumes of interest or co-registered and fused with CT images so that the superior tissue definition from MRI can be transferred to the CT data for treatment planning and subsequent treatment verification procedures. The main challenge is that of accurate co-registration given the difference in the two imaging modalities. With the introduction of MR simulation, synthetic CT has been developed to aid MR-only planning. With mpMRI, significant tumour within the gland, the dominant intraprostatic lesion (DIL) (Figure 14.6), can be identified which has led to studies where the DIL can be boosted to a higher dose than that of the rest of the prostate gland.

14.1.3.2 Brachytherapy

Brachytherapy is used in the treatment of prostate cancer both as a primary treatment and as a boost with external beam. Modern image guided brachytherapy is undertaken using a transperineal approach with real time transrectal imaging to accurately place radiation sources, typically I125 seeds, or afterloading catheters for High Dose Rate (HDR) brachytherapy. An example of a TRUS guided LDR seed implant is shown in Figure 14.7. HDR brachytherapy also uses TRUS to define the positioning of the afterloading applicators and guide implantation (Figure 14.8). The CTV is then defined using either TRUS, CT, or MRI (Figure 14.9). Non-rigid deformation registration programmes are now available which enable fusion of diagnostic MR with TRUS to improve CTV definition.

14.1.4 Therapeutic assessment and follow-up

The mainstay of response assessment following treatment for prostate cancer is serial PSA monitoring. Further evaluation, including imaging, is triggered by a rising PSA after treatment or in the case of post-prostatectomy a detectable PSA >0.2 ng/ml. In

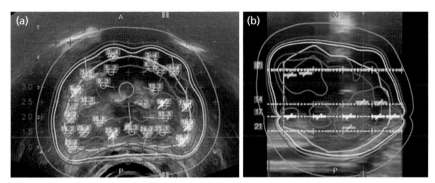

Fig. 14.7 Transrectal ultrasound images of LDR I125 implant showing (a) transverse and (b) sagittal ultrasound views with radiation distributions shown by coloured isodose lines.

patients who have had previous prostatectomy, MRI is used to detect local tumour recurrence. Recurrent disease is seen as asymmetrical soft tissue in the prostate bed or pelvis. TRUS in this setting may be used to obtain a biopsy and get pathological confirmation of recurrence.[13] Regional lymph node recurrence may also be seen.

After EBRT, detection of recurrent disease is made more difficult by post-radiotherapy change within the gland. Imaging is performed to assess the primary site, lymph nodes, and the skeleton. With the emergence of re-irradiation of the prostate and the treatment of oligometastatic disease, there is a move to image patients earlier on relapse with lower PSAs. mpMRI may demonstrate recurrent sites within the prostate as may choline or PSMA PET/CT to target with focal ablative techniques.

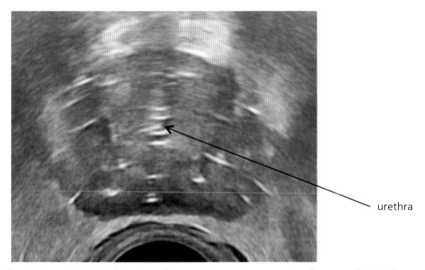

urethra

Fig. 14.8 TRUS image of implanted HDR catheters in preparation for HDR after loading brachytherapy.

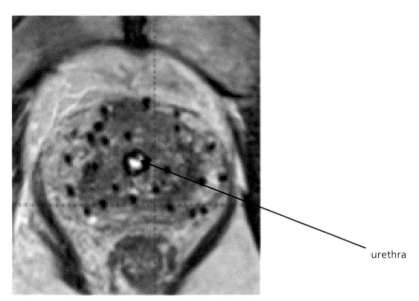

urethra

Fig. 14.9 Axial MRI image of implanted HDR catheters in preparation for HDR after loading brachytherapy.

Where such treatment is considered and where oligometastases are being considered for surgery or non-surgical ablation then further investigation to exclude other sites of disease is imperative.

CT for lymph node status and bone scintigraphy for skeletal imaging is most commonly repeated after treatment (Figure 14.4) where there is a rising PSA. The utility of bone scintigraphy in asymptomatic patients with biochemical disease relapse depends on PSA level. It is of no added diagnostic value unless the PSA serum levels are >20 ng/mL or unless the PSA velocity is >20 ng/mL/year. Whole body MRI has greater sensitivity for detection of bone metastases and where available is preferred. Patients with localized bone pain may be further investigated with plain X-ray or MRI of the relevant site.

PET/CT is recommended for suspected recurrence patients with rapidly rising PSA and negative or equivocal conventional imaging. Choline PET/CT may yield true positive findings in recurrent prostate cancer with serum PSA levels <5 ng/mL. PSMA PET/CT scans have been shown to detect recurrence in ~50% of men where the PSA level is <1.0 ng/ml, ~70% of patients where the PSA level is 1.0–2.0 ng/ml, and ~90% of patients where the PSA level is >2.0 ng/ml.

14.1.5 Summary

◆ The most important prognostic factors in prostate cancer are PSA level, tumour stage, and Gleason score.

◆ TRUS is used to direct systematic sampling of the prostate at present, but the use of MR-targeted biopsies is increasing.

- MRI is the imaging modality of choice for staging of the primary tumour.
- CT and MRI have a similar sensitivity and specificity for the detection of lymph node metastases. New PET/CT tracers (fluciclovine or PSMA) may aid this diagnosis.
- CT is the current standard for radiotherapy planning, but MRI-assisted planning can add complementary information.
- TRUS provides real time imaging for implantation and volume definition for brachytherapy.

14.2 **Bladder cancer**

14.2.1 Clinical background

Bladder cancer is the most common tumour of the urinary tract and comprises 6–8% of all male malignancies and 2–3% of all female malignancies.

14.2.2 Diagnosis and staging

14.2.2.1 Diagnosis

Diagnosis of bladder cancer is made at cystoscopy and biopsy. Imaging is used to assess upper urinary tracts with CT urography (CTU) used as standard. CTU images are obtained of the bladder and renal tract when contrast media has reached the renal collecting system and bladder. CTU protocols usually incorporate pre-contrast as well as images in the nephrographic phase of enhancement, that is, parenchymal enhancement of the kidney. These techniques therefore allow for detailed views of the renal parenchyma and the collecting systems. Mass lesions of the bladder and renal tract as well as pelvi-calyceal abnormality can all be evaluated simultaneously.

14.2.2.2 Staging

T stage Primary tumour staging with cystoscopy and transurethral resection (TUR) is accurate in the evaluation of superficial tumours.[14] For muscle-invasive tumours, however, clinical staging can understage by as much as 50%. In these cases, imaging will give added information to help assess the extent of tumour spread. US (Figure 14.10) may be useful in demonstrating a bladder tumour but is not routinely used in primary tumour staging, as the assessment of peri-vesical tumour spread is limited and it does not allow assessment of local lymph nodes.

MRI is the imaging modality of choice for local staging of bladder cancer. It is inaccurate in the evaluation of stage T1 and T2a tumours. However, there is some evidence to suggest that MRI can distinguish between T2a and T2b tumours. Invasion of the deep muscle layer by T2b tumours on T2-weighted imaging is demonstrated by disruption of the normal low-signal intensity bladder wall (Figure 14.11). Both T1- and T2-weighted sequences demonstrate T3b disease due to the contrast between tumour and perivesical fat. The staging error is similar for CT in the region of 30%. MRI is superior to CT in the assessment of local organ invasion due to superior contrast resolution and multiplanar imaging capability. Gadolinium-enhanced dynamic scanning techniques may improve visualization of depth of bladder wall and organ invasion (Table 14.3).

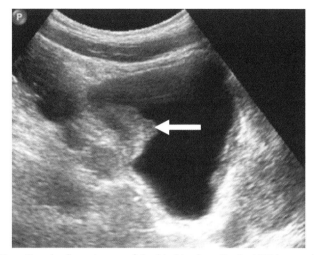

Fig. 14.10 Transitional cell carcinoma of the bladder. Longitudinal US image showing large mass (arrow) at the dome of the bladder.

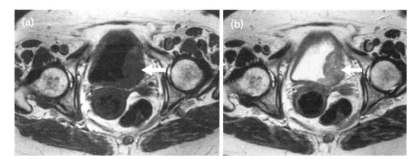

Fig. 14.11 Transitional cell carcinoma of the bladder. Axial (a) T1-weighted and (b) T2-weighted MR images showing a large intraluminal tumour (arrow) involving the left lateral bladder wall. The role of mp-MRI is yet to be determined in bladder cancer, but there has been an attempt to standardize the reporting in a way analogous to prostate, called the VIRADs system, using a composite of T2, DCE, and DW-MRI.

Table 14.3 VIRADs imaging reporting system for bladder cancer

VI-RADS 1	Muscle invasion is highly unlikely
VI-RADS 2	Muscle invasion is unlikely to be present
VI-RADS 3	Presence of muscle invasion is equivocal
VI-RADS 4	Muscle invasion is likely
VI-RADS 5	Invasion of muscle and beyond the bladder is very likely

Adapted with permission from Panebianco V et al. 'Multiparametric magnetic resonance imaging for bladder cancer: development of VI-RADS (Vesical Imaging-Reporting And Data System)'. *European urology*. Vol. 74, Issue 3, pp.294–306. Copyright © 2018 Elsevier Ltd.

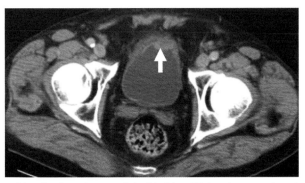

Fig. 14.12 Transitional cell carcinoma of the bladder. CT showing an enhancing soft tissue mass (arrow) arising from the anterior bladder wall with stranding in the peri-vesical fat suspicious of extra-vesical spread.

In patients who are unable to undergo MR imaging, CT imaging of the abdomen and pelvis is performed with a full bladder and intravenous contrast. Delayed images with contrast in the ureters and bladder are useful in defining the extent of tumour at the bladder base and dome and spread into the ureters. CT cannot differentiate between the bladder wall layers and therefore cannot differentiate between stage T1, T2a, and T2b tumours. In addition, residual bladder wall thickening following TURBT for T1 and T2a tumours is indistinguishable from muscle-invasive disease on CT. The main role of CT is to distinguish bladder tumours confined to the bladder wall from those that extend into the perivesical fat (Figure 14.12). However, the correlation between CT findings and tumour extent in cystectomy specimens is only 65–80%. Pelvic sidewall and local organ invasion is demonstrated by soft tissue extension from the main tumour.

N stage Lymphatic spread of bladder cancer occurs to the perivesical, presacral, hypo-gastric, obturator, and external iliac nodes, followed by common iliac and para-aortic nodes. Both CT and MR rely on nodal size to define abnormality and will therefore not detect early tumour infiltration without nodal enlargement. The use of FDG PET/CT in local staging is limited by urinary excretion of the tracer; however, it may be useful for staging of lymph node and distant metastases, with guidelines recommending its use prior to any extensive surgery.[15]

M stage Distant metastases occur in advanced disease to bone, lungs, brain, and liver. Chest, abdomen, and pelvis CT with contrast is routinely performed in all patients to assess distant sites. FDG PET/CT may have a role also but bone scintigraphy is not routinely indicated in asymptomatic patients,[16] but should be considered in high-risk patients and those with symptoms suggestive of bone involvement with suspicious findings confirmed on plain radiographs or MRI.

14.2.3 Imaging for radiotherapy planning

CT is the standard imaging method used for RTP whereby three-dimensional construction permits proper identification of the whole bladder in relation to the surrounding critical organs and normal tissue such as the bowel and rectum. Extra tumour localization information is also obtained from clinical maps of the bladder during cystoscopy and MRI. The main issue for bladder radiotherapy is that there is substantial variation on a day-to-day basis of bladder position and size due to bladder filling and emptying. This requires a larger planning margin of up to 1.5–2 cm to avoid a geographical miss. A variety of image guided radiotherapy (IGRT) methods are being evaluated to compensate for this bladder variation and can reduce the size of the planning margin needed. These methods use serial CT/MRI scans to assess a composite bladder volume (adaptive IGRT) or cine MR with cone beam CT to predict the daily volume bladder volumes (predictive IGRT). Fiducial markers have also been implanted into the bladder wall as another means of providing image guidance or to enable boosting of the bladder. Lipiodol is a radio-opaque contrast agent that can be injected into the bladder tumour bed at TURBT.

14.2.4 Therapeutic assessment and follow-up

After treatment of muscle-invasive bladder carcinoma with radical EBRT, follow-up serial cystoscopy and imaging is recommended. As recurrent disease may be local or metastatic, imaging of both the pelvis and abdomen is recommended Although retro-peritoneal recurrence usually occurs in association with pelvic node metastases, it may be an isolated finding in 10% of patients. Furthermore, these patients remain at risk of further metachronous tumours in the remaining urinary tract, which should be periodically evaluated using a CTU.

CT performed following EBRT has been shown to be relatively inaccurate in local tumour assessment due to the difficulty in distinguishing tumour from bladder wall thickening due to radiation fibrosis. MRI of the bladder performed following EBRT demonstrates abnormal signal intensity of the outer muscle layer on T2-weighted sequences and enhancement on contrast-enhanced T1-weighted images. Contrast enhancement cannot reliably distinguish between tumour recurrence and post-radiotherapy change. Residual or recurrent tumour has an earlier onset of enhancement than fibrotic tissue, which may be detected by DCE MRI in follow-up post-EBRT.

14.2.5 Summary

- Clinical staging is accurate in early stage disease, but inaccurate for evaluating invasive tumours spreading beyond the bladder.
- MR is superior to CT for staging early tumours.
- CT is unreliable for staging tumours confined to the bladder wall, but accurate for staging advanced disease.
- Radiotherapy uses CT for treatment planning. New adaptive strategies with IGRT are needed to deal with the substantial variation in bladder size and position from day to day.
- Serial cystoscopy with CT are used for monitoring response and detecting recurrent disease.

14.3 Upper urinary tract urothelial tumours

14.3.1 Clinical background

Tumours of the upper urinary tract urothelium are much less common than either bladder or renal cell carcinomas. Ureteric transitional cell carcinomas (TCCs) are less common still, arising most commonly in the distal ureter. Upper urinary tract TCCs are commonly multifocal. Multifocal, ipsilateral TCCs develop in 14–30% of patients.

14.3.2 Diagnosis and staging

The diagnostic evaluation of the upper tract urothelial cancer forms part of the assessment of haematuria as described for bladder tumours in section 14.2. Staging is performed with contrast enhanced CT. Though MRI is comparable to CT, it is not used in routine staging of TCC of the renal collecting system but is useful in assessing vascular invasion by infiltrating tumours. The multi-focal nature of the disease means the whole urinary tract needs to be studied. The accuracy of CT for staging upper tract TCC has been shown to be 50% or less and it is unable to differentiate T1 and T2 tumours. The lymphatic spread depends on the site of the primary lesion, which, due to the periureteric lymphatics, can be to nodes in the retroperitoneum or pelvis.

14.3.3 Imaging for radiotherapy planning

Radiotherapy has only a palliative role in controlling pain and haemorrhage associated with advanced disease using simple CT-based techniques.

14.3.4 Therapeutic assessment and follow-up

Post-surgery, follow-up CT of the abdomen and pelvis is performed to assess for evidence of tumour recurrence. The contralateral collecting system is studied radiographically with CTU.

14.3.5 Summary

- Urothelial tumours are often multi-focal and hence require imaging and evaluation of the whole renal tract using CTU.
- Staging is performed with CT but this is relatively inaccurate.

14.4 Testicular cancer

14.4.1 Clinical background

Testicular cancers comprise 1–1.5% of all male neoplasms but are the most common neoplasm in young men. They are important because >95% are curable. Germ cell tumours (GCT) comprise 95% of testicular neoplasms and are subdivided into seminomas (40%) and non-seminomatous germ cell tumours (NSGCT) (60%).

Patients with testicular tumours typically present with a painless scrotal mass, although occasionally they may present with features of metastatic disease.

14.4.2 Diagnosis and staging

14.4.2.1 Diagnosis

Diagnosis of testicular GCT is at biopsy or orchidectomy. Scrotal US is used to confirm diagnosis and look for other abnormalities such as microlithiasis in the contralateral testis. Scrotal US has a sensitivity of almost 100% for the detection of testicular tumours (Figure 14.13).[17]

14.4.2.2 Staging

Staging is based on the TNM classification[18] and patients are categorized into good, intermediate, and poor prognostic groups using the international germ cell cancer collaborative group (IGCCCG) classification (Table 14.4). Initial staging is with a contrast-enhanced CT of the thorax, abdomen, and pelvis.

Testicular GCT spreads via the lymphatics to the retroperitoneal nodes in a predictable pattern. Right-sided tumours initially spread to the aorto-caval nodes and nodes around the inferior vena cava. Left-sided tumours initially spread to the left para-aortic and pre-aortic nodes (Figure 14.14). Spread to the iliac and inguinal nodes usually occurs only in association with large volume retroperitoneal disease or with a history of testicular maldescent or surgery interfering with the lymphatic drainage, for example pelvic surgery.

Haematogenous spread occurs most commonly to the lungs; other sites include brain, bone, and liver. CT of the brain is indicated in those patients where there is clinical suspicion or with high-risk factors such as multiple lung metastases or HCG >10000 mIU/ml as brain metastases may be asymptomatic.

MRI is not used routinely in staging but has a role in the investigation of suspected brain metastases, meningeal disease, and spinal cord involvement, and in problem

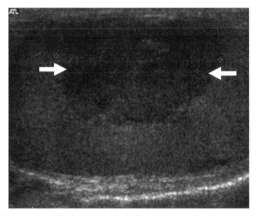

Fig. 14.13 Testicular cancer. US showing ill-defined hypoechoic intratesticular tumour (arrows).

Table 14.4 International Germ Cell Tumour Consensus Conference (IGCCCG) classification

NSGCT	Seminoma
Good prognosis—all of the following:	Good prognosis:
◆ AFP <1000ng/mL and HCG <5000IU/L (1000 ng/mL) and LDH <1.5 × N *and*	◆ No NPVM
◆ Non-mediastinal primary	◆ Any primary site
◆ No NPVM	◆ Normal AFP, any HCG, any LDH
Intermediate prognosis—all of the following:	Intermediate prognosis:
◆ AFP 1000–10,000 ng/mL, or HCG 5000–50,000 IU/L, or LDH 1.5–10 × N *and*	◆ NPVM present
◆ Non-mediastinal primary site *and*	
◆ No NPVM	
Poor prognosis—any of the following:	
◆ AFP >10,000 ng/mL or HCG >50,000 IU/L or LDH >10 × N *or*	
◆ Mediastinal primary site *or*	
◆ NPVM	

AFP, alpha feto-protein; HCG, human gonadotrophin; LDH, lactate dehydrogenase; N, upper limit of normal; NPVM, non-pulmonary visceral metastases.

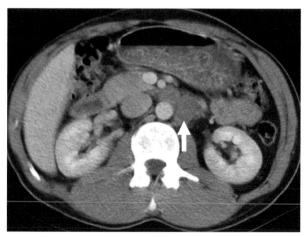

Fig. 14.14 Testicular germ cell carcinoma. CT shows enlarged left para-aortic lymph nodes (arrow) in a patient with non-seminomatous germ cell tumour.

solving if CT images are indeterminate. FDG PET/CT does not improve staging in patients with clinical stage I disease and is not recommended for primary staging.

14.4.3 Imaging for radiotherapy planning

Adjuvant radiotherapy has been replaced by high-dose carboplatin in most patients with stage I seminoma where there is a high risk of recurrence. Radiotherapy is used in exceptional cases where carboplatin is contraindicated, such as patients with impaired bone marrow function or severe cardiovascular morbidity. Radiotherapy has been the standard treatment of patients with stage IIA and IIB seminoma. An alternative to radiotherapy is cisplatin-based combination chemotherapy. Planning uses contrast-enhanced CT with the nodal CTV based on vascular anatomy. The renal outlines are used to identify the renal hilar lymph nodes as well as limit the dose to the kidneys.

14.4.4 Therapeutic assessment and follow-up

Men with low-risk testicular cancer after orchidectomy are offered surveillance. CT of the chest and abdomen is recommended unless the risk of pelvic relapse is high. The frequency of CT scans has been reduced to 3 and 12 monthly in the first year, and preliminary results from the Medical Research Council TRISST study suggest that reduced surveillance is non-inferior to standard surveillance and that MR is non-inferior to CT. CT is the main imaging modality used in routine follow-up of metastatic disease. Change in size or appearance of metastases and residual masses on CT are the main criteria used to assess response to therapy, alongside serum marker changes where detectable (Figure 14.15). Cystic and fatty change, which is readily assessed using CT, is associated with mature differentiated teratoma and may indicate the need for surgical removal.

Seminoma is extremely sensitive to chemo- and radiotherapy, such that a residual mass post-treatment usually represents fibrosis or necrosis. The CT findings may be allied to reduction in serum marker levels. In seminoma, FDG PET/CT may have a role in the assessment of residual masses after chemotherapy. A negative FDG PET/CT is 100% sensitive for absence of residual disease.[16]

In NSGCT, FDG PET/CT is less useful for evaluation of patients with residual masses as differentiated teratoma has variable low or no uptake and cannot be distinguished from fibrosis or necrosis.

Detection of recurrent disease relies on careful follow-up with a combination of clinical assessment, serum markers, chest radiographs, and abdominal CT.

14.4.5 Summary

- CT is the imaging modality of choice for staging testicular tumours.
- Regular CT monitoring is essential in the follow-up of testicular GCTs.
- FDG PET may have a role in the evaluation of a residual mass following treatment.

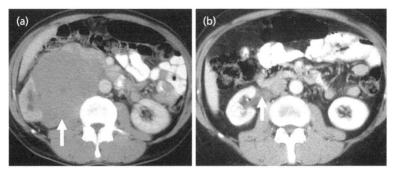

Fig. 14.15 Testicular germ cell carcinoma. CT (a) showing extensive paraaortic nodal disease (arrow) in a patient with metastatic seminoma. CT following chemotherapy (b) shows a significant reduction in the volume of nodal disease (arrow).

14.5 **Penile cancer**

14.5.1 **Clinical background**

Penile cancer is an uncommon malignancy with an incidence of 1.3 per 100,000 men in the UK in 2003.

14.5.2 **Diagnosis and staging**

14.5.2.1 Diagnosis

Diagnosis of the primary lesion is with a biopsy and imaging is not needed because the tumour is visible on examination.

14.5.2.2 Staging

Local staging is with US or MRI. Both can assist in identifying the depth of tumour invasion, particularly with regard to corpora cavernosa infiltration. US is often used as the initial imaging modality, with MRI as an alternative if US is inconclusive. MRI is more accurate at demonstrating corporal invasion or urogenital diaphragm involvement than US, and can help determine the extent of tumour along the surface of the penis, when the tumour is >2 cm.

Lymphatic spread occurs first to inguinal nodes then pelvic nodes. US allows evaluation of the inguinal nodes and gives an opportunity to sample them with fine needle aspiration. If inguinal lymph nodes are malignant then further imaging is required to look for metastases with CT of the chest, abdomen, and pelvis (Figure 14.16).

14.5.3 **Imaging for radiotherapy planning**

Most early stage penile cancers treatments include surgical removal and reconstruction. Only in those unfit for surgery or who refuse surgery will suitability for radiotherapy be assessed. EBRT or brachytherapy are used in the treatment of infiltrating tumours T1–2 <4 cm in diameter, with good results. Techniques typically use CT

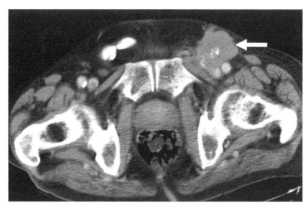

Fig. 14.16 Penile cancer. CT showing enlarged, partly calcified left inguinal nodal mass (arrow) in a patient with carcinoma of the penis.

planned volumes. Irradiation of regional lymph nodes is indicated postoperatively if there is extensive nodal involvement or in patients with recurrent or inoperable metastatic nodal disease.

14.5.4 Therapeutic assessment and follow-up

Regular clinical follow-up of all patients is recommended. Local recurrence is best visualized with MRI. CT of the abdomen and pelvis are performed in the follow-up of patients with positive nodes at pelvic node dissection.

14.5.5 Summary

- US is often the first imaging modality to assess disease extent, and allows for fine needle aspiration of the inguinal nodes.
- MRI provides the greatest anatomical definition of local disease extent especially with reference to cavernosa and urogenital diaphragm infiltration.

14.6 Renal cell carcinoma

14.6.1 Clinical background

Renal cell carcinoma (RCC) is the eighth most common malignancy. Renal tumours are often detected incidentally on imaging. This has resulted in increased incidence of renal tumours, which are also now smaller at presentation. For patients with renal tumour without evidence of metastases, surgery with radical nephrectomy is the treatment of choice. Imaging plays an important part in deciding the surgical approach. In patients that are poor surgical candidates, various image-guided ablation techniques have been described, with radiofrequency and cryoablation showing good long-term disease specific and overall survival for T1 tumours.

14.6.2 Diagnosis and staging

14.6.2.1 Characterizing renal mass lesions

In suspected RCC, the first investigation performed is CT. Traditionally, it has been thought that a solid lesion on contrast-enhanced CT most likely represents a RCC, allowing for differentiation between tumours and pseudotumours. However, there is now increasing evidence that not all solid lesions are RCC, especially smaller lesions <3 cm. The differential diagnosis of a solid renal lesion includes angiomyolipomas, oncocytomas, lymphoma, or metastases. Cystic lesions are also common. They are described using the Bosniak classification on a scale of I–IV (Table 14.5) according to their complexity and likelihood of malignant potential.

MR is particularly useful for identifying haemorrhage, with increased signal on T1, decreased signal on T2, and no enhancement with contrast. Most RCCs are hyperintense on T2-weighted sequences, with variable T1 signal intensity. An updated

Table 14.5 The Bosniak classification of renal cysts (proposed in 2019)

Bosniak class	Features
I	Pre-2019: simple cyst, no calcification or septa. Post-2019 CT: homogenous water content (<20 HU), no contrast enhancement. MR: homogenous signal enhancement similar to cerebrospinal fluid.
II	Pre-2019: benign cyst with fine calcification or thin septa. Post-2019 CT: six types, well defined (<2 mm or too small to characterize) with varying HU levels, including small cystic with small number of septa. MR: three types, well defined (<2 mm or too small to characterize) including small cystic with small number of septa. Can have calcification or markedly intense T1 or T2 weighted without contrast.
IIF	Pre-2019: multiple thin septa, coarse calcification, minimal wall thickening, >3 mm. Post-2019 CT: smooth thickening or enhancing wall with one or more enhancing septa. MR: two types, smooth thickening or enhancing wall with one or more enhancing septa or cystic masses heterogeneously hyperintense on unenhanced fat-saturated T1 weighted.
III	Pre-2019: thickened walls, contrast-enhanced, ~50% risk of malignancy. Post-2019 CT: one or more enhancing thick (>3 mm) or irregular wall or septa. MR: one or more enhancing thick (>3 mm) or irregular wall or septa.
IV	Pre-2019: enhancing soft tissue component, high risk of malignancy. Post-2019 CT: one or more enhancing nodules (>3 mm). MR: one or more enhancing nodules (>3 mm).

Source: data from Silverman SG, et al. 'Bosniak classification of cystic renal masses, version 2019: an update proposal and needs assessment'. *Radiology*. Vol. 292, Issue 2, pp.475–88. Aug 2019 RSNA.

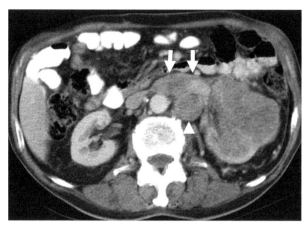

Fig. 14.17 Renal cell cancer. CT shows large left renal cancer with extension into the renal vein (arrows) and enlarged left para-aortic nodes (arrowhead).

Bosniak classification has been described which incorporates information from CT and MRI (Table 14.5); clinical validation is awaited. If, despite this, the lesion remains indeterminate then image-guided biopsy or surgical excision may be undertaken.

14.6.2.2 Staging

Staging in renal cancer is performed with CT (Figure 14.17), with US and MRI reserved for problem-solving, for example venous extension of tumour (stage T3b–c disease), when US is highly accurate at assessing tumour thrombus within the IVC if the examination is technically adequate. Transoesophageal echocardiography may be helpful if tumour thrombus is suspected to extend into the right atrium. MRI is useful in delineating the extent of IVC thrombus and tumoral invasion of the IVC wall.

The presence of lymph node disease is a poor prognostic factor. On both CT and MRI, the diagnosis of lymph node involvement is based on size criteria, which has well-known limitations. In the assessment of metastatic disease a combination of CT and MRI of the body and brain and bone scintigraphy are performed as clinically indicated. Distant metastases occur most frequently in the lungs, and other sites include bone, liver, contralateral kidney, adrenal, and brain. The role of FDG PET/CT in assessment for metastases in advanced renal cancer is limited as renal tumours have variable FDG uptake.

14.6.3 Imaging for radiotherapy planning

RCC are relatively radio-insensitive; therefore radiotherapy does not form part of the primary treatment. However, advances in radiotherapy have resulted in the use of stereotactic ablative techniques (SBRT) using extreme hypofractionation in an attempt to ablate the tumour. SBRT planning will be CT based.

Radiotherapy is effective in the palliation of local symptoms due to metastatic disease and has a role in the treatment of locally recurrent disease, usually based on CT imaging for localization of treatment volumes.

14.6.4 **Therapeutic assessment and follow-up**

Imaging following radical nephrectomy should be based on a risk assessment using one of the published nomograms.[17] Regular CT at six months and then annually to five years and two-yearly thereafter is recommended for high-risk patients; in contrast low-risk patients should have ultrasound at six months, followed by alternating CT and ultrasound for five years only.

14.6.5 **Summary**

- Renal mass lesions are best evaluated with CT; US, MRI, or biopsies are used where lesion remains indeterminate.
- Staging is with CT.
- Follow-up uses risk adapted US and CT.

14.7 **Urethral cancer**

14.7.1 **Clinical background**

Urethral cancer is very rare, occurring more commonly in women and has a peak incidence in the seventh decade.

14.7.2 **Diagnosis and staging**

Urethral cancer is diagnosed clinically with cystoscopy and transurethral biopsy. Local staging evaluation is best made using MRI, again due to its excellent soft tissue contrast resolution. T2-weighted sequences are used to define the primary tumour and local invasion. Contrast-enhanced T1-weighted sequences may be helpful and demonstrate a moderately enhancing tumour, local invasion, and fistulae. Urethral cancer principally spreads by local invasion and lymphatic spread is to the inguinal nodes if the distal urethra is involved and to the pelvic nodes if the proximal urethra is involved. Distant metastases are rare.

14.7.3 **Imaging for radiotherapy planning**

Local staging with MRI is used to assess tumour size, location, and local extension, and to plan radiotherapy treatment (Figure 14.18). Volume definition for radiotherapy is based on CT. For brachytherapy implantation, US-guided techniques are used.

14.7.4 **Therapeutic assessment and follow-up**

Regular MRI of the pelvis is performed post-treatment to assess for local tumour recurrence, treatment-related complications, or to evaluate treatment.

14.7.5 **Summary**

MRI is the imaging modality of choice for local staging and assists in treatment planning.

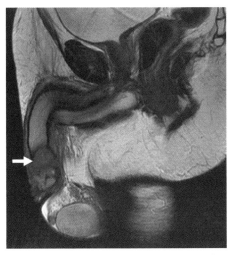

Fig. 14.18 Urethral carcinoma. Sagittal T2-weighted MR image of the penis showing locally invasive squamous cell cancer of the urethra (arrow).

References

1. **Ahmed HU, El-Shater Bosaily A, Brown LC, et al.** (2017). Diagnostic accuracy of multi-parametric MRI and TRUS biopsy in prostate cancer (PROMIS): a paired validating confirmatory study. *Lancet*, **389**(10071): 815–822.

2. **Petralia G, Padhani AR, Pricolo P, et al.** (2018). Whole-body magnetic resonance imaging (WB-MRI) in oncology: recommendations and key uses. *Radiol Med*, **124**(3): 218–233.

3. **Sonnad SS, Langlotz CP, Schwartz JS** (2001). Accuracy of MR imaging for staging prostate cancer: a meta-analysis to examine the effect of technologic change. *Academic Radiology*, **8**(2): 149–157.

4. **Engelbrecht MR, Jager GJ, Laheij RJ, Verbeek AL, van Lier HJ, Barentsz JO** (2002). Local staging of prostate cancer using magnetic resonance imaging: a meta-analysis. *European Radioliology*, **12**(9): 2294–2302.

5. **Husband JEaS SA** (1998). Prostate cancer. In: Husband JE RR, editor. *Imaging in Oncology*. Oxford: ISIS Medical Media. pp. 375–400.

6. **Oyen RH, Van Poppel HP, Ameye FE, Van de Voorde WA, Baert AL, Baert LV (1994).** Lymph node staging of localized prostatic carcinoma with CT and CT-guided fine-needle aspiration biopsy: prospective study of 285 patients. *Radiology*, **190**(2): 315–322.

7. **Jager GJ, Barentsz JO, Oosterhof GO, Witjes JA, Ruijs SJ** (1996). Pelvic adenopathy in prostatic and urinary bladder carcinoma: MR imaging with a three-dimensional TI-weighted magnetization-prepared-rapid gradient-echo sequence. *American Journal of Roentgenology*, **167**(6): 1503–1507.

8. **Thoeny HC, Barbieri S, Froehlich JM, Turkbey B, Choyke PL** (2017). Functional and targeted lymph node imaging in prostate cancer: current status and future challenges. *Radiology*, **285**(3): 728–743.

9. **Woo S, Suh CH, Kim SY, Cho JY, Kim SH** (2018). The diagnostic performance of MRI for detection of lymph node metastasis in bladder and prostate cancer: an updated

systematic review and diagnostic meta-analysis. *American Journal of Roentgenology*, **210**(3): W95–W109.

10. **Herlemann A, Wenter V, Kretschmer A, et al.** (2016). (68)Ga-PSMA positron emission tomography/computed tomography provides accurate staging of lymph node regions prior to lymph node dissection in patients with prostate cancer. *European Urology*, **70**(4): 553–557.

11. **O'Donoghue EP, Constable AR, Sherwood T, Stevenson JJ, Chisholm GD** (1978). Bone scanning and plasma phosphatases in carcinoma of the prostate. *British Journal of Urology*, **50**(3): 172–177.

12. **Rasch C, Barillot I, Remeijer P, Touw A, van Herk M, Lebesque JV** (1999). Definition of the prostate in CT and MRI: a multi-observer study. *International Journal of Radiation Oncology. Biology. Physics*, **43**(1): 57–66.

13. **(NICE) NIfHaCE. Bladder cancer: diagnosis and management (Guidelines).** Available from: https://www.nice.org.uk/guidance/ng2.

14. **Alfred Witjes J, Lebret T, Comperat EM, et al.** (2017). Updated 2016 EAU guidelines on muscle-invasive and metastatic bladder cancer. *European Urology*, **71**(3): 462–475.

15. **Schmoll HJ, Souchon R, Krege S, et al.** (2004). European consensus on diagnosis and treatment of germ cell cancer: a report of the European Germ Cell Cancer Consensus Group (EGCCCG). *Annals of Oncology*, **15**(9): 1377–1399.

16. **De Santis M, Becherer A, Bokemeyer C, et al.** (2014). 2-18fluoro-deoxy-D-glucose positron emission tomography is a reliable predictor for viable tumor in postchemotherapy seminoma: an update of the prospective multicentric SEMPET trial. *Journal of Clinical Oncology*, **22**(6): 1034–1039.

17. **Ljungberg B, Bensalah K, Canfield S, et al.** (2015). EAU guidelines on renal cell carcinoma: 2014 update. *European Urology*, **67**(5): 913–924.

18. **Sobin LH, Gospodarowicz MK, Wittekind CH** (2017). *UICC TNM Classification of Malignant Tumours* (eighth edn). Oxford: Wiley Blackwell.

Chapter 15

Gynaecological cancers

Kate Lankester and Lavanya Vitta

15.1 Introduction

Gynaecological cancers account for only 5% of cancer cases in the UK. However, there has been an increasing incidence in older age groups, with the exception of invasive cervical carcinoma, which has been declining since 1990, and vaginal cancer, which has remained stable. Imaging has become integrated into the management pathways for patients with suspected gynaecological malignancy. Imaging investigations inform treatment decisions, although evidence that they alter management in ways that impact on outcome measures, such as disease-free and overall survival, is still lacking. Combined molecular and anatomical imaging modalities such as ^{18}F-fluorodeoxyglucose positron emission tomography/ computed tomography (FDG PET/CT) are becoming more accessible. Imaging also aids radiotherapy planning and is used during treatment to match bony and soft-tissue anatomy to the original planning CT scan to ensure accurate treatment set-up.

15.2 Ovarian cancer

Ovarian cancer is treated with a combination of surgery and chemotherapy. Radiotherapy has only a limited role but can be useful in the palliative setting, for example for a symptomatic pelvic mass or if a patient develops brain metastases. Imaging for ovarian cancer is not discussed further in this chapter.

15.3 Uterine cancer

15.3.1 Clinical background

Uterine cancer is the fourth most common malignancy in UK women, with an incidence of ~30 per 100,000. The majority are adenocarcinomas arising from the endometrium. Most women (94%) are over the age of 50 years. Early stage presentation is the norm, reflected by an overall five-year survival of 79%. However, an improving survival rate has been offset by a rise in incidence since the early 1990s. Other uterine cancers such as carcinosarcomas (malignant mixed Müllerian tumours) and malignant myometrial tumours (e.g. leiomyosarcoma) are uncommon or rare.

15.3.2 Diagnosis and staging

Staging is defined by the International Federation of Gynaecology & Obstetrics (FIGO) system (2009) shown in Table 15.1). Endometrial cancer typically presents with postmenopausal bleeding (PMB), seen in 90%, resulting in early detection. Initial investigation often utilizes transvaginal ultrasound (TVUS) to establish the endometrial thickness. It has been shown to be a cost-effective means to determine the need for sampling, as an endometrial thickness of ≤4 mm indicates a low risk of malignancy, with a sensitivity of 90.6%; which can be maximized to 96.9% using a threshold of 3 mm. Although TVUS is able to locally stage endometrial tumours with accuracy similar to MRI, it is usual practice for patients to undergo MRI staging once a cancer diagnosis has been made.

MRI is the preferred modality for treatment planning: to assess the depth of myometrial invasion, cervical stromal invasion, lymph node involvement, and advanced disease.[1] Diffusion-weighted MRI (DWI) improves the differentiation of malignant from benign pathologies[2] and also improves the accuracy of assessment of depth of myometrial invasion.

The endometrium, junctional zone, and myometrium have high, low, and intermediate signal intensity, respectively, on T2-weighted MRI. This differential anatomy allows substaging of stage I tumours. Endometrial cancer initially penetrates the junctional zone to invade the myometrium, which can be depicted with an accuracy of 90–95% on fusion MRI combining T2-weighted and DWI. DWI measures the random

Table 15.1 FIGO staging (2009) for carcinoma of the endometrium

Stage I	Tumour confined to the uterus
IA	≤50% myometrial invasion
IB	≥50% myometrial invasion
Stage II	Tumour invades cervical stroma, but does not extend beyond the uterus
Stage III	Local and/or regional spread of the tumour
IIIA	Tumour invades the uterine serosa and/or adnexae
IIIB	Vaginal and/or parametrial involvement
IIIC	Metastasizes to pelvic and/or para-aortic lymph nodes
IIIC1	Pelvic lymph node involvement
IIIC2	Para-aortic lymph node involvement, (with or without pelvic lymph nodes)
Stage IV	Tumour invades bladder and/or bowel mucosa, and/or distant metastases
IVA	Tumour invasion of bladder and/or bowel mucosa
IVB	Distant metastases, including intra-abdominal metastases and/or inguinal lymph nodes

Adapted with permission from Pecorelli S, 'Revised FIGO staging for carcinoma of the vulva, cervix, and endometrium', *International Journal of Gynecology & Obstetrics,* Vol. 105, Issue 2, pp. 103–4. Copyright © 2009 John Wiley & Sons.

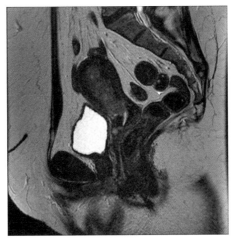

Fig. 15.1 Sagittal T2-weighted MRI of a large endometrial cancer invading the cervical stroma—FIGO stage II.

Brownian motion of water molecules in tissues and can aid differentiation between tumour and normal tissue, as highly cellular tumours and swollen cells show restricted diffusion and a lower diffusion coefficient. The tumour may grow caudally to invade the mucosa or stroma of the cervix (FIGO stage II) (Figure 15.1).

Dynamic contrast enhanced MR and DWI is able to define cervical involvement with an accuracy of imaging 95%.[3] Difficulties in tumour staging arise when the junctional zone is indistinct or abnormal (as in adenomyosis) and when the myometrium is thin. Gadolinium enhancement can be of particular value in these cases as the tumour typically enhances less than the normal myometrium, improving tumour to muscle contrast.

Uterine carcinoma usually metastasizes initially to the loco-regional lymph nodes. However, anatomical imaging remains limited in its ability to stage nodal disease and depends mainly on the presence of enlarged lymph nodes. Detection of metastases within normal sized lymph nodes is limited. If the nodes look normal on imaging, then tumour grade and the extent of myometrial invasion may be used to stratify patients into risk groups in order to decide whether lymphadenectomy is needed for staging purposes.[4] Sentinel lymph node sampling can be used to detect involved lymph nodes peri-operatively by injecting a blue dye or radiotracer.

MRI is also effective where advanced disease is clinically suspected (Figure 15.2).

Uterine sarcomas are rare tumours, comprising approximately 3–7% of all uterine malignancies.[5] They are subdivided into leiomyosarcomas, carcinosarcomas (malignant mixed Müllerian tumours), and endometrial stromal tumours. The diagnosis is established histologically for uterine leiomyosarcomas as there is no pelvic imaging modality that can reliably differentiate between a leiomyoma (benign) and a uterine leiomyosarcoma (malignant). They appear similar on imaging: both are focal masses within the uterus and can have central necrosis. If a sarcoma is suspected on

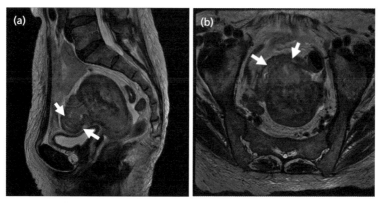

Fig. 15.2 Sagittal (a) and para-axial (b) T2-weighted MRI of an advanced endometrial cancer extending through the anterior uterine serosa to invade the sigmoid colon (arrows) confirmed on histology—FIGO stage IVA.

imaging or proven pathologically, a staging body CT is recommended as these tumours have a greater propensity for metastasizing to the lungs. Both leiomyomas and leiomyosarcomas are known to show focal uptake of 18 FDG on PET scanning and demonstrate restricted diffusion on DWI and ADC (Apparent Diffusion Coefficient) maps (Figure 15.3).

15.3.3 Imaging for radiotherapy planning

Surgery is the primary treatment for uterine cancer, which comprises a total laparoscopic hysterectomy and bilateral salpingo-oophorectomy, as well as a pelvic lymphadenectomy in higher risk groups. To aid decision making regarding adjuvant treatment, patients can be stratified into risk groups (low, intermediate, high-intermediate, high, and advanced) depending on tumour stage, grade, and the presence of multifocal lymphovascular space invasion.[4] Adjuvant radiotherapy to the pelvis is recommended to reduce the risk of local recurrence for patients with stage I disease with poor prognostic features (deep myometrial invasion, grade 3, multifocal lymphovascular space invasion), and for patients with higher stages.[4] Adjuvant brachytherapy to the vaginal vault is recommended on its own for intermediate risk patients or in conjunction with pelvic radiotherapy for patients who have cervical involvement.[4] Guidelines and imaging atlases have been developed to aid outlining of organs at risk (OAR) and clinical target volumes for treatment with Intensity Modulated Radiotherapy (IMRT).[6,7] Patients are planned using a CT scan with IV contrast (to help distinguish blood vessels from bowel loops), with reference to the pre-op MRI imaging. Patients are scanned and treated with a comfortably full bladder and bowel preparation (e.g. sodium citrate enemas) may be used to minimize internal organ movement.

Imaging during radiotherapy (e.g. cone beam CT imaging) is used to ensure accurate set-up and adequate target coverage, by matching soft tissue and bony anatomy to the planning CT scan images. Image quality is not as good as diagnostic CT imaging

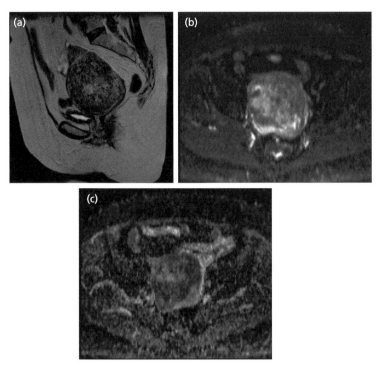

Fig. 15.3 Sagittal T2-weighted image (a) showing a large heterogenous mass within the uterus with ill-defined margins, confirmed as leiomyosarcoma at histology. Corresponding axial DWI (b) and ADC (c) images show restricted diffusion within the mass.

due to the inherent geometry of the system (increased scatter) causing increased noise, resulting in low contrast resolution. A bladder ultrasound scan before the radiotherapy planning CT scan and before treatment to ensure consistency of bladder filling may also be useful.

15.3.4 Therapeutic assessment and follow-up

As uterine cancer is generally a surgically treated disease, post-treatment imaging is reserved for those patients who present with inoperable disease where palliative treatment (radiotherapy and/or chemotherapy) and response monitoring is deemed appropriate. Relapse can affect many sites—the most frequent being the vaginal vault, pelvic lymph nodes, peritoneum, and the lungs. Patient education is an important part of post-treatment surveillance as the majority of relapses are symptomatic, particularly those at the vaginal vault (causing vaginal bleeding). If local recurrence is discovered, or disseminated disease clinically suspected, body imaging, usually with CT (and/or MRI for assessment of local recurrence) is undertaken to establish the extent of disease for treatment planning. PET/CT may be useful where a radical surgical approach is proposed.

15.4 **Cervical cancer**

15.4.1 **Clinical background**

The incidence of invasive cervical cancer in the UK is 10 per 100,000. The majority are squamous cell carcinomas, though adenocarcinomas, adenosquamous carcinomas, and other rare histological types may also occur.

15.4.2 **Diagnosis and staging**

The FIGO staging (2018) for cervical cancer is presented in Table 15.2. Previous versions were based mainly on clinical examination, but the 2018 staging system has been revised to allow imaging and pathological findings to assign stage. The TNM staging system is also useful if using MRI to stage as it separates out primary tumour (T) from regional nodal involvement (N).

If not detected at screening, presentation with vaginal bleeding and discharge is usual. Gynaecological examination, colposcopy, and biopsy are used to establish the diagnosis.

Most of the published literature regarding cervical cancer imaging refers to the evaluation of patients with macroscopically visible tumours (FIGO ≥IB). (By definition, stage IA cancers are microscopic, so cannot be reliably detected by any of the available imaging modalities.)

Imaging, especially MRI, has been shown to be superior to clinical examination alone for correctly evaluating cervical carcinoma stage (Figure 15.4 demonstrates a stage IB3 tumour). A meta-analysis reported a pooled sensitivity for detection of parametrial invasion of 84% versus 40% for MRI, compared to clinical examination (specificity was similar: 92% vs. 93%).[8] The preferred imaging method for local cervical cancer evaluation is MRI but CT is equally effective for evaluation of extra-uterine spread of the disease. PET-CT shows high diagnostic performance for the detection of tumour relapse and metastatic lymph nodes.[9]

Imaging aids treatment planning in terms of choice of treatment between surgery and radiotherapy. Standard surgical management of cervical cancer is a radical hysterectomy plus pelvic lymphadenectomy. However, fertility-sparing surgery may be possible for small stage I tumours: a cone biopsy alone for a stage IA tumour or a radical trachelectomy (which removes the cervix and upper vagina, leaving the uterine body *in situ*) for a small IB tumour. Endovaginal MRI, although not widely available, may be useful in selecting patients for trachelectomy by improving accuracy in staging, particularly where early parametrial invasion is suspected on external coil imaging.

For stage ≥IB tumours, decisions regarding whether a patient should be offered either surgery or radical chemoradiation depend on tumour size, the presence of parametrial invasion, and whether regional lymph nodes are involved. MRI can accurately exclude parametrial invasion, with a negative predictive value ranging from 94% to 100%.[9] An intact hypointense stromal ring around the cervix on T2-weighted axial imaging represents the main sign for excluding parametrial invasion. DWI further improves the assessment of parametrial invasion when it is added to conventional T2-weighted MRI. DWI also improves the detection of lymph nodal metastases.

Table 15.2 FIGO staging for cervical cancer

Stage I	The carcinoma is strictly confined to the cervix (extension to the corpus would be disregarded)
IA	Invasive carcinoma that can be diagnosed only by microscopy, with maximum depth of invasion <5 mm
IA1	Measured stromal invasion of <3 mm in depth
IA2	Measured stromal invasion of ≥3 mm and <5 mm in depth
IB	Invasive carcinoma with measured deepest invasion ≥5 mm (greater than stage IA), lesion limited to the cervix uteri
IB1	Invasive carcinoma ≥5 mm depth of stromal invasion, and <2 cm in greatest dimension
IB2	Invasive carcinoma ≥2 cm and <4 cm in greatest dimension
IB3	Invasive carcinoma ≥4 cm in greatest dimension
Stage II	The carcinoma invades beyond the uterus, but has not extended onto the lower third of the vagina or to the pelvic wall
IIA	Involvement limited to the upper two-thirds of the vagina without parametrial invasion
IIA1	Invasive carcinoma ≤4 cm in greatest dimension
IIA2	Invasive carcinoma >4 cm in greatest dimension
IIB	With parametrial involvement, but not up to the pelvic wall
Stage III	The carcinoma involves the lower third of the vagina and/or extends to the pelvic wall and/or causes hydronephrosis or non-functioning kidney and/or involves pelvic and/or para-aortic lymph nodes
IIIA	The carcinoma involves the lower third of the vagina, with no extension to the pelvic wall
IIIB	Extension to the pelvic wall and/or hydronephrosis or non-functioning kidney (unless known to be due to another cause)
IIIC	Involvement of pelvic and/or para-aortic lymph nodes, irrespective of tumour size and extent
IIIC1	Pelvic lymph node metastasis only
IIIC2	Para-aortic lymph node metastasis
Stage IV	The carcinoma has extended beyond the true pelvis or has involved (biopsy proven) the mucosa of the bladder or rectum (a bullous oedema, as such, does not permit a case to be allotted to stage IV)
IVA	Spread to adjacent pelvic organs
IVB	Spread to distant organs

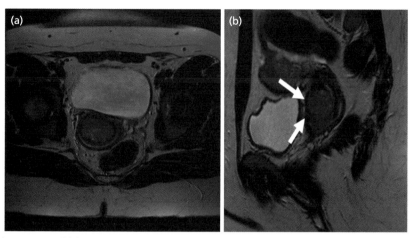

Fig. 15.4 Axial (a) and sagittal (b) T2-weighted MRI in the anterior lip of the cervix with a thin rim of intact low signal cervix shown by arrows—stage IB3.

The addition of DWI may increase the diagnostic performance of MRI compared with PET/CT. It is reported that MRI including the DWI sequences is more precise than FDG PET/CT for detecting pelvic lymph node metastases, with a sensitivity, specificity, and diagnostic accuracy of 67%, 84%, and 81% compared to 33%, 92%, and 81% for PET/CT; although the differences were not as pronounced for para-aortic lymph nodes.[10] Although the addition of DWI clearly improves sensitivity of MRI for the detection of nodal metastases, PET/CT still has a higher specificity of up to 97%.[11] Especially in cases of advanced disease, PET/CT has a high sensitivity (75–100%) and specificity (87–100%)[9] and can help demonstrate sites of unexpected disease such as supraclavicular lymph nodes. However, neither PET/CT nor MRI is sufficiently accurate to replace lymphadenectomy (or biopsy) as the definitive assessment of lymph node status.[10,11]

15.4.3 Imaging for radiotherapy planning

If a cervical cancer is too advanced for a radical hysterectomy (e.g. stage IB3 or above), then radical radiotherapy with concomitant chemotherapy (chemoradiation) is recommended. Radical radiotherapy comprises external beam radiotherapy followed by intrauterine brachytherapy. Guidelines (e.g. for the substitute EMBRACE II trial) have been developed which define clinical target volumes for the primary tumour and the pelvic nodes and give recommendations regarding appropriate CTV-PTV margins for both conventional 3D radiotherapy and IMRT. Image fusion with the diagnostic MRI scan may help delineate the GTV.

In some patients, the uterus is very mobile and its position varies depending on the degree of bladder filling. As described in section 15.3.3, measures to minimize internal organ movement (by treating with a comfortably full bladder and using enemas to reduce rectal filling) and imaging during treatment to ensure consistent bladder filling

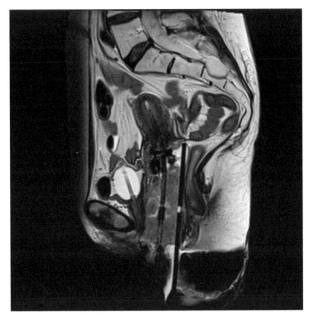

Fig. 15.5 MRI pelvis in sagittal plane with intra-uterine tube and vaginal ovoids, rectal retractor *in situ* for brachytherapy. Bladder catheter balloon and vaginal gauze packing also shown.

are important to ensure accurate treatment, particularly for IMRT. Some centres are able to create a series of radiotherapy plans (with varying bladder volumes) and so, with daily image guidance, select the best 'plan of the day'. This approach enables a decrease in CTV-PTV margins and consequent reduction of dose to the bowel, rectum, and bladder.

A repeat MRI scan performed during the final week of external beam radiotherapy is useful to aid planning for brachytherapy.

For brachytherapy, the advent of MRI- and CT-compatible applicators means that 3D treatment planning is now possible as cross-sectional imaging can be performed with the applicators *in situ*. Recommendations for the definition and delineation of the 'high-risk CTV' have been published by the ICRU (report 89) and the EMBRACE II group.[12,13] 3D planning, particularly with T2-weighted MRI, allows tumour dose escalation, while maintaining dose to bladder, bowel, and rectum within tolerance levels.[13] MRI is superior to CT as, while OAR can be clearly identified on CT images, MRI provides more accurate tumour definition (Figure 15.5).[14]

15.4.4 Therapeutic assessment and follow-up

Following chemoradiation, MRI is repeated at three months to assess treatment response. If the cervix demonstrates uniform low signal, residual tumour is effectively excluded. A residual mass is usually a sign of persistent disease. However, persistent

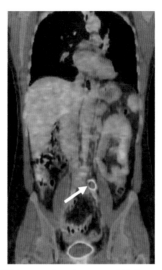

Fig. 15.6 Coronal FDG PET/CT image showing an avid left common iliac lymph node in a patient with relapsed cervical cancer.

high signal in the cervix is more problematic for distinction between residual disease and radiation effect, usually resulting in multidisciplinary discussion as to whether follow-up imaging (e.g. after another three months) or biopsy is most appropriate.

Depending on the results of MRI ± biopsy, CT may be utilized to evaluate potential distant sites. FDG PET/CT may be a useful adjunct or replacement to anatomical imaging as it has the potential to differentiate local recurrence from fibrosis, to more accurately detect distant metastases and to alter management in a significant proportion of patients. However, to date, evidence for the addition of PET/CT to MRI and CT in women with suspected recurrent/persistent cervical cancer and in asymptomatic women as surveillance remains scarce. Nevertheless, it has been recommended for patients with a local recurrence prior to considering a pelvic exenteration (Figure 15.6).

15.5 **Vaginal cancer**

15.5.1 **Clinical background**

Vaginal cancers are rare, comprising <1% of gynaecological malignancies. The incidence increases with age, with 38% arising in patients who are 75 or older in the UK in 2013–2015. The majority are squamous cell carcinomas, though rarely vaginal melanomas may occur. Secondary vaginal cancers are more common than primary vaginal cancers and most vaginal metastases occur by means of direct spread from the cervix, uterus, or rectum. Five-year survival has improved across all age groups and was 64% for 2009–2013. Pelvic examination continues to be the most important tool for evaluation of the local extent of the disease, but imaging is required to detect lymph node involvement, the extent of tumour infiltration, and metastatic spread.

15.5.2 Diagnosis and staging

Clinical presentations include discharge, bleeding, itching, and dyspareunia. Initial investigation comprises an examination under anaesthetic and biopsy. Staging is defined by the FIGO system (2009) (Table 15.3). MRI (Figure 15.7) is able to depict the majority of tumours and in doing so can aid treatment planning by evaluating the size, location, and local extent of vaginal tumours and demonstrating the degree of lymph node involvement. The differential anatomy of the three vaginal layers is best appreciated on T2-weighted images: vaginal mucosa is hyperintense; the submucosa and muscularis layers are hypointense; and the adventitial layer is hyperintense. The tumour is best assessed on T2-weighted images and shown as intermediate to high signal abnormality. Contrast enhanced T1-weighted fat saturated sequences may improve accuracy. MRI is superior for defining the anatomical relationships of the primary tumour, whilst FDG PET/CT will be more accurate for detection of metastatic disease and also provide prognostic information—which may have a particular bearing when local radical treatment is contemplated.

15.5.3 Imaging for radiotherapy planning

Radiotherapy is usually recommended for vaginal cancer, enabling organ preservation. As vaginal cancer is rare, there is limited data regarding the benefit of chemoradiation, but it is thought reasonable to extrapolate from the cervical cancer data and weekly cisplatin is used in combination with radiotherapy for patients with a good performance status. For the phase II boost, a brachytherapy boost (with a vaginal cylinder +/- interstitial needles) may be appropriate. As with cervical and endometrial cancer radiotherapy planning, a diagnostic MRI scan aids outlining the primary tumour and regional nodes. MRI also guides planning for a phase II brachytherapy boost—particularly if interstitial needles are used in addition to a vaginal cylinder.

15.5.4 Therapeutic assessment and follow-up

Once again, extrapolating cervical cancer practice to the rare vaginal cancer group, MRI will aid clinical assessment of treatment response and local recurrence with the

Table 15.3 FIGO staging for vaginal cancer

I	Tumour confined to the vaginal wall
II	Tumour invades paravaginal tissues but does not extend to pelvic wall
III	Tumour extends to pelvic wall
IVA	Tumour invades mucosa of the bladder or rectum and/or extends beyond the true pelvis
IVB	Distant metastasis

Adapted with permission from 'Current FIGO staging for cancer of the vagina, fallopian tube, ovary, and gestational trophoblastic neoplasia'. *International Journal of Gynecology & Obstetrics*, Vol.105, Issue 1, pp.3–4. Copyright © 2009 John Wiley & Sons.

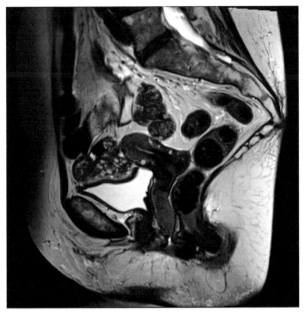

Fig. 15.7 Sagittal T2-weighted MRI of a stage I vaginal cancer.

attendant difficulties of distinguishing tumour from fibrosis—where FDG PET/CT and biopsy are likely to be useful adjuncts.

15.6 Vulval cancer

15.6.1 Clinical background

Vulval cancers are also rare (<1% of cancers in women). It is strongly related to age, with 44% of cases arising in women aged 75 and above. Overall five-year survival is 64%; 90% of vulval cancers are squamous cell carcinomas. The vast majority are treated surgically with a radical vulvectomy +/- inguinal lymph node sampling or resection.

15.6.2 Diagnosis and staging

Clinical presentation is typically with localized soreness, irritation, and a lump or ulcer. Tumours may also be detected during surveillance of vulval intra-epithelial neoplasia (VIN) or lichen sclerosis. Staging is defined by the FIGO system (2009) (Table 15.4).

The primary tumour is assessed clinically but cross-sectional imaging can help staging of the tumour, assessing extent of disease, and selecting operable versus inoperable patients (Figure 15.8).

15.6.3 Imaging for radiotherapy planning

The majority of cancers are managed surgically. Adjuvant radiotherapy is recommended for close margins and lymph node-positive disease. Inoperable locally

Table 15.4 FIGO staging for vulval cancer

Stage I	Tumour confined to the vulva
IA	Lesions ≤2 cm in size, confined to the vulva or perineum and with stromal invasion ≤1.0 mm, no nodal metastasis
IB	Lesions >2 cm in size or with stromal invasion >1.0 mm, confined to the vulva or perineum, with negative nodes
Stage II	Tumour of any size with extension to adjacent perineal structures (the lower third of the urethra or the vagina or the anus) with negative nodes
Stage III	Tumour of any size with or without extension to adjacent perineal structures (the lower third of the urethra or the vagina or the anus) with positive inguino-femoral lymph nodes
IIIA	(i) With 1 lymph node metastasis (≥5 mm), or
	(ii) 1–2 lymph node metastasis(es) (<5 mm)
IIIB	(i) With 2 or more lymph node metastases (≥5 mm), or
	(ii) 3 or more lymph node metastases (<5 mm)
IIIC	With positive nodes with extracapsular spread
Stage IV	Tumour invades other regional (the upper two-thirds of the urethra or the vagina), or distant structures
IVA	Tumour invades any of the following: (i) upper urethral and/or vaginal mucosa, bladder mucosa, rectal mucosa, or fixed to pelvic bone, or
	(ii) fixed or ulcerated inguino-femoral lymph nodes
IVB	Any distant metastasis including pelvic lymph nodes

Reproduced with permission from Pecorelli S, 'Revised FIGO staging for carcinoma of the vulva, cervix, and endometrium', *International Journal of Gynecology & Obstetrics*, Vol. 105, Issue 2, pp. 103–4. Copyright © 2009 John Wiley & Sons.

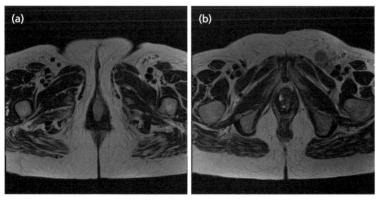

Fig. 15.8 (a) axial T2-weighted MRI of a vulval cancer, (b) Axial MRI of the same patient showing a pathological left groin node.

advanced primary disease may be referred for radiotherapy. In these cases, an MRI scan of the pelvis will aid assessment of the extent of the primary tumour, and inguinal and pelvic lymph node involvement. As in vaginal cancer, with extrapolation from the cervical cancer data, weekly cisplatin is used in combination with radiotherapy for patients with good performance status.

As discussed above, preparation for the CT planning scan is important (e.g. a comfortably full bladder). Clinician review prior to the CT planning scan is helpful—so that visible tumour, the introitus, and groin scars can be outlined with wire to aid target volume delineation. Consensus guidelines have been developed to aid outlining of the GTV and give recommendations regarding which areas should be included in the CTV.[15]

15.6.4 Therapeutic assessment and follow-up

Pathological staging determines completion or otherwise of resection and hence the need for further surgery or radiotherapy. Recurrence is usually clinically apparent.

15.7 Summary

- Imaging is integral to the management of the majority of gynaecological cancer patients from diagnosis through treatment to follow-up.
- Functional imaging, using both MRI and FDG PET/CT, plays a major role in all points of the patient care pathway, strengthening the case for ever closer collaboration between all members of the multidisciplinary team.

References

1. **Nougaret S**, **Horta M**, **Sala E, et al.** (2019). Endometrial cancer MRI staging: updated guidelines of the European society of urogenital radiology. *European Radiology*, **29**(2): 792–805.

2. **Addley H**, **Moyle P**, **Freeman S** (2017). Diffusion-weighted imaging in gynaecological malignancy. *Clinical Radiology*, **72**(11): 981–990.

3. **Lin G**, **Huang YT**, **Chao A, et al.** (2017). Endometrial cancer with cervical stromal invasion: diagnostic accuracy of diffusion-weighted and dynamic contrast enhanced MR imaging at 3T. *European Radiology*, **27**(5): 1867–1876.

4. **Concin N, Matias-Guiu X, Vergote I , et al.** (2021). ESGO/ESTRO/ESP guidelines for the management of patients with endometrial carcinoma. *Int J Gynecol Cancer,* **31**(1): 12–39.

5. **Mbatani N, Olawaiye AB, Prat J** (2018). Uterine sarcomas. *International Journal of Gynaecological Obstetrics*, **143**(2): 51–58.

6. **Taylor A, Rockall AG, Powell ME** (2007). An atlas of the pelvic lymph node regions to aid radiotherapy target volume definition. *Clinical Oncology* (Royal College of Radiologists), **19**(7): 542–550.

7. **Gay HA, Barthold HJ, O'Meara E, et al.** (2012). Pelvic normal tissue contouring guidelines for radiation therapy: a Radiation Therapy Oncology Group consensus panel atlas. *International Journal of Radiation Oncology. Biology. Physics*, **83**(3): e353–362.

8. Thomeer MG, Gerestein C, Spronk S, van Doorn HC, van der Ham E, Hunink MG (2013). Clinical examination versus magnetic resonance imaging in the pretreatment staging of cervical carcinoma: systematic review and meta-analysis. *European Radiology*, **23**(7): 2005–2018.

9. Sala E, Rockall AG, Freeman SJ, Mitchell DG, Reinhold C (2013). The added role of MR imaging in treatment stratification of patients with gynecologic malignancies: what the radiologist needs to know. *Radiology*, **266**(3): 717–740.

10. Monteil J, Maubon A, Leobon S, et al. (2011). Lymph node assessment with (18)F-FDG-PET and MRI in uterine cervical cancer. *Anticancer Research*, **31**(11): 3865–3871.

11. Choi HJ, Ju W, Myung SK, Kim Y (2010). Diagnostic performance of computer tomography, magnetic resonance imaging, and positron emission tomography or positron emission tomography/computer tomography for detection of metastatic lymph nodes in patients with cervical cancer: meta-analysis. *Cancer Science*, **101**(6): 1471–1479.

12. ICRU (2016). Report 89: Prescribing, recording and reporting brachytherapy for cancer of the cervix *J ICRU*, **13**(1–2):NP.

13. Haie-Meder C, GYNAE GEC ESTRO working group (2005). 3D image based concepts in brachytherapy for cervical cancer. *Gynecologic Oncology*, **99**(3, Suppl 1): S176.

14. Viswanathan AN, Dimopoulos J, Kirisits C, Berger D, Pötter R (2007). Computed tomography versus magnetic resonance imaging-based contouring in cervical cancer brachytherapy: results of a prospective trial and preliminary guidelines for standardized contours. *International Journal of Radiation Oncology. Biology. Physics*, **68**(2): 491–498.

15. Gaffney DK, King B, Viswanathan AN, et al. (2016). Consensus recommendations for radiation therapy contouring and treatment of vulvar carcinoma. *International Journal of Radiation Oncology. Biology. Physics*, **95**(4):1191–1200.

Chapter 16

Head and neck cancers

Gill Barnett and Tilak Das

16.1 Clinical background

Head and neck cancers are the sixth most common cancer worldwide, with an incidence of more than 650,000 cases per year (11,900 in the UK) and a mortality of 330,000 cases per year (4000 in the UK).[1]

16.2 Head and neck squamous cell carcinoma

16.2.1 Diagnosis

A full clinical assessment which includes flexible fibre-optic naso-endoscopy will reveal the primary site in the majority of head and neck squamous cell carcinoma (HNSCC) patients. In some patients, the primary site will be only apparent on computed tomography (CT) or magnetic resonance imaging (MRI). ^{18}F-fluorodeoxyglucose (FDG) positron emission tomography (PET/CT) is performed if the primary tumour is not present on clinical examination and may guide biopsies at examination under anaesthesia (EUA). PET-CT has a higher detection rate than a combination of contrast-enhanced CT and MRI.[2] In a small number of patient with no obvious primary tumour on PET/CT, EUA will identify suspicious areas, and biopsy will diagnose the primary site in 16–26% of cases; tonsillectomy on the same side as the nodal disease will establish the primary site in a further percentage. Blind biopsies from the nasopharynx, palatine tonsil, tongue base, and pyriform sinus were commonly performed in the past, but this is not currently standard practice in patients with radiologically and clinically normal findings.[2]

Recent studies of inclusion of PET/CT in the work-up of patients with an unknown primary show that a primary site is detected in up to 87% (Figure 16.1).[3] The effectiveness of FDG PET/CT depends to some extent on the investigations prior to FDG PET/CT. The ultimate role of FDG PET/CT is to reduce the number of patients where a primary site cannot be identified.

Locating the primary site in HNSCC can markedly alter the treatment plan to direct treatment with a high dose to the primary cancer and a lower dose to surrounding normal tissue, so reducing morbidity. The human papillomavirus (HPV) status of the tumour is also important as an HPV positive tumour is most likely to have originated from the oropharynx.[4] Irradiation of the oropharynx may be considered in patients with HPV positive disease who present as a carcinoma of unknown primary.

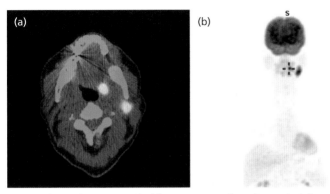

Fig. 16.1 Patient who presented with squamous cell carcinoma in left neck nodes. Full clinical assessment including flexible fibre-optic nasoendoscopy, showed no primary site. FDG PET/CT demonstrated intense uptake in the left oropharynx and neck. The patient underwent EUA, bilateral tonsillectomies and directed biopsies and squamous cell carcinoma was found in the left tonsil.

PET/CT is best performed before EUA to minimize false positive results. In addition to identifying the primary site, FDG PET/CT may detect unexpected nodal disease in the contralateral neck, undiagnosed nodal disease within the mediastinum, metastatic disease, and synchronous second cancers, including cancers linked by a common aetiology such as head and neck, oesophageal and lung cancer, and also other common cancers such as colorectal cancer.[4] PET/CT is therefore recommended in patients with more advanced stage head and neck cancer.[5]

16.2.2 **Staging**

16.2.2.1 Primary site

In patients with the established diagnosis of HNSCC the main purpose of imaging is to determine the deep extent of local tumour involvement and the presence of nodal disease. Only very occasionally does imaging suggest an alternative or unexpected diagnosis.

Initial choice between CT and MRI as the main imaging tools will depend on a number of factors, including availability and team preference. In many centres, MR is the preferred modality for imaging oral cavity, nasopharyngeal, and oropharyngeal tumours. High-resolution CT with intravenous contrast may be preferred for patients with primary hypopharyngeal, and laryngeal cancer. CT scanning is very helpful for patients who are unable to tolerate MRI.[6]

The MRI protocol used will vary considerably, partly related to: (1) time available on the scanner; (2) the preferences of the head and neck team; and (3) the make of the MRI scanner. In general, high-quality multi-planar data of the primary site, potential sites of direct invasion, and areas of predicted nodal drainage are included.[6] MR sequences typically performed include a coronal short tau inversion recovery (STIR) or fat-saturated T2-weighted (T2W) sequence which encompasses the primary tumour and neck, and coronal and/or axial T1-weighted (T1W) images specifically for primary tumour evaluation. Additional information is gained by using intravenous gadolinium, scanning in other planes, and additional sequences. Many centres include one or more of the following: post-gadolinium fat-saturated T1W sequence in the coronal and axial planes ± sagittal plane, fat-saturated T2W sequence in the sagittal ± axial ± coronal planes.

Initial assessment of laryngeal cartilage invasion, as with cortical bone and marrow involvement, will be made on the initial staging examination. Imaging may show clearly either no tumour involvement or alternatively definite invasion of tumour through laryngeal cartilage. Laryngeal cartilage calcifies in an irregular manner and it can be particularly challenging to distinguish uncalcified cartilage from early cartilage destruction. The literature suggests that MRI is more sensitive but less specific, that is, occurrence of false negatives is less with MRI compared with CT, but false positives are higher with MRI compared with CT. CT and MRI complement each other; if one is equivocal then the other can be performed.

16.2.2.2 Neck

The presence of metastatic tumour within cervical nodes has a major influence on the treatment plan and determines the likely prognosis in patients with HNSCC. The neck is assessed routinely with the primary site on CT or MRI and imaging will diagnose neck disease in 20% of patients who are thought to have no disease on clinical assessment.

Ultrasound (US) with fine needle aspiration cytology (FNAC) is a useful adjunct to CT and MRI for detection of nodal disease. In expert hands, an accuracy in excess of 90% can be achieved. When compared with diagnostic imaging, FDG PET/CT is similar or slightly superior for detecting abnormal cervical lymph nodes, but is generally reserved for patients with nodes not accessible to US, for example mediastinal and retropharyngeal nodes, and in cases where US does not provide the diagnosis.[6]

16.2.2.3 Distant metastases

CT scan of the thorax is usually performed to look for evidence of metastatic disease. In patients with a high risk of distant metastases, such as locally advanced disease (T3/4, N2/3) and tumours arising from subsites that have a particular predilection to metastasize, for example nasopharyngeal cancer, FDG PET/CT is recommended (Figure 16.2).[6] PET/CT should be included in the routine diagnosis of patients with stages II–IV HNSCC, as it significantly improves staging accuracy and also has a marked impact on management plans. In addition, PET/CT is an accurate method of detecting second primaries with a high negative predictive value. However, additional diagnostic methods are necessary to exclude false-positive results.[6]

16.2.3 Radiotherapy planning

Localization of tumour volume and delineation of normal structures is based on CT complemented by MRI. The inclusion of FDG PET/CT may result in substantial change in CTV definition compared to conventional CT alone, leading to more accurately targeted radiotherapy fields. There is also evidence that FDG PET/CT improves consistency in volume definition between different operators. There is, however, at

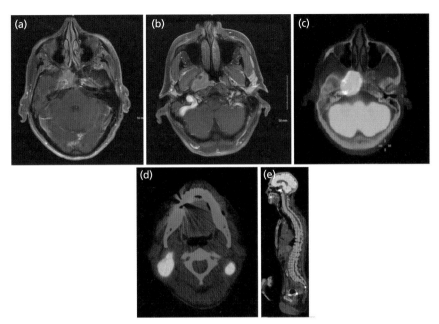

Fig. 16.2 Patient with a poorly differentiated nasopharynx carcinoma and bilateral neck nodes. MRI showed a right nasopharyngeal mass that extends superiorly into the right head of the clivus and right cavernous sinus, surrounding the inferior carotid siphon and anterior petrous carotid canal, extending into the right sphenoid sinus (a–b). FDG PET/CT showed uptake at the primary site and in the neck on both sides (c–d). It also showed unexpected focal uptake in the sacrum (e). MRI pelvis confirmed a lesion in S3. The RT treatment plan was modified as a result of the FDG PET/CT.

present a paucity of evidence to show that this translates into improvements in local control or toxicity.

Tumour edge definition using FDG PET/CT has not yet been standardized.[6] The main limitation is that it is a highly operator-dependent process, and it is influenced by window-level settings. Isocontouring based on a fixed standardized uptake value (SUV), such as 2.5 -3 gl^{-1} or relative thresholds such as percentage of the maximum tumour intensity (e.g. 40% SUVmax) may be used. More elaborate methods are being developed such as those based on signal-to-noise ratios, tumour dimension and grade, and gradient-based detections to refine delineation of tumour margins.

Recent studies have shown that functional imaging with MR and PET/CT may be used to provide information on the biological status of regions within HNSCC and to identify radio-resistant subregions that could be targeted for higher doses of radiation using intensity modulated radiotherapy (IMRT).[7]

16.2.4 Therapeutic assessment and follow-up

On CT and MRI the features which suggest residual tumour or recurrence include the presence of one or more soft tissue masses enlarging on sequential scans, especially if associated with bone or cartilage destruction. Other features, although less specific, that raise the suspicion of recurrence include focal soft tissue swelling >1 cm, that cannot be readily explained by post-surgical appearances, such as those due to a reconstruction flap and any abnormal soft tissue which shows enhancement with intravenous contrast 6 weeks or more after surgery and 12 weeks or more after radiotherapy.

Because many changes that follow intervention may be confused with or mask tumour recurrence, many experts consider a baseline CT or MRI during the interval when most alterations due to treatment have resolved and there is only little chance of tumour recurrence. Four to eight weeks post-treatment seems to be the best compromise, but there is a lack of published guidelines. Even with a baseline scan in many patients the early diagnosis of recurrent disease while it is still amenable to treatment remains a challenge.

PET/CT is very useful in assessing response to treatment. The negative predictive value (NPV) is very high, so a negative study is very suggestive of absence of residual disease. PET/CT should ideally be performed 12 weeks after treatment is complete. The PET-NECK study showed that PET-CT-guided surveillance resulted in fewer neck dissections, similar survival outcomes, and improved cost effectiveness compared with planned neck dissections.[8,9] In addition to more accurate assessment of the post-treatment head and neck, FDG PET/CT detects unexpected distant metastases and will from time to time diagnose synchronous cancers.

16.2.5 Surveillance

Preliminary studies show FDG PET/CT can detect subclinical recurrent disease. One of the largest studies included 388 patients who had undergone radical chemoradiotherapy. In this study 95% of asymptomatic recurrences occurred within two years of follow-up.[10] Further work needs to be done to clarify the role of FDG PET/CT in the surveillance of HNSCC patients, including the optimal time points when FDG PET/CT should be considered and especially in those with a high risk of relapse.[6]

16.3 Salivary gland tumours

US is the usual initial investigation for patients with suspected tumours of the salivary glands; it is quick, cheap, and often no further imaging will be required. This is especially the case when the mass is small, clinically benign, easily localized, and delineated, as with the classic and common pleomorphic adenoma lying superficially in the parotid gland. US will determine the location of the lesion, particularly whether or not it lies within a major salivary gland or outside it (e.g. a lymph node or asymmetric masseteric muscle hypertrophy). It will also often provide a confident diagnosis of the nature of the lesion, based on its US anatomy, echogenicity, and marginal definition. US-guided biopsy can be performed. The main limitation of US is its inability to accurately assess the extent of disease deep to the parotid gland, beyond the stylomandibular canal. CT and MRI are useful in this situation and MRI has the additional benefit of more accurate assessment of skull base invasion.

As a general rule, the vast majority of benign tumours are well-defined on all modalities. Salivary gland malignancies show a broad spectrum of appearances from relatively well-defined benign appearing masses to ill-defined clearly invasive lesions. The commonest salivary gland malignancy encountered is the mucoepidermoid carcinoma. These lesions show a variable degree of malignancy. Low-grade tumours appear similar to benign lesions, showing well-defined margins and a signal intensity on MRI similar to pleomorphic adenomas. They may be associated with cystic areas which may be complicated by rupture and inflammation, necrosis, and haemorrhage. In keeping with cystic lesions anywhere in the body these processes can alter the appearances on MRI. Generally, the presence of blood or a significant amount of protein or mucin will produce high signal on both T1W and T2W sequences. There may be a layering effect with blood products and debris settling posteriorly. High-grade carcinomas are ill-defined and more cellular, appearing more homogeneous and with a lower signal intensity on the T2W sequence. FDG PET/CT is of limited value for distinguishing between benign and malignant salivary gland tumours as both can be intensely avid for FDG.

Adenoid cystic carcinomas, in common with other malignancies in the head and neck may show some variable reduction in signal on the T2W sequence and there is some evidence that the degree of reduction correlates with increased cellularity and a higher grade of malignancy. Regardless of site of origin (major salivary gland or ectopic salivary gland tissue) adenoid cystic carcinomas show a predilection for perineural invasion and classically extend into skull base foramina and then intracranially. Where extension is gross, CT may demonstrate tumour along the cranial nerves and widened foramina. More subtle perineural/neural invasion is better seen with MRI following intravenous gadolinium.

Diagnosis of recurrent adenoid cystic carcinoma can be a challenge on imaging, including FDG PET/CT. In this situation a positive scan is useful but a negative scan cannot exclude recurrent disease. Perineural invasion cannot be reliably diagnosed on FDG PET/CT, and MRI with gadolinium is usually superior.

Adenocarcinoma within the parotid typically has ill-defined margins and is locally invasive. It can be a primary tumour of the gland or a metastatic deposit within lymph nodes in the salivary gland. Consequently, imaging should be extended to search for possible primary sites with CT chest (for carcinoma of the bronchus), abdomen, and pelvis (for gastrointestinal, pancreatic, and renal carcinomas), and, where appropriate, clinical or mammographic assessment of the breasts.

Squamous cell carcinoma within the parotid, with its typically similar imaging appearance to adenocarcinoma, is more likely to be metastatic. It is most often due to spread from a local primary site such as the scalp and external auditory canal. However, if the primary site is not obvious clinically, CT of the chest should be considered, as likely primary sites include the bronchus and thoracic oesophagus.

16.4 **Thyroid cancer**

16.4.1 **Background**

Thyroid cancer is a relatively uncommon condition but most countries have shown a significant increase in thyroid cancer over the last 30 years. Thyroid cancer is responsible for 567,000 cases worldwide, ranking in ninth place for incidence. The global incidence rate in women of 10.2 per 100,000 is three times higher than in men.

16.4.2 Diagnosis

The vast majority of thyroid cancer is differentiated and will present with a mass or swelling in the neck. US is the key imaging modality for diagnosis, usually combined with fine needle aspiration or core biopsy. Features suggestive of papillary carcinoma, the commonest cancer, include ill-defined margins, reduced echogenicity, microcalcification (25–40%) (Figure 16.3), and, in up to 30% of cases, cystic areas, irregular margin, and 'taller than wide' shape (anterior/posterior (AP) > transverse (TR) diameter when imaged in the axial plane).[11]

Follicular carcinoma is notoriously non-specific in appearance at US, usually appearing well-defined and similar to a benign adenoma (Figure 16.4). Colour flow Doppler of a thyroid nodule may be of some assistance. Chaotic intranodal vascular flow suggests a malignant lesion, while benign nodules typically have absent or only peripheral flow.

For more overtly invasive carcinomas of all types (including the rare undifferentiated carcinomas) US features are more obviously malignant, with the tumour being ill-defined and invasive both within the thyroid gland and extending into adjacent structures.

16.4.3 Staging

Most patients do not require further preoperative staging investigations. A minority, however, will have clinically (or ultrasonographically) locally advanced tumour at initial presentation. In these circumstances, preoperative staging is indicated, either in those cases for whom thyroidectomy is likely to be unfeasible or inappropriate

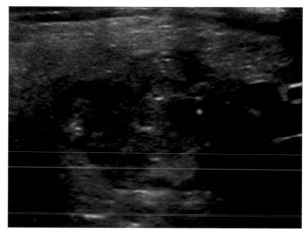

Fig. 16.3 Longitudinal US image through the left lobe of thyroid shows an ill-defined predominantly hypoechoic mass with areas of punctuate calcification.

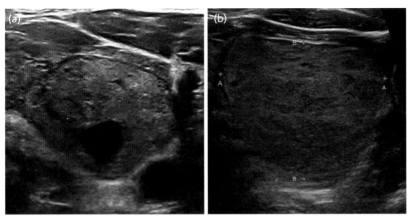

Fig. 16.4 Two patients with follicular carcinoma. (a) Transverse US image through the left lobe of thyroid shows an echogenic nodule with well-defined hypoechoic margins and a small cystic focus. (b) Transverse US image through the left lobe of thyroid shows a large solid echogenic nodule and lack of cystic change. Both were classified as indeterminate (U3) nodules.

(advanced undifferentiated carcinoma) or to guide the surgery (Tables 16.1 and 16.2). In these situations imaging is required to describe as accurately as possible the local invasion. Tumour may extend into adjacent critical structures (trachea, larynx, pharynx, oesophagus, and the carotid arteries) and inferiorly into the mediastinum.

The recommended pathological staging is by the TNM staging system. There are a number of other postoperative staging systems in use for differentiated thyroid cancers which are used for assessing prognosis. The TNM and MACIS have been shown to be the best predictors of outcome in validation studies. Recent updates mean that more patients will be classified as lower stage in the eighth edition compared to the seventh edition. This reflects the low risk of death from thyroid cancer for the majority of patients.

Either MRI or CT may be used to assess the neck (Figure 16.5). Protocols are based on the recommendations of the UK Royal College of Radiologists.[13]

Intravenous iodine containing contrast media interferes with radioactive iodine uptake by the thyroid for several weeks. It is therefore important to establish with the referring clinician if this is planned before using intravenous contrast.

MRI and CT have a similar accuracy for predicting local invasion of the oesophagus, trachea, larynx, and recurrent laryngeal nerve (RLN).[14] The main sign of tracheal or oesophageal invasion is a mass contacting 180° or more of the circumference of these organs. Other findings suggesting tracheal invasion are deformity of the lumen, focal mucosal irregularity or thickening, and soft tissue within the trachea. The oesophageal wall is more difficult to evaluate than the trachea because it is not usually distended with air. On MRI, the most suspicious finding for oesophageal invasion is a focal T2 signal in the outer layer of the oesophageal wall. On CT, there may be loss of the normal oesophageal wall and lumen. Invasion of the RLN can be predicted on MRI

Table 16.1 TNM classification of papillary, follicular, poorly differentiated, Hurthle cell and anaplastic thyroid cancer

T primary tumour*	
TX	Primary tumour cannot be assessed
T0	No evidence of primary tumour
T1	Tumour 2 cm or less in greatest dimension, limited to the thyroid
T1a	Tumour 1 cm or less in greatest dimension, limited to the thyroid
T1b	Tumour more than 1 cm but not more than 2 cm in greatest dimension, limited to the thyroid
T2	Tumour more than 2 cm but not more than 4 cm in greatest dimension, limited to the thyroid
T3	Tumour more than 4 cm in greatest dimension, limited to the thyroid or gross extrathyroidal extension invading only strap muscles (sternohyoid, sternothyroid, or omohyoid muscles)
T3a	Tumour more than 4 cm in greatest dimension, limited to the thyroid
T3b	Tumour of any size with gross extrathyroidal extension invading strap muscles (sternohyoid, sternothyroid, or omohyoid muscles)
T4a	Tumour extends beyond the thyroid capsule and invades any of the following: subcutaneous soft tissues, larynx, trachea, oesophagus, recurrent laryngeal nerve
T4b	Tumour invades prevertebral fascia, mediastinal vessels, or encases carotid artery
Note	
*Including papillary, follicular, poorly differentiated, Hurthle cell and anaplastic carcinomas	
N regional lymph nodes cervical and upper mediastinal	
NX	Regional lymph nodes cannot be assessed
N0	No regional lymph node metastasis
N1	Regional lymph node metastasis
N1a	Metastasis in Level VI (pretracheal, paratracheal, and prelaryngeal/Delphian lymph nodes) or upper/superior mediastinum
N1b	Metastasis in other unilateral, bilateral, or contralateral cervical (levels I, II, III, IV, or V) or retropharyngeal
M distant metastases	
M0	No distant metastasis
M1	Distant metastasis

Reproduced with permission from Sobin LH, Gospodarowicz MK, Wittekind CH. *UICC TNM Classification of Malignant Tumours*. 8th ed. © 2017 Wiley Blackwell.

Table 16.2 Staging of differentiated and anaplastic thyroid cancer

Papillary or follicular carcinoma	Under 55 years	55 years and older		
Stage I	Any T, Any N, M0	T1	N0	M0
		T2	N0	M0
Stage II	Any T, Any N, M1	T1	N1	M0
		T2	N1	M0
		T3a/T3b	Any N	M0
Stage III		T4a	Any N	M0
Stage IVA		T4b	Any N	M0
Stage IVB		Any T	Any N	M1
Anaplastic or undifferentiated carcinoma				
Stage IVA	T1–T3a	N0/Nx	M0	
Stage IVB	T1–T3a	N1	M0	
	T3b–T4	Any N	M0	
Stage IVC	Any T	Any N	M1	

Source: data from Sobin LH, Gospodarowicz MK, Wittekind CH. *UICC TNM Classification of Malignant Tumours.* 8th ed. © 2017 Wiley Blackwell.

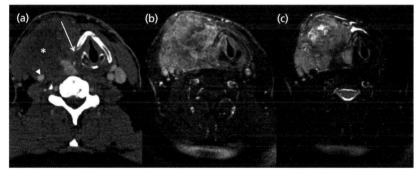

Fig. 16.5 (a) Post-contrast CT of the neck demonstrates a large right-sided anaplastic thyroid carcinoma (*) involving the right thyroid lamina (arrow) with cartilage destruction and partially encasing the right internal carotid artery (arrowhead). (b) Axial fat-suppressed T2-weighted and (c) axial fat-suppressed post-contrast T1-weighted images of the same patient demonstrating the large right-sided thyroid mass involving the right thyroid lamina and extending into the posterior larynx.

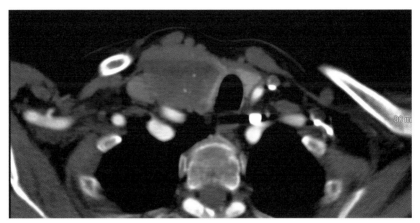

Fig. 16.6 CT scan demonstrating a large anaplastic carcinoma of the right thyroid lobe containing foci of calcification. There is posterior displacement of the right common carotid artery but no evidence of arterial invasion.

and CT by effacement of fat in the tracheoesophageal groove where the nerve courses. Other imaging features of RLN invasion are signs of vocal cord dysfunction and 25% or more of the circumference of the primary tumour abutting the capsule at the posterior portion of the thyroid (sign of posterior extracapsular invasion). Contact of the thyroid tumour with 270° or more of the circumference of the vessel is a highly specific sign for common carotid artery and internal jugular vein invasion on CT and MRI. Arterial compression or deformation or loss of the fat plane are also radiological signs of vessel involvement.[14]

CT may produce better quality images than MRI when patients have respiratory distress and have difficulty lying flat due to compromise of the airway by tumour invasion (Figure 16.6). CT is also quicker and superior for the detection of pulmonary metastases.

Lymphatic drainage from the thyroid gland is extensive and includes deep and superficial cervical, para- and pretracheal, paraoesophageal, paralaryngeal, supraclavicular, submandibular, and anterior mediastinal lymph nodes. The lymph node groups at highest risk of metastases are the central compartment (level VI, pre- and paratracheal), lower deep cervical (levels III and IV), and the lower half of the posterior triangle (level Vb). Papillary carcinoma has the highest rate of lymph node metastases, in excess of 75% of cases at presentation. The rate of early lymph node spread is also high with both anaplastic and medullary carcinoma, >50%, whereas the rate is low with follicular carcinoma, <20%.

Papillary carcinoma lymph node metastases may show multiple discrete foci of calcification on CT and areas of reduced (cystic or necrotic change) or increased (intra-nodal haemorrhage or areas of high thyroglobulin concentration) density (Figure 16.7).[14]

On MR these changes may appear as high signal on the T2W and low, intermediate, or high signal on T1W sequences. Papillary carcinoma may present with abnormal lymph nodes without a primary thyroid lesion demonstrable on imaging.

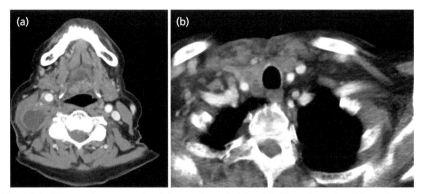

Fig. 16.7 CT scan demonstrating (a) an enlarged right-sided lymph node with cystic change characteristic of papillary carcinoma metastasis. (b) CT image through the thyroid gland of the same patient demonstrating a region of low density corresponding to the primary tumour.

Lymph node metastases from medullary and anaplastic carcinoma also often show necrotic changes. Consequently MRI and CT are reasonably accurate in the detection of involved lymph nodes both at the time of presentation and in recurrent disease.[14] Accuracy is less for follicular carcinoma, due to the lower incidence of morphological changes in the affected lymph nodes.

16.4.4 Therapeutic assessment and follow-up

Dynamic risk stratification should be performed 6–9 months after radioiodine ablation for all patients with R0 disease. This allows potential modification of the post-surgical risk; so, for example, some patients who were deemed high risk after their surgery may be lower risk after a good response to RRA. This facilitates a more personalized approach to treatment, follow-up, and prognosis. Stimulated thyroglobulin is measured and neck ultrasound is performed. Cross-sectional or diagnostic uptake scans may be performed if indicated. The response to initial therapy may thus be divided into excellent, indeterminate, or incomplete.

In patients with an excellent response to treatment, the serum TSH should be suppressed to between 0.3 mU/l and 2 mU/l. In patients with an indeterminate response to treatment, the serum TSH should be suppressed to between 0.1 mU/l and 0.5 mU/l for 5–10 years, at which the need for continuing TSH suppression should be re-evaluated. In patients with an incomplete response to treatment, the serum TSH should be suppressed to <0.1 mU/l indefinitely. These high-risk patients need lifelong follow-up, both because of the risk of curable late relapses and to monitor and manage the toxicity of supra-physiological thyroid replacement.

The commonest site of recurrence of thyroid cancer is cervical lymph nodes; recurrence outside the neck is most often in the chest, usually in the form of pulmonary metastases which are often multiple tiny metastases with a relatively indolent course. The only other common metastases are skeletal.

Routine follow-up of patients with differentiated thyroid cancer includes examination of the neck or other relevant systems, clinical and biochemical assessment of thyroid status, and serum thyroglobulin measurement (calcitonin levels for medullary thyroid cancer).[12] Abnormal masses in the neck should trigger further investigations, which may include FNA cytology (FNAC). If the thyroglobulin level rises, US of the neck (with biopsy if appropriate) is indicated in the first instance.[12] MRI or CT may then be further used to evaluate positive findings in the neck. CT may also be indicated to assess the chest for metastases. FDG-PET/CT is useful in this setting.

16.5 **Summary**

- ♦ MRI and CT offer good demonstration of the local extent of head and neck tumours; MRI offers better delineation of soft tissue invasion. MRI is the modality of choice for assessing skull base invasion.
- ♦ FDG PET/CT may improve detection of occult primary tumours, is a cost-effective single staging investigation in tumours at high risk of metastases, and superior to MRI and CT for detection of recurrent disease.
- ♦ Superficial salivary tumours and thyroid tumours are best assessed initially with ultrasound.

References

1. **CancerStats from Cancer Research UK. Available at:** http://info.cancerresearchuk.org/cancerstats and Global cancer statistics 2018

2. **Rassy E, Nicolai P and Pavlidis N.** (2019). Comprehensive management of HPV-related squamous cell carcinoma of the head and neck of unknown primary *Head & Neck*, **41**: 3700–3711.

3. **Albertson M, Chandra S, Sayed Z, Johnson C.** (2019). PET-CT evaluation of head and neck cancer of unknown primary. *Seminars in Ultrasound, CT, and MRI*, **40**(5): 414–423.

4. **Hohenstein NA, Chan JW, Wu SY, et al.** (2020). Diagnosis, staging, radiation treatment response assessment, and outcome prognostication of head and neck cancers using pet imaging: a systematic review. *PET Clinic*, **15**: 65–75.

5. https://www.nice.org.uk/guidance/qs146/chapter/Quality-statements

6. **Royal College of Radiologists (2014).** *Recommendations for Cross-Sectional Imaging in Cancer Management.* London: RCR.

7. **Cacicedo J, Navarro A, Del Hoyo O, et al.** (2016). Role of fluorine-18 flourodeoxyglucose PET-CT in head and neck oncology: the point of view of the radiation oncologist. *British Journal of Radiology*, **89**: 20160217.

8. **Grégoire V, Thorwarth D, Lee JA.** (2018). Molecular imaging-guided radiotherapy for the treatment of head-and-neck squamous cell carcinoma: does it fulfill the promises? *Seminars in Radiation Oncology*, **28**(1): 35–45.

9. **Mehanna H, Wong WL, McConkey CC, et al.** (2016). PET-CT surveillance versus neck dissection in advanced head and neck cancer. *New England Journal of Medicine*, **374**: 1444–1454.

10. **Beswick DM, Gooding WE, Johnson JT, Branstetter BF** 4th (2012). Temporal patterns of head and neck squamous cell carcinoma recurrence with positron-emission tomography/computed tomography monitoring. *Laryngoscope*, **122**(7): 1512–1517.

11. **Bray F, Ferlay J, Soerjomataram I, Siegel RL, Torre LA, Jemal A.** (2018). **Global Cancer Statistics** 2018: GLOBOCAN Estimates of Incidence and Mortality Worldwide for 26 Cancers in 185 Countries. CA: A *Cancer Journal for Clinicians*, **68**: 394–424.

12. **Perros P, Boelaert K, Colley S, et al.** (2014). **British Thyroid Association guideline for the management of thyroid cancer.** *Clinical Endocrinology*, **81**(Supp1): 1–122 https://onlinelibrary.wiley.com/doi/pdf/10.1111/cen.12515.

13. **Tuttle RM, Haugen B, Perrier ND.** (2017).The updated AJCC/tnm staging system for differentiated and anaplastic thyroid cancer (eighth edition): what changed and why? *Thyroid*, **27**(6): 751–756.

14. **Hoang JK, Branstetter BF** 4th, **Gafton AR, Lee WK, Glastonbury CM.** (2013). Imaging of thyroid carcinoma with CT and MRI: approaches to common scenarios. *Cancer Imaging*, **13**(1):128–139.

Chapter 17

Central nervous system

Sara C. Erridge, Gerard Thompson, and David Summers

17.1 Introduction

The purpose of imaging is to try to determine the nature, anatomical extent, and histological type of an intracranial lesion (solitary or multiple; intra-parenchymal or extra-axial; benign or aggressive). The demonstration of the relationship between the lesion and the adjacent neuroanatomy allows more precise surgical planning and accurate targeting of radiotherapy treatment volumes. Imaging is also used to assess treatment response. Multidetector computed tomography (CT) and magnetic resonance imaging (MRI) permit detailed, non-invasive, structural, and morphological analysis of masses within the brain and spine. More recent developments in imaging such as MR spectroscopy, CT and MR perfusion, and MR diffusion imaging are providing further insights into tumour subtype, behaviour, and spread. At present none of the available imaging tools can predict the histological tumour type with sufficient certainty, and pathological confirmation is obtained whenever practicable. Conversely, a small biopsy of a heterogeneous lesion may yield histological appearances compatible with low-grade tumour, when the imaging suggests a more aggressive neoplasm. Best practice requires the correlation of imaging and pathological findings, usually in the context of a multidisciplinary meeting.

The choice of imaging modality in the assessment of a probable tumour depends greatly on the issues which imaging is being asked to resolve. Both CT and MRI have strengths and weaknesses. MRI provides the best soft tissue contrast, displaying excellent definition of intracerebral structures, and shows anatomic detail and subtle contrast enhancement not visible on CT. The panoply of modern MR techniques such as perfusion and diffusion imaging, spectroscopy, and functional studies may provide useful additional information beyond the macroscopic structure of an abnormality. These sequences are more complex and time consuming and are usually undertaken at tertiary centres. They may also require greater patient cooperation, so standard structural MRI is the preferred modality for tumour imaging under most circumstances.

CT is often the first examination performed, as multidetector CT is now fast, readily accessible, and allows multi-planar image reconstruction akin to MR, although the tissue contrast and the distinction between normal brain and tumour remains inferior. CT may be all that is required, for example in planning the resection of a skull vault meningioma, or acute assessment for hydrocephalus or bleed. CT has additional advantages in the skull base where the quality of bone imaging is considerably better than MRI. CT can demonstrate lesion calcification that may not be readily visible on MRI. The two modalities are often complementary, for example in the assessment of a skull base tumour where high-resolution CT provides bone detail and MRI shows the extent of soft tissue involvement, or for detection of macroscopic calcification.

17.2 Advanced imaging techniques

Over the last decade there has been extensive investigation of the role of advanced MRI and nuclear medicine techniques to improve the accuracy of initial radiological diagnosis, to identify the extent of tumour spread, guide biopsies, and to assess the post-treatment tumour status.

17.2.1 Magnetic resonance imaging techniques

MR spectroscopy examines the presence of specific metabolites in tissues, and in brain tumours has primarily been used to examine the levels of N-acetylasparate (NAA), creatine, choline, and lactate. The ratio of these compounds, for example NAA to choline, may help differentiate normal brain from tumour infiltration. The presence of the amino acid alanine has also been identified as a marker of meningioma. However, at present the low spatial resolution (6–10 mm) limits the use in target definition.

Diffusion weighted imaging (DWI) measures the ability of water to move primarily in the extracellular space, which in broad terms may become restricted in higher grade and cellular tumours, although the biological specificity remains uncertain. As with enhancement, it is non-specific, and diffusion restriction can be seen in infarct and postoperative tissue handling. As with other MRI techniques, interpretation can become challenging once blood products are present. Diffusion tensor imaging (DTI) examines the microarchitecture of tumours and white matter tracts, and these may be disrupted by tumour before macroscopic lesions are visible on standard MR sequences Figure 17.1a–c. This may be useful in the planning of radiotherapy, but whilst DWI is now part of standard brain tumour imaging protocols, DTI still requires additional time and expert image processing to perform well, is subject to technique and processing variability, and its availability is limited in many current clinical settings.

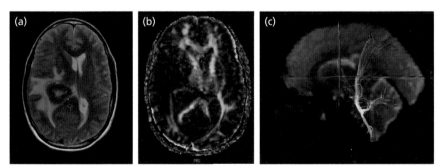

Fig. 17.1. (a) DTI T2 map. (b) DTI structural map. (c) DTI fibre track.

Perfusion/permeability MR imaging attempts to measure the degree of angiogenesis and capillary permeability. There are a number of techniques in use. The role of perfusion imaging has yet to be fully established although it may be helpful in determining grade of astrocytic (but not oligodendroglial) lesions. Perfusion MRI may help differentiate post-treatment changes from tumour progression in conjunction with radiological interpretation (see below).

17.2.2 Computed tomography techniques

CT perfusion is a more robust technique than MR, with a linear relationship between contrast density and cerebral blood flow and volume parameters, but like MR perfusion requires significant post-processing time. It also uses an ionizing radiation dose significantly higher than standard CT head imaging and is therefore less suited for follow-up imaging; newer systems with whole head coverage and reductions in ionizing radiation dose may yet bring CT perfusion into more widespread clinical use.

17.2.3 Nuclear medicine techniques

Single photon emission tomography (SPECT) and positron emission tomography (PET) scanning examine physiological parameters rather than structure. Although relatively low-resolution structural detail is captured they have been extensively investigated in brain tumours. SPECT scanning uses a number of different radioisotope tracers, for example ^{99m}Tc-HMPAO (hexamethylpropylene amine oxime) to examine brain blood flow or ^{201}thallium chloride to identify areas of increased metabolism. However, the spatial resolution is inferior to CT-PET which has largely superseded SPECT as metabolic imaging of choice for research into brain lesions.

^{18}Flourodeoxyglucose (FDG) PET scanning can be used in the evaluation of brain tumours with the degree of uptake correlating with tumour grade and survival, but the high level of glucose metabolism in normal grey matter makes differentiation from tumour difficult. Other tracers, which identify increased amino acid uptake or increased protein or DNA synthesis, have also been developed. Amino acid PET in neuro-oncology has recently been appraised by the RANO initiative. The most commonly used tracer in brain imaging is ^{11}C-methionine (MET), but the very short half-life of ^{11}carbon makes this tracer difficult to use. So other tracers using ^{18}fluoride have been developed, principally ^{18}fluorothymidine (FLT), which measures cell proliferation rates, and ^{18}fluroethyl-L-tyrosine (FET) that assesses amino acid uptake. FLT is robust at grading tumours and predicting prognosis and FET may also prove useful in differentiating normal brain from tumour.

Although these techniques appear promising, whether or not these will prove useful and cost effective in routine practice requires prospective, ideally randomized, studies with health economic assessment.

17.3 How to review imaging of the CNS

Having excluded a finding requiring immediate action, such as acute hydrocephalus or significant haemorrhage, the most important consideration, whether reviewing CT or MR, is to decide on the anatomical location of the lesion. In particular, is it *intra-parenchymal* (within the substance of the brain) or *extra-axial* (outside the brain itself, and arising from vault, dura, or other meninges). The differential diagnoses are distinct between these two groups, and making this distinction allows the possible causes to be narrowed considerably.

17.3.1 Intraparenchymal

A solitary intra-axial lesion may be either a primary tumour of the CNS, most commonly a glioma, or a metastasis. The relative likelihood depends upon the patient's age and the lesion site; for example a solitary posterior fossa lesion in a middle-aged adult is most likely to be a solitary metastasis (and 50% of brain metastases are solitary).

Intra-axial lesions expand or outwardly displace the cortical grey matter, narrowing the subarachnoid and extra-axial cerebrospinal fluid (CSF). The outer margins of the lesion may be distinct and sharp (as in a metastasis or gliosarcoma) or ill-defined and irregular (as in glioblastoma multiforme). As a gross generalization, more fast-growing lesions enhance more avidly, and the absence of central enhancement raises the possibility of necrosis or tumour cyst, although it should be noted that contrast enhancement is an epiphenomenon of blood-brain barrier disruption and vascularity as discussed below. Intra-axial tumours provoke varying degrees of surrounding white matter change. This is demonstrated as high signal on T2-weighted sequences and FLAIR imaging. It may be due to vasogenic tumour oedema, tumour infiltration, or both. This is a particular problem for intra-axial primary tumours, where definition of the tumour margin is important for planning radiotherapy and an area of active discussion and research.

17.3.2 Extra-axial

Extra-axial masses are commonly benign, with meningiomas forming the largest group. Typical features include a sharp cleft of CSF between the lesion and the cortical surface, and a broad base on the dura or the skull. Inward displacement of cortical vessels is also a useful imaging sign. Other lesions include bone and dural metastases, and tumours of nerve sheathes such as vestibular schwannomas. This latter group is usually easily identifiable by their anatomical location. The presence of a tail of enhancement along the dura is a feature of extra-axial lesions, but is not specific to meningioma.

17.3.3 Other features

In addition to location, other factors, such as the degree of enhancement following the injection of contrast media, can help differentiate between types of tumour. Tumour enhancement, whether on MRI or CT, reflects either disruption of the normal blood-brain barrier, significantly increased vascularity of a lesion, or a combination of both. Assessment of contrast enhancement characteristics is an essential part of the diagnostic study so only patients with a known allergic reaction to contrast media or significantly impaired renal function should not receive contrast. The enhancement characteristics do not necessarily directly correlate with tumour grade. For example, meningiomas usually enhance uniformly and avidly, whilst some moderately aggressive gliomas may demonstrate only minor enhancement.

17.4 **Role of imaging in treatment planning**

Imaging now plays a central role in the planning of surgery and radiotherapy for all CNS lesions.

Prior to surgery most patients will have a volumetric MRI scan performed, which can be used in conjunction with a neuro-navigation system to help guide surgery. This enables the surgeon to perform framed or frameless stereotactic craniotomies and biopsies, guiding them to a specific area on a scan which is co-registered with the patient in theatre. Surgical instruments are tracked in three dimensions by this system and matched to the imaging volume. These systems are used during a resection in combination with anatomical knowledge and preoperative functional imaging planning to establish how much tumour tissue can be removed safely. Some larger neurosurgical centres have intra-operative MRI scanners, usually in a room adjacent to the neurosurgical theatre, which perform a scan during the procedure to assess whether the planned extent of resection has been achieved and to guide any further surgery, allowing account to be taken of brain shift during the procedure.

When the tumour is close to an eloquent area of brain, a preoperative functional MRI (fMRI) may be performed to assess the potential impact of a resection. This can be used in conjunction with neuro-navigation and an awake craniotomy. For example, if the lesion is close to eloquent speech/language cortex the patient can be instructed to perform naming tasks during the operation to maximize preservation of eloquent brain areas.

When planning radiotherapy for CNS lesions, though the planning CT scan can provide information on tumour location, the inferior tissue contrast makes the images less suitable for target delineation than MRI. Therefore, when defining radiotherapy target volumes for CNS tumours fused CT/MRI images should be used. The accuracy of alignment varies so this should always be inspected carefully, and repeated or adjusted if necessary.

17.5 **Intra-parenchymal tumours**

Intra-parenchymal tumours arise from neuroglial progenitor cells and demonstrate features relating to two distinct lineages of glial cells: oligodendrocytes, which form and maintain the myelin sheath around axons, and astrocytes, which undertake a number of functions for maintaining CNS function, for example metabolic support for neurons, interacting with vasculature as a component of the blood-brain barrier, formation of synapses, and interaction with the immune system. They can also exhibit behaviours present during neurodevelopmental processes such as migration, in addition to uncontrolled proliferation. These properties are postulated to contribute to the treatment resistance and heterogeneity demonstrated by gliomas. Ependymomas are also considered in this category.

17.6 **Astrocytomas**

17.6.1 **Glioblastoma (grade IV)**

These fast-growing tumours account for around half of all malignant tumours and occur most frequently between the ages of 45 and 70 and are more common in men. Glioblastomas (GBM) are rare in children, but if they do occur, they may be infra-tentorial.

GBM with IDH mutations have transformed from a lower grade tumour, occur in younger people, and have a better prognosis than GBH with IDH wildtype. Glioblastomas are also classified by the presence or absence of methyl-guanine methyl transferase (MGMT) promoter methylation; so-called 'methylated glioblastomas' have a better prognosis and are more likely to respond to alkylating chemotherapy, such as temozolomide (TMZ). MGMT promoter methylation silences the MGMT enzyme, which is a key DNA repair mechanism for alkylation and therefore impedes the effectiveness of TMZ.

Infiltrative growth is characteristic, with spread along white matter tracts, for example across the corpus callosum, the internal capsule, fornix, or anterior commissure. Multifocal lesions occasionally occur and have a worse prognosis. Spread via the CSF is relatively rare (slightly more common in 'glioblastoma with PNET features') and extraneural metastases are even rarer, but are occasionally observed in long-term survivors.

17.6.1.1 Imaging features

See Figures 17.2a and 17.2b.

- Complex-looking tumour
- Cystic or necrotic centre, but with some enhancing structures within
- Irregular thick enhancing walls on T1-weighted MRI following gadolinium (Gd) chelate
- Usually moderate mass effect
- Moderate surrounding white matter high signal on T2-weighted/FLAIR
- Predilection for white matter tracts, for example cross corpus callosum/ commissures
- Haemorrhage uncommon but can precipitate clinical deterioration
- Calcification rare

17.6.1.2 Radiotherapy target definition

Radiotherapy target delineation should be performed on a contrast enhanced CT scan (slice thickness 3 mm or less) performed in an immobilization mask. The preoperative and postoperative MRI scans should be fused to the CT scan. The preoperative imaging can be helpful in locating all areas of disease, but when a resection has been performed the shift of structures can result in movement of the target, hence the need for a postoperative MRI also to be fused. However, sometimes postoperative scans can have enhancement due to surgical changes, so having both pre- and postoperative MRI scans fused can aid identification of all areas at risk. Immediate postoperative MRI is generally recommended within 48–72 hours. The most commonly utilized sequences are gadolinium enhanced volumetric T1w and volumetric FLAIR. Volumetric sequences are acquired with reduced distortion and have more slices, enabling more accurate fusion. In general, isotropic voxels should be acquired to permit multiplanar reformatting. The T1w image with gadolinium demonstrates

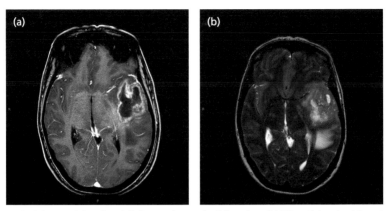

Fig. 17.2. (a) T1-weighted gadolinium enhanced axial section. (b) T2-weighted axial section.

any residual enhancing tumour and the resection cavity. A pre-contrast T1-weighted volume using the same sequence parameters is useful to distinguish genuine enhancement from postoperative blood products. The FLAIR shows areas of infiltrative tumour, though will also include areas of oedema, particularly on the preoperative scan acquired prior to commencing steroids.

The gross target volume (GTV) should consist of the area of residual enhancing tumour or resection cavity defined on T1-weighted with gadolinium, adjusted to take into account any areas of new enhancement on the planning CT scan.[1]

The clinical target volume (CTV) should include areas of greatest likelihood of microscopic spread, created by adding a 2 cm margin to the GTV, edited to remove anatomical barriers to spread (e.g. tentorium cerebelli, the falx cerebri, or the contralateral ventricle). The recommendation of a 2 cm margin is based on a number of single-centre retrospective analyses of recurrence patterns which have shown that around 80% occur within this margin. This volume should then be inspected to consider areas of potential spread as glioma cells migrate along white matter tracts and in perineural and perivascular spaces. The FLAIR sequence can help identify these areas, as can enlargement of gyri when compared to contralateral side. The subventricular region has been identified as a site harbouring neural stem cells and some authors recommend including this region in the CTV. Studies are ongoing to see if MRI sequences such as DTI or physiological imaging such as PET will enable more individualized targets to be created.

17.6.2 Anaplastic astrocytoma (grade III non-codeleted glioma)

In the 2016 WHO reclassification of brain tumours, grade III lesions have been defined by the presence or absence of loss of the short arm of the first chromosome (1p) and long arm of chromosome 19 (19q) as either co-deleted (anaplastic oligodendroglioma) or non-codeleted (anaplastic astrocytoma).[2] Anaplastic astrocytoma represents around 20% of astrocytomas, and occurs at a slightly younger age than glioblastomas. There may be evidence of progression from a grade II diffuse astrocytoma when there is usually IDH mutation and ATRX mutation. They are diffuse lesions with marked cellular atypia and mitotic activity but without frank or geographic necrosis. They have a similar growth pattern to glioblastoma

17.6.2.1 Imaging features

See Figure 17.3.

- Infiltrative mass, predominantly along white matter tracts
- Uniformly high signal on T2-weighted sequences
- Often of considerable size with local mass effect
- Typically, does not enhance, but small focal areas of enhancement may occur

17.6.2.2 Radiotherapy target definition

Similar target volumes to GBM are used with most neuro-oncologists recommending a 1.5–2 cm margin to be added to the contrast enhancing region demonstrated on T1-weighted postoperative MRI but as they often derive from lower grade glioma and are less likely to have oedema, any changes on the FLAIR sequence are likely to represent tumour infiltration so should be included in the CTV.

17.6.3 Diffuse astrocytoma (grade II non-codeleted glioma)

These lesions represent around 15% of all astrocytomas and are diagnosed most frequently in early adulthood. They can occur anywhere in the brain, with the temporal

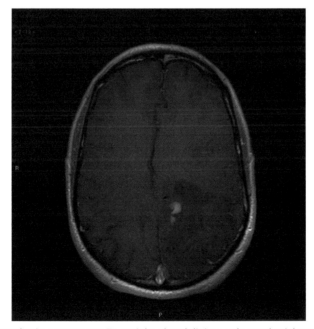

Fig. 17.3 Anaplastic astrocytoma T1-weighted gadolinium enhanced axial section.

and frontal lobes most commonly affected. Histologically there is increased cellularity and nuclear atypia but mitotic activity is low. The majority have IDH mutation
present and the absence of this, after full sequencing, raises the concerns that the
lesion may behave more like a higher-grade glioma (pre-GBM). Diffuse astrocytoma
by definition do not have 1p/19q co-deletion.

Certain features suggest a more 'aggressive' clinical course:

1) Size >5 cm

2) Crossing mid-line

3) Age >40 years

4) Localizing clinical signs

5) Shorter history of symptoms

17.6.3.1 Imaging features

See Figure 17.4.

◆ Bland homogeneous lesions, usually in frontal or temporal lobes

◆ Usually uniform T2-weighted high signal

◆ Infiltrate along white matter tracts

◆ Contrast enhancement absent or minimal

◆ Often less mass effect than expected for lesion size

◆ May be indistinguishable from anaplastic astrocytoma

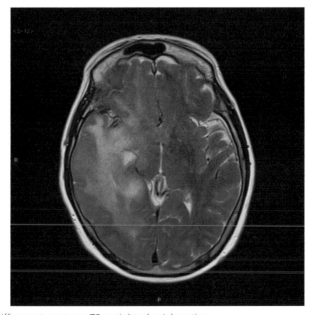

Fig. 17.4 Diffuse astrocytoma T2-weighted axial section.

17.6.3.2 Radiotherapy target definition

When defining the target for a low-grade glioma it is particularly important to use fused MRI images. The FLAIR sequence can be particularly useful to generate the GTV as the areas of high signal are likely to represent tumour. To create the CTV, a margin of 1.0–1.5 cm is added. As the prognosis of this group of patients, particularly when IDH mutation is present, is good, then the CTV should be edited to remove any regions where tumour spread is unlikely.

17.6.4 **Pilocytic astrocytoma (grade I)**

These well-circumscribed, slow-growing tumours usually occur in children and young adults, but can occur at any age. They can occur anywhere throughout the neuraxis but frequently occur in the cerebellar hemispheres (60%) ('cerebellar astrocytoma'), optic pathway (30%) ('optic pathway glioma' OPG, particularly seen in patients with neurofibromatosis type 1 (NF1)), third ventricle, and hypothalamus (also associated with NF1). They have heterogeneous histology, including areas of compact bipolar cells with long processes and other regions with microcysts.

17.6.4.1 Imaging features

See Figure 17.5.

◆ Avid enhancement of mural nodule

◆ Rounded cyst or cysts

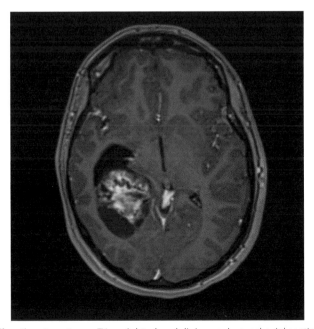

Fig. 17.5 Pilocytic astrocytoma, T1-weighted gadolinium enhanced axial section.

- Variable size of cyst(s), usually without enhancement in cyst wall
- Sharply defined margins with normal brain

17.6.4.2 Radiotherapy target definition

Most pilocytic astrocytomas can be successfully treated with resection, requiring no additional therapy. However, occasionally a lesion grows or recurs locally or even seeds along the neural axis. When local radiotherapy is required the GTV is the enhancing tumour nodule and cyst with a small margin 0.3–0.5 cm used to create the CTV.

17.7 **Oligodendrogliomas (codeleted glioma)**

17.7.1 **Oligodendrogliomas (grade II)**

In the revised WHO 2016 classification, oligodendrogliomas are defined by a codeletion of the short arm of chromosome 1 (1p) and long arm of chromosome 19 (19q), and IDH mutation. If these are not present then the lesion is classified as a non-codeleted glioma (astrocytoma). If the molecular characterization is not available then WHO 2016 allows for the traditional histological phenotype to be employed carrying the suffix NOS for not otherwise specified but, whenever available, the molecular marker supersedes the histological appearances.

Oligodendroglioma are slow-growing infiltrative gliomas usually occurring supratentorially. They are typically located peripherally in the frontal lobe. One of the pathognomonic features is the presence of dense foci of macrocalcification. Historically they were often diagnosed in the early to mid-40s, but the routine use of imaging in the investigation of seizures means many are now diagnosed at a younger age. The classic histological features are of tumour cells with clear cytoplasm ('fried egg cells'), a branching network of capillaries (chicken wire appearance), and microcalcification.

As with diffuse astrocytoma, the management of co-deleted grade II glioma has changed in recent years, with more undergoing surgical resection followed by immediate postoperative radiotherapy and adjuvant PCV chemotherapy, particularly if the postoperative characteristics meet the RTOG 9802 entry criteria.

17.7.1.1 Imaging features

See Figure 17.6.

- Peripheral location
- Most commonly frontal
- Nodular calcification in 80%+, best seen on CT
- Margins often relatively well-defined
- May contain cystic areas
- Variable enhancement, usually heterogeneous within tumour and can wax and wane
- Haemorrhage in 20%
- Skull vault may be scalloped

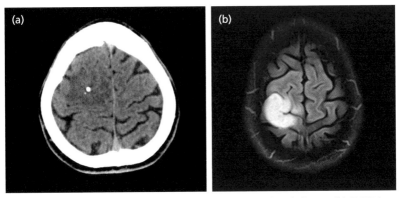

Fig. 17.6 (a) CT scan showing calcification in grade 2 co-deleted glioma. (b) FLAIR image of grade 2 co-deleted glioma.

17.7.1.2 Radiotherapy target definition

When defining the target for oligodendroglioma, the FLAIR sequence can be particularly useful to identify all the infiltrating tumour and then a margin of 1.0–1.5 cm is added to create the CTV. In light of the likelihood of prolonged survival there should be every effort to minimize the volume of normal brain, editing out areas where tumour spread is unlikely.

17.7.2 Anaplastic oligodendroglioma (grade III)

These lesions usually occur on the background of a grade II codeleted lesion and are diagnosed at a slightly older age. The features of a grade II oligodendroglioma are present, along with marked nuclear atypia, high mitotic activity, and sometimes the presence of vascular proliferation and necrosis. Standard management of these tumours is maximal safe debulking followed by radiotherapy and then adjuvant (or neo-adjuvant) PCV chemotherapy.

17.7.2.1 Imaging features

See Figures 17.7a and 17.7b.

◆ Similar to grade II oligodendroglioma but more aggressive features include:
◆ Avid enhancement, or new areas of enhancement, which continue to enlarge
◆ Increasing mass effect
◆ Extensive cystic change

17.7.2.2 Radiotherapy target definition

As these often occur in the background of a low-grade lesion the GTV consists of postoperative cavity and all enhancing disease on T1-weighted gadolinium enhanced MRI and all areas of high signal on the FLAIR. To create the CTV a margin of 1.5–2 cm is added, but as these lesions can also have a good prognosis the volume should be carefully edited to remove areas where spread is unlikely.

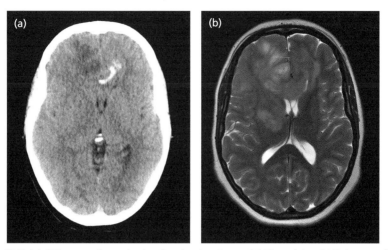

Fig. 17.7 (a) CT image of anaplastic oligodendroglioma. (b) T2-weighted MR image of anaplastic oligodendroglioma.

17.8 **Mixed gliomas**

With improved molecular profiling using 1p/19q and ATRX, true mosaic oligo-astrocytomas are very rare.

17.8.1 **Gliomatosis cerebri**

Historically this term was used to define tumours involving three or more lobes but this entity was removed in the WHO 2016 reclassification. Instead the tumour is defined by its morphological and molecular features and the growth pattern only mentioned as a description.

17.8.2 **Gliomas of the spinal cord**

See Figure 17.8.

These are relatively rare, principally diffuse astrocytoma and anaplastic astrocytoma, though glioblastomas do occasionally occur.

17.8.2.1 Follow-up imaging for glioma

The interpretation of images acquired following surgery or radiotherapy can be challenging and result in a degree of uncertainty during follow-up. For patients in whom a gross total tumour resection was intended, an immediate postoperative MRI is useful for estimation of extent of resection. Postoperative MRI should be performed within 72 hours of surgery to minimize the enhancement due to surgical reaction and granulation tissue which generally becomes more prominent after this time. Imaging may, however, be confounded by post-surgical haematoma and mass effect. Alternatively, imaging after several weeks may be performed when such postoperative changes have generally resolved.

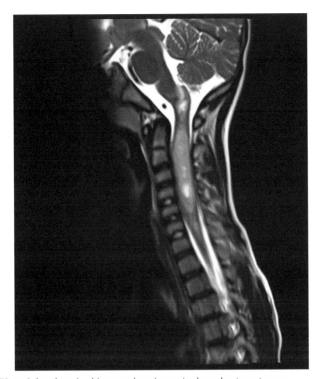

Fig. 17.8 T2-weighted sagittal image showing spinal cord astrocytoma.

Following radiotherapy there are marked changes, particularly in the white matter, with high T2-weighted and FLAIR signal with facilitated diffusion which can take a number of months to resolve or may result in permanent microvascular-related changes. The appreciation of these changes is particularly important following concurrent chemo-radiation as they can be falsely interpreted as tumour progression.

Radiation necrosis is unusual, but when it occurs there is often mass effect, irregular peripheral enhancement and necrosis, and it is difficult to distinguish from recurrent high-grade tumour on structural imaging alone. MR perfusion demonstrates reduced relative cerebral blood volume (rCBV) areas within radiation necrosis (as compared with generally increased relative blood volume in recurrent tumour)(Figure 17.9a and 17.9b), and MR spectroscopy shows an increase in lipid/lactate peak with decreases in all other metabolites in radiation necrosis, unlike recurrent tumour. Other modalities such as PET-CT with FDG can demonstrate the hypometabolism of radiation necrosis.

The optimal follow-up schedule for high-grade glioma has not been established and depends on the patient's fitness for treatment at progression. Some centres perform imaging every 3–4 months in order to detect small recurrences amenable to re-resection, whereas other neuro-oncologists feel that the early detection of asymptomatic recurrence is unlikely to be beneficial.

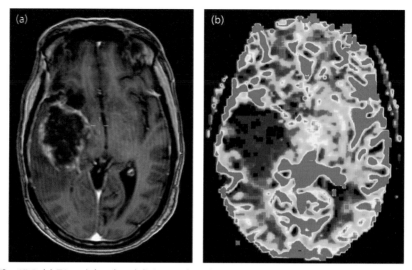

Fig. 17.9 (a) T1-weighted gadolinium enhancing imaging showing radiation necrosis. (b) MR perfusion showing rCBV within radiation necrosis.

For patients with low-grade lesions, especially where there are more treatment options, patients are usually followed with routine MRI scanning, initially every 3–6 months to assess growth characteristics and then annually.

17.9 Ependymoma

These tumours arise from the ependymal lining of the cerebral ventricles and from the central canal of the spinal cord.

Ependymomas account for around 3% of CNS lesions, and although they occur mainly in children and young adults they are seen at any age. They commonly develop in the posterior fossa, spinal cord, or lateral ventricles. They can spread along the neuraxis, so whole brain and spine imaging should be performed. They can be either grade I (myxopapillary), II, or III (anaplastic). Lesions in the brain, particularly supratentorial are associated with an inferior outcome, as is age over 40 years of age, grade III lesions, and subtotal excision.

17.9.1 Imaging features

See Figure 17.10.

- Typically arise from the *floor* of the fourth ventricle
- Conform to shape of ventricle
- Extend through foramina of Luschka and Magendie
- Enhancement variable, often mild and heterogeneous
- 'Drop metastases' into spine and CSF spaces are common

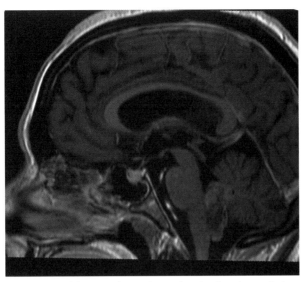

Fig. 17.10 T1-weighted gadolinium enhanced MRI showing fourth ventricular ependymoma.

17.9.2 Target definition

Immediate postoperative radiotherapy is usually recommended for ependymoma, except for grade II lesions when a complete resection has been performed and surveillance can be adopted. Historically, because of the propensity for CSF seeding, craniospinal radiotherapy was recommended, especially for the anaplastic lesions. However, there is now a clear body of evidence that provided whole neuraxis imaging and CSF are clear then focal radiotherapy can be utilized.

The GTV is delineated on gadolinium enhanced T1-weighted MRI to include resection cavity and any residual disease. The CTV consists of a margin of 1–2.5 cm depending on grade and location.

17.10 Spinal cord myxopapillary ependymoma (grade I)

These low-grade lesions principally occur in the conus and cauda equina, growing very slowly over years. CSF spread has been documented but is uncommon.

17.10.1 Imaging features

♦ Well demarcated mass centred on conus or filum terminale/cauda equina (key feature)

♦ Haemorrhage common

♦ Enhancement typical

♦ Bony canal may be expanded

17.10.2 **Radiotherapy target definition**

As complete surgical resection is difficult, often a combination of subtotal resection and radiotherapy is used and has very good long-term control rates.[3] The target should encompass the whole spinal canal extending from 2cm to 3 cm above the lesion to the thecal sac.

17.10.3 **Follow-up of ependymal lesions**

These patients usually undergo MRI imaging every 3–6 months.

17.11 **Embryonal tumours**

This group of undifferentiated round-cell tumours occur principally in children and young adults. Medulloblastomas, which occur in the cerebellar region, are the most common type of lesion.

17.11.1 **Medulloblastoma**

These are typically midline tumours arising from the roof of fourth ventricle posteriorly (unlike fourth ventricular ependymoma) growing to occupy the ventricle. In older age groups the lesion may arise laterally in the cerebellar hemispheres. Medulloblastomas are now grouped into four subtypes depending on the presence or absence of sonic hedgehog (SHH), WNT, and p53 mutations.

17.11.1.1 Imaging features

See Figure 17.11.

- Usually solid, rounded, slightly heterogeneous mass
- Small intralesional cysts common, large tumour cyst rare
- Well-defined margins, little oedema
- Do not grow through foramina of fourth ventricle (unlike ependymoma)
- Heterogeneous enhancement in more than 80% cases
- Early leptomeningeal spread so post-contrast imaging of the whole of the brain and spine is required for complete staging
- Diffusion restriction (lower ADC values than normal hindbrain)
- Lateral epicentre in cerebellum more likely to be SHH mutated
- Cerebellar peduncle epicentre more likely to be WNT mutated

17.11.1.2 Radiotherapy target definition

Because of their tendency to disseminate throughout the neuraxis, patients with medulloblastoma should be treated with craniospinal irradiation encompassing the whole of the meninges. Particular attention should be paid to the cribriform plate, the optic nerve reflection, the temporal lobe reflection, and any post-surgical meningocele. The inferior limit of the thecal sac (sacral cul-de-sac) should be defined individually using the MRI imaging of the spine. The boost usually consists of the whole

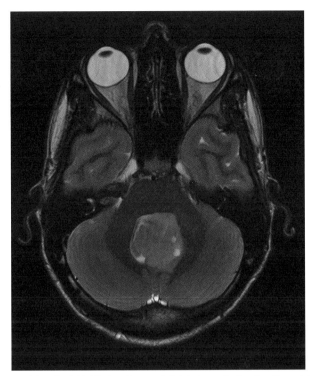

Fig. 17.11 T2-weighted axial MRI showing medulloblastoma in the fourth ventricular region.

of the posterior fossa, defined using fused MRI scan with the inferior border at C2/3 junction.

17.11.1.3 Follow-up of patients with embryonal tumours

Most patients are followed up by routine post-contrast MRI of the CNS axis every 3–6 months for five years and then annually.

17.12 Primary CNS lymphoma

PCNSL are usually B cell lymphomas, though T cell lesions are well recognized. They occur most commonly in the supratentorial white matter, usually in periventricular regions or in the deep grey matter nuclei. They may cross the corpus callosum, extending along ventricular ependyma and may be multifocal. Though normally occurring in older patients, PCNSL also occurs in patients with immunosuppression either from HIV-AIDS or post-transplantation, when they can appear more heterogeneous.

17.12.1 Imaging features

See Figures 17.12a and 17.12b.

- Usually enhances avidly and uniformly

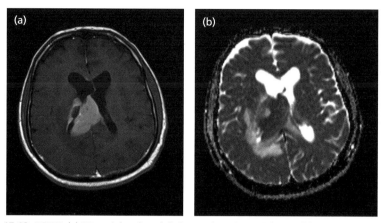

Fig. 17.12 PCNSL (a) T1-weighted gadolinium enhancing axial MRI. (b) ADC imaging.

- Necrosis or cyst formation rare unless immune-compromised
- High density on pre-contrast CT, and restricted diffusion on DWI MR—reflects tumour cellularity and packing
- Minor oedema for lesion size
- Calcification rare pre-treatment
- In immunocompromised patients the appearances are very different—often appearing as ring enhancing lesions

17.12.2 Radiotherapy target definition

The role of post-chemotherapy radiotherapy, particularly in older patients, is controversial because of concerns about late neurocognitive toxicity. However, when radiotherapy is delivered, the whole of the cranial meninges encompassing the optic nerve reflection, base of temporal lobes, and taking the inferior border to the C2/3 junction should be treated and any residual disease boosted with a margin of 1–2 cm.

17.12.3 Follow-up imaging following treatment for PCNSL

This is highly dependent on the clinical condition of the patient and if radiotherapy has been used. If it has been decided to defer radiotherapy then routine imaging every 3–6 months is usually performed to detect any asymptomatic recurrence at an early stage when radiotherapy maybe more effective.

17.13 Pineal lesions

Lesions in this region can either arise from the pineal parenchyma itself or represent metastases.

1) Pineoblastoma—embryonal lesions which can disseminate throughout the neuraxis.

2) Pineocytoma—relatively benign, slow-growing lesions.

3) Pineal tumour of intermediate differentiation.

4) Germ cell lesions (germinoma (akin to seminoma of testes), teratoma, yolk sac tumours, embryonal carcinoma, or choriocarcinoma). The pineal gland is the commonest site of intracranial germ cell tumours, though they can occur anywhere, most often in the midline.

17.13.1 Imaging features

17.13.1.1 Pineocytoma

◆ Well defined
◆ Generally, under 3 cm
◆ Homogeneous signal
◆ Avid homogeneous enhancement
◆ May be cystic and can resemble pineal cyst
◆ Obstructive hydrocephalus rare
◆ Pineal calcification pushed peripherally

17.13.1.2 Pineoblastoma

◆ Aggressive, heterogeneous appearance
◆ Generally, over 4 cm reflecting growth rate
◆ Infiltration into nearby structures
◆ Enhancement often only moderate
◆ Multi-cystic/necrotic change
◆ Obstructive hydrocephalus common
◆ Pineal calcification pushed peripherally

17.13.1.3 Germ cell tumours

See Figure 17.13.

◆ Germinoma—homogeneous and often low T2-weighted signal with avid homogeneous enhancement
◆ Calcification often remains central within tumour mass
◆ 'Mature' teratoma may show differentiation into fat and dense calcification

17.13.1.4 Radiotherapy target definition

Classically pineoblastoma and germ cell lesions disseminate throughout the CSF. They have been classically treated with craniospinal irradiation with a boost to the local tumour with a 1–2 cm margin. However, clinical trials have been conducted to establish whether or not equivalent results can be achieved with chemotherapy followed by more focal radiotherapy, but the final results are awaited.

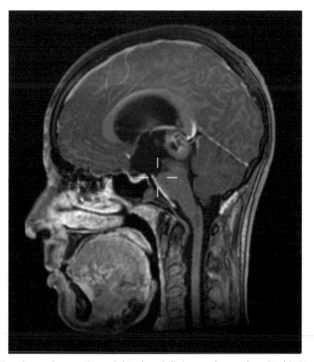

Fig. 17.13 Pineal germinoma T1-weighted gadolinium enhanced sagittal MRI.

17.13.1.5 Follow-up imaging for patients with pineal lesions

Most patients undergo craniospinal axis imaging every 3–6 months to detect recurrences which could be treated with chemotherapy.

17.14 Brain metastases

Secondary spread to the brain is common, with some autopsy series finding up to a quarter of cancer patients have intracranial spread. Classically, the commonest primary tumours to spread to the brain are lung (11% at initial diagnosis), renal, melanoma, and breast cancers. With better systemic local control, the brain is becoming a more frequent site of late relapse for patients.

For many years, whole brain radiotherapy was the mainstay of treatment for brain metastases, but concerns about neurotoxicity and efficacy have led to a reduction in its use. Focal treatment using stereotactic radiosurgery (SRS) has been shown to improve overall survival for patients with one metastasis and stabilize neurological function in those with up to four metastases. The use of SRS when more than four metastases are present is controversial and trials are ongoing for this group, comparing SRS with whole brain radiotherapy.

17.14.1 Imaging appearance

See Figure 17.14.

- Well defined lesions, sharp interface with brain parenchyma
- Usually located peripherally at grey-white junction
- Posterior fossa lesions common
- May be cystic, solid, or mixed
- Often provoke marked adjacent white matter oedema for lesion size
- Look carefully for subtle, additional lesions which may inform management

17.14.2 Radiotherapy target definition

For SRS, the GTV is delineated on a fused volumetric T1-weighted gadolinium enhanced MRI encompassing all areas of enhancement. The addition of a margin to create a CTV is debated; historically 1–3 mm were added but one study has suggested that this may not be required.

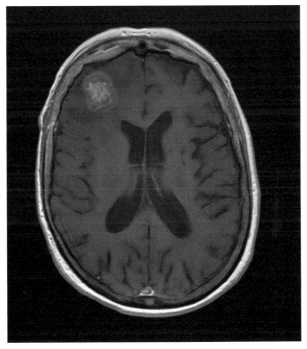

Fig. 17.14 Brain metastasis on T1-weighted gadolinium enhanced MRI.

17.15 **Extra-axial tumours**

17.15.1 Meningioma

These are the commonest extra-axial lesions, accounting for around 38% of all CNS tumours. They present most frequently in the fifth and sixth decades of life and are the only CNS lesion to occur more frequently in women. Most intracerebral meningiomas are associated with the falx cerebri or dura over the cerebral convexity, but they also occur around the orbit and base of skull. Spinal meningiomas are most common in the thoracic region.

The majority of meningiomas are WHO grade I lesions with a low mitotic rate, but around 20% are atypical (grade II) with increased cellularity and mitotic activity. Around 2% are malignant lesions (grade III) with fast growth rates. The presence of brain invasion is associated with reduced local control, so tumours with this are now classified as grade II or III.

17.15.1.1 Imaging features

See Figure 17.15.

- Well defined extra-axial mass
- Broad dural base
- CSF cleft between lesion and brain
- Inward displacement of cortical vessels

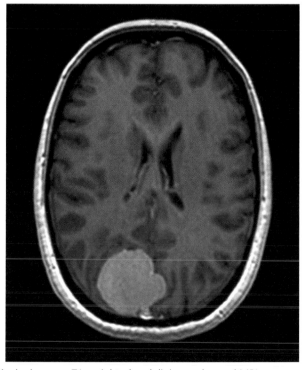

Fig. 17.15 Meningioma on T1-weighted gadolinium enhanced MRI.

- Uniform avid enhancement
- Adjacent bony hyperostosis
- Radial vessel 'spokes' within, from a point towards the base
- Parenchymal vasogenic oedema/white matter gliosis
- A 'tail' of enhancement may extend along the adjacent dura (non-specific)

17.15.1.2 Radiotherapy target definition

The GTV should consist of the enhancing tumour on T1-weighted MRI. The inclusion of the thickened enhancing dural tails and hyperostotic bone remains controversial, but they are usually included.[4] The margin for the CTV depends on the tumour grade, with grade I lesions treated with 0–3 mm margin, but grade II or III lesions a margin of 5–10 mm is added.

17.15.1.3 Follow-up imaging for meningioma

To detect recurrences when they are potentially amenable to salvage surgery most patients undergo MR imaging three months after surgery or six months after radiotherapy and then annually for three years for grade I lesions and five years for grade II lesions and then alternate years to ten years after treatment. Grade III lesions are usually imaged more frequently.

17.16 Tumours of the sellar region

There are three principal neoplastic lesions which occur at this location; pituitary adenomas, craniopharyngiomas, and meningiomas.

17.16.1 Pituitary adenomas

These benign lesions present either with hormonal effects or local symptoms such as visual disturbance. They are defined as either microadenomas (<1 cm) or macroadenomas (>1 cm). and can be functioning or non-functioning, dependent on clinical presentation and pituitary function results.

17.16.1.1 Imaging features

Pituitary microadenoma

- Intra-pituitary mass
- Enhance less rapidly than normal pituitary (i.e. hypointense on post-Gd imaging)
- Distortion of superior border of gland
- May be difficult or impossible to see despite biochemical abnormality

Pituitary macroadenoma
See Figure 17.16.

- Large sellar mass with suprasellar extension
- 'Cottage loaf' or 'snowman' appearance
- Usually enhance avidly
- May contain cysts or haemorrhage

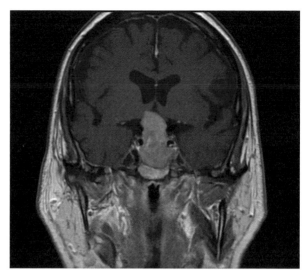

Fig. 17.16 Pituitary macroadenoma on T1-weighted gadolinium enhanced MRI.

♦ May invade cavernous sinuses, pituitary fossa floor

♦ Infundibular displacement away from epicentre of mass

♦ Suprasellar component may threaten chiasm

17.16.1.2 Radiotherapy target definition

Radiotherapy is usually offered to patients with an enlarging postoperative residuum or in whom surgery has not cured a functional lesion. The treatment should be planned using T1w gadolinium enhanced MRI scan using preoperative and postoperative images. The target for macroadenomas includes the whole of the pituitary fossa, paying particular attention to any areas of cavernous sinus invasion, and to the roof of the sphenoid sinus following trans-sphenoidal surgery.

For microadenomas it may be possible to target just the lesion but anatomical distortion following surgery can make this challenging.

17.16.2 **Craniopharyngiomas**

These occur mainly in children, but they may also diagnosed in adulthood. Patients present commonly with visual disturbance or hormonal problems (such as diabetes insipidus) but children may present with a non-specific cognitive change.

17.16.2.1 Imaging features

See Figure 17.17.

♦ Mixed cystic and solid mass centred on suprasellar cistern

♦ Enhancement of solid components and cyst walls

♦ Calcification occurs in 90%, best seen on CT

♦ The pituitary may be visible separate from the mass

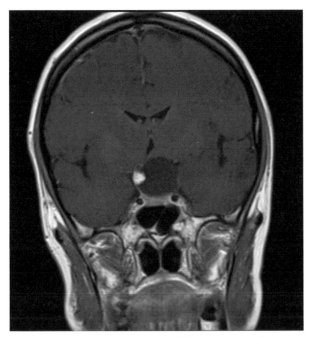

Fig. 17.17 Craniopharyngioma on T1-weighted gadolinium enhanced MRI (coronal section).

17.16.2.2 Radiotherapy target definition

Radiotherapy should be planned using a postoperative gadolinium enhanced T1w MRI. The GTV is any residual solid tumour and cyst. No margin is required for the CTV.

17.16.2.3 Follow-up imaging

Following radiotherapy, the cyst may enlarge so the patient should be followed carefully in the immediate post-treatment period and if they develop any new symptoms (such as reduced visual fields) an urgent MRI should be requested. In the absence of such symptoms patients usually have MRI imaging 3–4 months following radiotherapy and then annually.

17.17 Benign nerve sheath tumours of the CNS

Schwannomas are the most common lesions occurring on the cranial nerves, particularly the vestibulocochlear nerve ('vestibular schwannoma', also previously erroneously called acoustic neuroma) or the spinal nerves. There are seen more frequently in patients with neurofibromatosis 2 (NF2) for which vestibular schwannomas are considered pathognomonic if bilateral. Proper neurofibromas can occur on the spinal nerve roots but do not occur on the cranial nerves. These are connected with neurofibromatosis 1 (NF1). The presenting symptoms reflect the nerve involved, with, for example, patients with vestibular schwannoma presenting with dizziness and ipsilateral hearing loss.

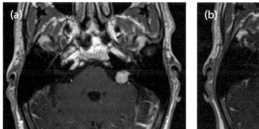
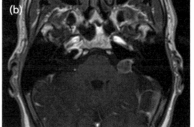

Fig. 17.18 Vestibular schwannoma (a) MRI before SRS. (b) MRI after SRS.

17.17.1 Imaging features

See Figure 17.18a (pre-SRS) and Figure 17.18b (post-SRS).

- Extra-axial mass centred on internal auditory canal (IAC)
- May be intracanalicular or extend into cerebellopontine angle cistern
- May expand IAC
- Avid uniform enhancement
- 'Ice cream cone' appearance typical
- Can extend to fundus and vestibulocochlear labyrinth

17.17.2 Radiotherapy target definition

Radiotherapy, delivered either as radiosurgery or a fractionated stereotactic radiotherapy is often used to treat schwannomas not amenable to surgical resection. The target should be defined on a T1-weighted contrast enhanced MRI scan with the GTV encompassing the enhancing lesion. Check the cochlear aperture and basal turn carefully. No CTV margin is required.

17.17.3 Follow-up imaging

These patients undergo annual MRI scanning for 5–10 years to detect recurrences which might be amenable to surgery. On follow-up imaging following stereotactic radiosurgery, around a third of lesions enlarge on the first post-treatment MRI and then the size stabilizes. Over time, lesions may be slow to reduce in size, but often develop central cystic change with corresponding with loss of enhancement.

17.18 Orbital lesions

A number of tumours or other lesions can occur in the orbits, potentially threatening sight. The most common lesions seen by an oncologist are:

17.18.1 Dysthyroid eye disease/thyroid orbitopathy

See Figure 17.19.

Swelling of the intra-orbital muscles (usually bilateral) associated with thyroid dysfunction. The extra-ocular muscle enlargement typically spares the tendinous

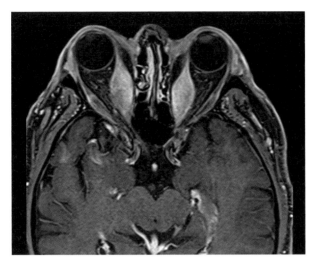

Fig. 17.19 Thyroid orbitopathy.

insertions. Proliferation of orbital fat is also usually seen. This condition is sometimes treated with radiotherapy where the ocular muscles are treated to reduce the inflammatory infiltrate.

17.18.2 Pseudo-tumour

These are usually asymmetrical or unilateral diffuse inflammatory change within the orbital tissues, which are often painful. The aetiology is unknown, but this can occasionally require radiotherapy if systemic treatments fail.

17.18.3 Orbital lymphoma

These usually involve unilateral swelling of the orbital tissues, including the adnexa/lacrimal glands. These lesions are often MALTomas or other types of non-Hodgkin lymphoma (NHL) as part of a systemic disease.

17.18.4 Metastases

These occur either to the soft tissues, resulting in proptosis or diplopia, or choroid, producing reduced visual acuity and eventually blindness. These are treated palliatively, encompassing the orbit either unilaterally or bilaterally depending on the patient's general condition and previous treatment.

17.18.5 Meningioma

This can affect either the optic nerve or an extension of a parasellar lesion. These can be successfully treated with radiotherapy, sometimes with improvement of vision. The classical description of optic nerve meningioma radiologically is of a 'tram track' appearance.

Further reading

NICE guideline [NG99] Brain tumours (primary and brain metastases in adults https://www.nice.org.uk/guidance/ng99

References

1. **Niyazi M, Brada M, Chalmers AJ,** (2016). ESTRO-ACROP guideline 'target delineation of glioblastomas'. *Radiotherapy & Onco*logy, **118**(1): 35–42.
2. **Louis DN, Perry A, Reifenberger G, et al.** (2016). The 2016 World Health Organization Classification of Tumors of the Central Nervous System: a summary. *Acta Neuropathology*, **131**(6): 803–820.
3. **Weber DC, Wang Y, Miller R, et al.** (2015). Long-term outcome of patients with spinal myxopapillary ependymoma: treatment results from the MD Anderson Cancer Center and institutions from the Rare Cancer Network. *Neuro-oncology*, **17**(4): 588–595.
4. **Maclean J, Fersht N, Short S** (2014). Controversies in radiotherapy for meningioma. *Clinical Oncology* (Royal College of Radiologists), **26**(1): 51–64.

Chapter 18

Soft tissue sarcomas

Morag Brothwell, Sarah Prewett, Gail Horan,
and Emma-Louise Gerety

18.1 Introduction

Soft (connective) tissue sarcomas are a rare, heterogeneous group of malignancies constituting less than 1% of all adult cancers. There are over 50 different histological subtypes according to the 2013 World Health Organization classification, with pleomorphic sarcoma, liposarcoma, leiomyosarcoma, synovial sarcoma, and malignant peripheral nerve sheath tumours accounting for over 75% cases.

They can arise almost anywhere in the body, but approximately 75% affect the extremities (legs > arms), with other common sites being the trunk wall, retroperitoneum, and head and neck. The dominant pattern of metastatic spread is haematogenous to the lungs, and less commonly bone and liver. Lymphatic spread is rare, but may be more common in certain subtypes such as epithelioid and synovial sarcomas.

The mainstay of radical treatment includes radiotherapy and surgery, the order depending on factors such as the site and histology of the primary. Biopsy of suspected soft tissue sarcoma should be planned and performed at a specialist sarcoma centre, so that the biopsy site can be marked and the tract then incorporated into the surgery and/or radiotherapy field, minimizing the risk of seeding. This chapter will discuss the different imaging modalities involved in the diagnosis, staging, response to treatment, and follow-up for soft tissue sarcomas, with an emphasis on those arising in the extremities or superficial tissues.

18.2 Diagnosis and staging

Ultrasound (US) and magnetic resonance imaging (MRI) are the most important imaging modalities for characterizing soft tissue lesions. However, radiographs, computed tomography (CT) and positron emission tomography (PET)/CT using 18-fluoride labelled fluorodeoxyglucose (FDG) can all play a role in diagnosis and staging (Table 18.1). Superficial sarcomas such as angiosarcomas may have significant skin involvement, often best appreciated clinically, and in these cases photography and clinical assessment are also crucial.

Table 18.1 The use of different imaging modalities in the diagnosis, staging, and follow-up of patients with soft tissue sarcomas

Imaging modality	Location of soft tissue lesion	
	Extremity/superficial layers of the trunk/head and neck	**Deep thorax/abdomen/pelvis**
Ultrasound (with Doppler)	First-line imaging	May be first-line imaging (pelvis)
MRI	Definitive imaging/follow-up	First-line/definitive imaging/follow-up
CT	Staging/follow-up	May be first-line imaging/staging/follow-up
[18F]-FDG-PET	Staging/follow-up	Staging/follow-up
Radiograph	Staging (lung metastases), follow-up	Staging (lung metastases), follow-up

Imaging is important for determining the size of the primary and categorizing it as superficial or deep, detection of lymph node involvement and distant metastases. The stage grouping (I–IV) then incorporates TNM staging and histological grade.

Source: data from Sobin LH, Gospodarowicz MK, Wittekind CH (2017). *UICC TNM Classification of Malignant Tumours* (eighth edn). Oxford: Wiley Blackwell.

18.2.1 Ultrasound

US utilizes subtle differences in acoustic impedance of different soft tissues to ultra-high frequency sounds waves. US is recommended for first-line evaluation of soft tissue masses in the trunk wall and extremities and also for investigation of female pelvic masses.

Tumours are measured in three planes to assess their size and precise location, in addition to their internal sonographic characteristics. Additional use of Doppler US allows evaluation of the vascularity of the tumour and involvement of adjacent vessels (Figure 18.1). There is some evidence that contrast-enhanced Doppler ultrasound may be more sensitive than Doppler ultrasound alone in determining hypervascularity and the likelihood of malignancy.

Dynamic US (scanning whilst the patient moves) can help assess tumours of the distal extremities and their relationship with tendons and small muscles of the hand.

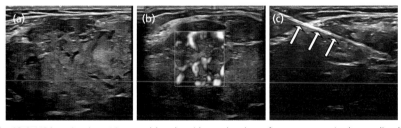

Fig. 18.1 US imaging in a 19-year-old male with an alveolar soft part tumour in the popliteal fossa. B-mode grey-scale US image (a) of the popliteal fossa mass and corresponding Doppler US (b) demonstrates hypervascularity within the mass. US-guided core biopsy of the mass (c) shows the hyper-echoic, linear biopsy needle (arrows) within the mass.

The initial US may rule out the need for further investigation if the findings strongly support a benign process such as a lipoma or a simple cyst. Caution and close follow-up may be needed with the interpretation of trauma-related haematoma to ensure that it is not due to haemorrhagic sarcoma.

Lipomatous lesions appear hyperechoic (brighter) on US, whereas fluid and fresh blood appear anechoic (dark), with posterior acoustic enhancement (a brighter shadow deep to the lesion). Sonographic features of concern for malignancy include a maximum diameter >7 cm (for lipomatous lesions), hypervascularity, heterogeneity, and involvement of the deep tissues. Clinical features are also important, such as pain or rapid growth. In these situations, further characterization with MRI is required.

Biopsies are usually US-guided for superficial masses and CT-guided for deep, intra-abdominal masses. Endoscopic US may be used to biopsy lesions close to the bronchi, oesophagus, or distal bowel. Uterine masses are usually biopsied via hysteroscopy under direct visualization. Although rarely required, echocardiograms can be used to characterize soft tissue sarcomas arising from the myocardium or pericardium and assess their effect on cardiac function.

Although very useful as an initial and rapid investigation, there are limitations of US as a modality. These include reduced resolution with increased lesion depth and significant inter-operator variability. Therefore, if US is concerning for malignancy, or the deep extent of the lesion cannot be completely determined, MRI is performed.

18.2.2 Magnetic resonance imaging

MRI provides definitive imaging for both superficial and deep soft tissue tumours which have been demonstrated by US or CT. Table 18.2 shows the different MRI sequences commonly used for imaging of soft tissue sarcomas.

MRI is performed in at least two planes, according the location and shape of the mass (Figure 18.2). T1-weighted images and fat suppressed T2-weighted images are acquired first. The T1-weighted image is used for the assessment of fat content; fat is high signal (bright) and water is low signal (dark). Non-lipomatous tumour and muscle typically have a similar intermediate T1-weighted signal and are difficult to differentiate.

On T2-weighted images, fat, water, and cellular material all have high signal. Fat suppression can be applied, using techniques such as spectral fat saturation or short T1 inversion recovery (STIR). On fat saturated T2-weighted sequences, water is of high

Table 18.2 MRI sequences for characterization of soft tissue sarcomas

Sequence	Demonstrates
T1-weighted	Fat (also blood products, melanin, high protein content fluid)
T2-weighted with fat saturation (fs)	Fluid (fat signal suppressed)
T1-weighted fs post IV gadolinium	Enhancement of vascular/solid masses; non-enhancement of fluid—differentiation of cystic areas

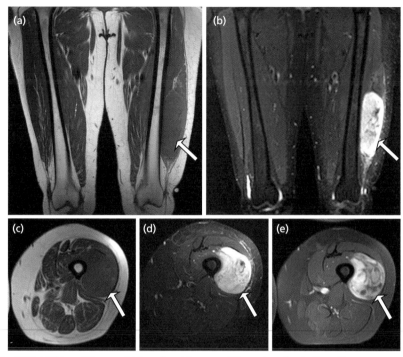

Fig. 18.2 MRI in a 63-year-old female with an undifferentiated spindle cell/
pleiomorphic sarcoma (arrow) in the vastus lateralis muscle. Coronal T1-weighted image
(a) demonstrates the mass as isointense to muscle with no internal fat signal. Coronal
T2-weighted fat saturated image (b) demonstrates the lesion is of heterogeneous, high
fluid-sensitive signal. Corresponding axial T1-weighted (c), axial T2 fat saturated (d) and
axial T1 fat saturated post IV gadolinium (e) images.

signal (bright). It may not be possible to determine whether the high signal is due to
high intra-cellular water content in a solid lesion or cyst.

Intravenous para-magnetic contrast agents containing gadolinium can be administered which will be preferentially distributed to vascular structures, such as solid
sarcomas, inflammatory lesions, and normal structures such as synovium. If the initial
MRI shows that the lesion is of high T1-weighted signal, the lesion contains fat and
gadolinium is not required.

If the lesion is of high T2-weighted signal, it may not be clear whether this represents water or high water-containing cellular material. Therefore, fat suppressed
T1-weighted pre- and post-intravenous gadolinium images may be acquired. Of note
there is growing concern that the gadolinium used in MRI leads to long-term gadolinium deposition in the brain, liver, and skin, the consequences of which are unknown. Long-term data is needed, but the potential risks of intravenous gadolinium
are currently outweighed by the benefit of accurate diagnosis and follow-up.

MRI allows determination of the size, character, location, and involvement of surrounding structures and fascial planes. MRI characteristics are similar for many

histological subtypes of soft tissue sarcoma. They are typically heterogeneous masses composed of cellular, myxoid, necrotic, and/or haemorrhagic components. Contrast enhancement is often more pronounced in the cellular tumour periphery. They may be lobulated and have septations and they can exert pressure on surrounding structures. They also have a tendency to grow along fascial planes on a path of least resistance. Biopsy and clinical correlation are always needed for a definitive diagnosis, which allows determination of the sarcoma subtype and grade; both important prognostic indicators.

Despite the similar MRI-characteristics seen across many histological subtypes of sarcoma, there are some specific imaging features which are associated with particular sarcoma subtypes, such as fat content, cerebral metastases, lymph node metastases, and anatomical location. These are considered separately below. Calcification and bone involvement are best appreciated on CT and are covered later in the chapter.

18.2.2.1 Fat content

Fat shows a high signal intensity on T1- and T2-weighted MRI but loss of signal on fat-suppressed images (Figure 18.3). Soft tissue sarcomas that typically contain fat include the adipocytic subtypes: well-differentiated, dedifferentiated, pleomorphic, and myxoid liposarcomas. The differential for a fat-containing lesion also includes benign lesions such as lipoma, haemangioma, or teratoma. Well-differentiated liposarcomas are often oval, round, or lobulated. At MRI, the amount of fat generally corresponds to the degree of differentiation, with dedifferentiated liposarcomas containing less, or sometimes no discernible fat on MRI. The presence of septations or solid enhancing elements may suggest dedifferentiation.

18.2.2.2 Anatomical location

Anatomical location may provide clues as to the sarcoma subtype. Sarcomas which tend to be superficially located include myxofibrosarcoma, angiosarcoma, epithelioid sarcoma, leiomyosarcoma, and epithelioid haemangioendothelioma. Subtypes associated with tendons include synovial sarcoma, clear cell sarcoma, and epithelioid sarcoma. Synovial sarcomas are typically multilobulated, septated masses of the extremities, often found in the deep soft tissues around the knee and adjacent to joints and tendon sheaths. Peripheral nerve sheath tumours (PNSTs) tend to be fusiform masses with tapered ends, continuous with a nerve and possibly associated with muscular atrophy. In contrast to benign PNSTs, malignant lesions tend to be larger, with more ill-defined margins and surrounding oedema.

Retroperitoneal sarcomas are most commonly found to be liposarcomas or leiomyosarcomas. Retroperitoneal leiomyosarcomas may appear on imaging as a large, heterogeneous, necrotic mass contiguous with a vessel (usually the inferior vena cava below the level of the hepatic veins). Uterine leiomyosarcomas are commonly large infiltrating myometrial masses with low-intermediate signal intensity on T1-weighted images and high signal on T2-weighted images. Although a detailed consideration of retroperitoneal and uterine sarcomas is outside the scope of this chapter, diffusion weighted imaging in MRI may be useful in differentiating uterine leiomyomas from leiomyosarcomas.

18.2.2.3 Lymph node metastasis

Lymph node metastasis is rare but can occur in epithelioid sarcoma, synovial sarcoma, rhabdomyosarcoma, clear cell sarcoma, and angiosarcoma. This may be evaluated on

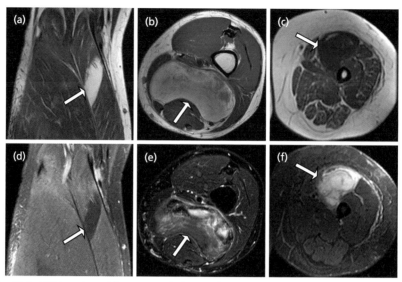

Fig. 18.3 MRI imaging of lipomatous lesions with T1 weighted, fat-sensitive images (a, b, c) and T2-weighted water-sensitive, fat suppressed images (d, e, f). Coronal images (a, d) of a benign, intramuscular lipoma (arrow) in the medial gastrocnemius of a 58-year-old male with complete loss of signal on fat suppressed images. Axial images (b, e) of a low grade, well differentiated liposarcoma (arrow) in the posterior thigh of a 50-year-old male with partial fat, partial water-sensitive signal. Axial images (c, f) of a myxoid liposarcoma (arrow) in the anterior thigh of a 60-year-old female with minimal fat-sensitive signal and high T2-weighted signal.

the MRI if local lymph node groups are included in the field of view, but are better assessed by a staging CT.

18.2.2.4 Central nervous system metastasis

Clear cell sarcoma, alveolar soft part sarcoma, angiosarcoma, and myxoid liposarcoma are at greatest risk of CNS spread and may warrant MRI of the head as part of staging. T1-weighted images post intravenous gadolinium are acquired as there is little fat in the brain and so enhancement is not obscured by fat signal (Figure 18.4).

18.2.3 Computed tomography

High resolution, isotropic CT images are acquired which can be reformatted in the coronal and sagittal planes. Lesions in the thorax, abdomen, or pelvis may be discovered on CT performed to investigate symptoms when there is no palpable mass (Figure 18.5). Significant findings are usually then evaluated with MRI.

CT may be helpful in characterization of primary lesions which are calcified or eroding adjacent bone and also in patients in whom MRI is contraindicated. Calcification often arises in a chronic, benign lesion but can also be seen in soft tissue sarcomas. It is best appreciated on CT or radiograph. It occurs most commonly in liposarcomas, undifferentiated pleomorphic sarcomas, and synovial sarcomas. Calcification in a liposarcoma

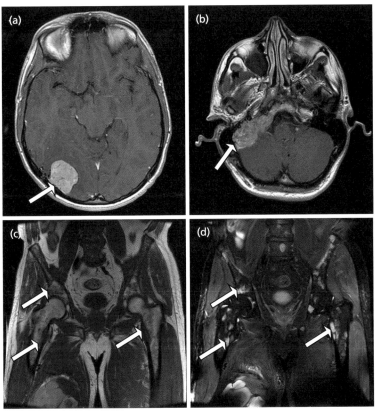

Fig. 18.4 MRI detection of metastases. Axial T1-weighted contrast enhanced images showing (a) brain metastasis (arrow) and (b) dural metastasis (arrow) in a 19-year-old male with alveolar soft part tumour in the popliteal fossa. Coronal T1-weighted (c) and coronal T2-weighted fat saturated (d) image of multiple femoral and pelvic bone metastases (arrows) in a 24-year-old male with synovial sarcoma in the thigh. The metastases replace the normal fatty marrow and return low T1-weighted signal and high T2-weighted signal compared to normal bone marrow.

can be large and coarse and may represent dedifferentiation with poor prognosis (Figure 18.5) but can also indicate inflammatory or sclerosing variants of well differentiated liposarcomas. Calcification in synovial sarcomas can be fine and stippled.

Bone may be eroded by pressure effect of a high-grade tumour growing in a confined space, or by direct invasion (Figure 18.5). This is associated with higher grade sarcomas and is most typically seen in dedifferentiated liposarcoma, undifferentiated pleomorphic rhabdomyosarcomas, and synovial sarcomas.

CT is routinely used for staging of soft tissue sarcoma, usually scanning the chest, abdomen, and pelvis (Figure 18.6). Lung is the most common site of metastasis and pulmonary metastases are present in around 10% of patients at presentation. CT thorax without intravenous contrast detects lung metastases which are dense compared to the low-density, air-filled normal pulmonary tissues. Liver metastases may

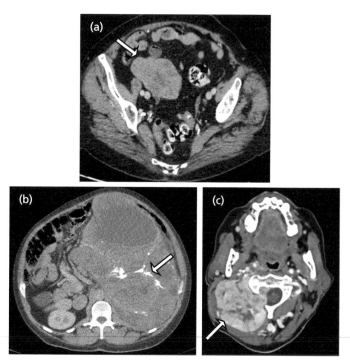

Fig. 18.5 CT characterization of primary soft tissue sarcomas. Axial CT post IV contrast medium (a) in the portal venous phase in an 83-year-old female showing a heterogeneous, soft tissue mass in the pelvis (arrow), likely originating from the right ovary, histologically a leiomyosarcoma. Axial CT post iv contrast medium (b) in the portal venous phase in a 53-year-old male showing a large, retroperitoneal, heterogeneous mass with internal calcified septations (arrow), histologically a dedifferentiated liposarcoma. Axial CT post IV contrast medium (c) of a solitary fibrous tumour in an 89-year-old female. There is a large, heterogeneous mass in the right neck (arrow), with destruction of the right posterior arch of the C1 vertebra and extending into the spinal canal.

not be demonstrated without IV contrast medium, without which they may be of similar density to liver parenchyma. Lung metastases may be nodular, cavitating, or have a ground glass 'halo' appearance if there is surrounding haemorrhage, characteristic of lung metastases from epithelioid angiosarcoma (Figure 18.6).

18.2.4 Radiographs

Radiographs remain important in oncological imaging as they are easily obtained, inexpensive, and quick to acquire. Those sarcomas that become calcified may be first detected by radiograph. Even a non-calcified, large soft tissue mass will be evident on a radiograph although it is usually difficult to precisely localize the mass on the 2D image. For low-grade sarcomas with a low risk of metastasis, a chest radiograph alone may be used to screen for lung metastases (Figure 18.7). Occasionally chest symptoms may the first presentation. Radiographs are also used as a simple screen for bone metastases if patients develop significant bone pain.

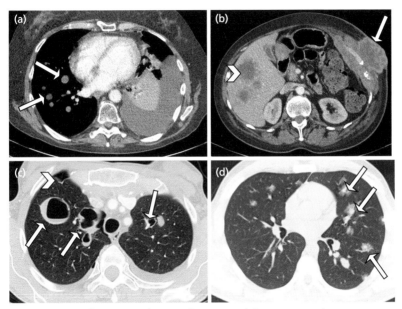

Fig. 18.6 Detection of metastases by CT. Pulmonary nodular metastases (a, arrows; mediastinal windowing) and liver metastases (b, arrowhead; abdominal windowing) and left rib synovial sarcoma recurrence (arrow) in a 24-year-old female. Cavitating lung metastases (c, arrows; lung windowing) with a small pneumothorax (arrowhead) in a 56-year-old female with endometrial stromal sarcoma. Solid/ground glass metastases (d, arrows; lung windowing) in a 29-year-old male with an epithelioid angiosarcoma in the deltoid muscle.

18.2.5 Nuclear imaging

Nuclear imaging uses radionuclides attached to molecules (radiolabelling with tracers) which are injected intravenously prior to imaging. This radioactivity is subsequently detected and then reported as SUV: standard uptake value. There are a variety of different radioactive tracers in use but FDG is most often used in soft tissue sarcoma imaging and is taken up by metabolically active tissues.

There is currently no routine role for FDG PET/CT in the diagnosis and staging of soft tissue sarcomas, but it may be useful in certain circumstances. Many soft tissue sarcomas are FDG-avid, but uptake is variable. FDG PET/CT can usually distinguish benign tumours from high-grade soft tissue sarcomas, but cannot reliably distinguish them from low or intermediate grade sarcomas. One notable exception is malignant PNSTs, which show consistently high uptake in contrast to benign PNSTs, with a high sensitivity and specificity for malignant change (Figure 18.8).

Small-scale studies and retrospective analyses of mixed soft tissue sarcoma subtypes suggest that SUV_{max} may correlate with the probability of recurrence and prognosis and that variation in SUV can provide information about the heterogeneity of the tumour which might be of use at biopsy. With the exception of malignant PNSTs, there is only a small proportion of cases in which FDG PET/CT can add value to the staging and follow-up in patients with soft tissue sarcomas. This is likely because the typical pattern of spread is haematogenous to the lungs and CT chest is currently very

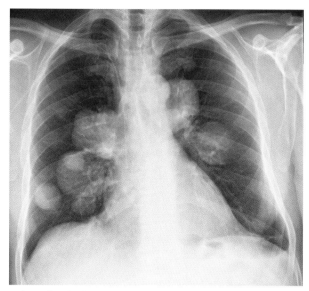

Fig. 18.7 Detection of multiple pulmonary metastases by chest radiograph of a 24-year-old male with synovial sarcoma in the thigh.

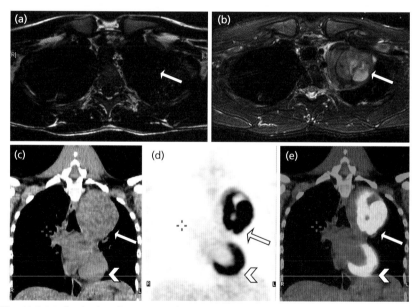

Fig. 18.8 Mediastinal malignant peripheral nerve sheath tumour (arrow) in a 25-year-old male. Axial T1-weighted MRI (a) shows no fat within the lesion. Axial T2-weighted fat saturated MRI (b) shows water content of the lesion. Coronal non-contrast CT (c), FDG PET (d) and fused FDG PET/CT image (e) shows tumour uptake with background uptake also in the heart (arrowhead).

sensitive for pulmonary metastases. There is therefore inadequate evidence that the adoption of routine FDG PET/CT would significantly alter management or prognosis.

In line with the above findings, the Royal College of Radiologists (RCR) gave guidance (2016) for indications for FDG PET/CT for soft tissue sarcoma as certain high-grade soft tissue sarcomas, such as pleomorphic undifferentiated sarcomas, rhabdomyosarcomas, leiomyosarcomas, synovial sarcomas, and myxoid liposarcomas with FDG PET/CT in search of metastatic disease not seen on staging CT thorax. The guidance also supports the use of FDG PET/CT in distinguishing MPNSTs from benign neuromas in patients with neurofibromatosis type 1. The UK guidelines for soft tissue sarcoma (2016) adds that FDG PET/CT may be particularly useful in situations in which extra-thoracic metastases would change management significantly, for example prior to an amputation (Figure 18.9).

Whole body bone scintigraphy with 99m-technetium-methyldiphosphonate is not commonly used in the management of soft tissue sarcomas, due to the relative rarity of bone metastases. However, 18F-NaF PET/CT has shown some promise in the detection of skeletal metastases in bone and soft tissue sarcoma which is an area for future investigation.

18.3 **Vascular imaging and interventional radiology**

CT and MR angiography (CTA and MRA) are rarely performed but can be useful in determining the vascular anatomy around a lesion for the purpose of embolization and surgical planning. In general, CTA has a better spatial resolution and lower cost compared to MRA (Figure 18.10). Given that the majority of soft tissue sarcoma metastases

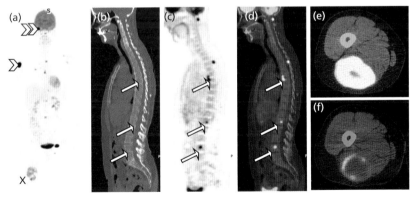

Fig. 18.9 A 60-year-old female with spindle cell sarcoma in the posterior right thigh. FDG PET MIP image (a) demonstrates the right thigh primary lesion (X) and metastases (arrowheads). Background uptake also noted in the brain, heart, bowel and renal system. Sagittal CT image of the spine (b), corresponding FDG PET (c) and fused PET/CT (d) image shows uptake in lesions in the T6/7, L1, L4 vertebral bodies; posterior elements of the T4 vertebral body; and skull base. Axial FDG PET/CT image (e) of the right thigh lesion and three months later (f) shows reduced FDG uptake and only at the periphery of the necrotic mass post radiotherapy.

are in the lung, and this is an area that lends itself well to radiofrequency ablation. There are a number of series demonstrating the acceptability and good local control rates allowed by this technique, but larger scale, randomized studies are needed.

18.4 **Response to treatment**

Response to treatment may be assessed following primary chemotherapy or radiotherapy or following the definitive surgery as a baseline prior to routine follow-up. This is usually assessed with MRI. Following radiotherapy, the size of the sarcoma may increase due to necrosis and there may be local oedema. The size may conversely decrease following radiotherapy (Figure 18.11). Small-scale studies have suggested that FDG PET/CT may be useful in evaluating response to chemotherapy and radiotherapy, but further studies are needed for clarification.

18.5 **Follow-up**

A combination of clinical assessment, radiograph, CT, and MRI is used during follow-up to assess for recurrence, which can be in the form of local or distant metastatic disease.

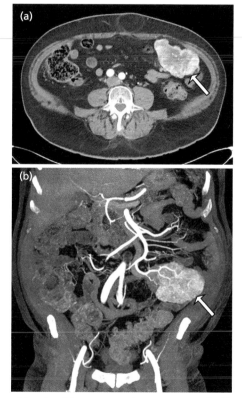

Fig. 18.10 A 61-year-old male with a mesenteric sarcoma supplied by a large hypertrophied ileal branch arising from the main trunk of the superior mesenteric artery. CT angiography images in the arterial phase in axial (a) and coronal (b) planes demonstrate the enhancing tumour and feeding vessels.

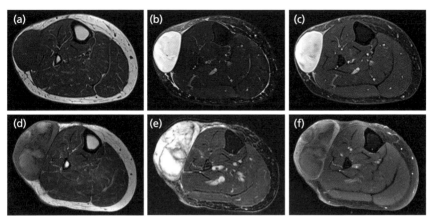

Fig. 18.11 T1-weighted axial (a, d), T2-weighted fat saturated axial (b, e) and T1-weighted post contrast fast-saturated axial MRI images (c, f) of a myxofibrosarcoma in the lateral lower leg in a 69-year-old female pre- (a–c) and post- (d–e) radiotherapy. Whereas the sarcoma initially enhances almost homogenously post IV gadolinium, following radiotherapy there is central necrosis with central, non-enhancing fluid, and only residual peripheral enhancing sarcoma.

The choice of imaging depends on the risk of recurrence, the age of the patient (in view of the risks of secondary malignancy from radiation), and the site of the primary.

18.5.1 Local recurrence

Recurrence following radical treatment is usually nodular, with signal characteristics of the original sarcoma. MRI post intravenous gadolinium can aid differentiation of recurrence from post-surgical changes such as scarring, infection, or fluid collections (Figure 18.12). FDG PET/CT can also be useful in addition to MRI if the primary was known to have a high SUV, and as a problem-solving tool with MRI to investigate

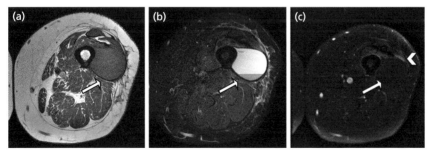

Fig. 18.12 T1-weighted axial (a), T2-weighted fat saturated axial (b), and T1-weighted post contrast fast-saturated axial (c). MRI images demonstrate post-surgical change in this 60-year-old female following surgical excision of a spindle cell/pleiomorphic sarcoma in the vastus lateralis muscle. There is a postoperative seroma (arrow). Anteriorly, a small focus of enhancement post IV gadolinium is concerning for local recurrence (arrowhead).

equivocal cases. There should be interval imaging of the primary site (in general this is MRI for primaries of the extremity and CT for primaries of the trunk).

18.5.2 Metastatic disease

A chest radiograph may be sufficient to screen for pulmonary metastases in low-risk disease or elderly patients, but a CT thorax may be preferable for high-risk histology or following a pulmonary metastatectomy.

18.6 Summary

- US, CT, and MRI all play a major role in the investigation of soft tissue sarcomas, with MRI the most influential in terms of diagnosis, treatment planning, and follow-up.
- Biopsy is always needed to determine histological subtype and grade.
- Further studies will clarify the role of FDG PET/CT in the diagnosis and staging of soft tissue sarcomas.

Further reading

Amini B, Jessop A, Ganeshan D, Tseng W, Madewell J (2014). Contemporary imaging of soft tissue sarcomas. *Journal of Surgical Oncology*, **111**(5): 496–503. https://doi.org/10.1002/jso.23801

Chee D, Peh W, Shek T (2011). Pictorial essay: imaging of peripheral nerve sheath tumours. *Canadian Association Radiologists Journal*, **62**(3): 176–182.

Dangoor A, Seddon B, Gerrand C, Grimer R, Whelan J, Judson I (2016). UK guidelines for the management of soft tissue sarcomas. *Clinical Sarcoma Research*, **6**(1): 20. doi:10.1186/s13569-016-0060-4.

De Baere T, Tselikas L, Gravel G, et al. (2018). Interventional radiology: role in the treatment of sarcomas. *European Journal of Cancer*, **97**: 148–155.

De La Hoz Polo M, Dick E, Bhumbra R, Pollock R, Sandhu R, Saifuddin A (2017). Surgical considerations when reporting MRI studies of soft tissue sarcoma of the limbs. *Skeletal Radiology*, **46**(12): 1667–1678.

Jackson T, Mosci C, von Eyben R, et al. (2015). Combined 18F-NaF and 18F-FDG PET/CT in the evaluation of sarcoma patients. *Clinical Nuclear Medicine*, **40**(9): 720–724.

Levy A, Manning M, Al-Refaie W, Miettinen M (2017). Soft-tissue sarcomas of the abdomen and pelvis: radiologic-pathologic features, Part 1—Common sarcomas: from the Radiologic Pathology Archives. *RadioGraphics*, **37**(2): 462–483. doi:10.1148/rg.2017160157

Messiou C, Moskovic E, Vanel D, et al. (2017). Primary retroperitoneal soft tissue sarcoma: Imaging appearances, pitfalls and diagnostic algorithm. *European Journal of Surgical Oncology*, **43**(7): 1191–1198.

Roberge D, Vakilian S, Alabed Y, Turcotte R, Freeman C, Hickeson M (2012). FDG PET/CT in initial staging of adult soft-tissue sarcoma. *Sarcoma*, 2012: 1–7.

Sobin LH, Gospodarowicz MK, Wittekind CH (2017). *UICC TNM Classification of Malignant Tumours* (eighth edn). Oxford: Wiley Blackwell.

van Vliet M, Kliffen M, Krestin G, van Dijke C (2009). Soft tissue sarcomas at a glance: clinical, histological, and MR imaging features of malignant extremity soft tissue tumors. *European Radiology*, **19**(6): 1499–1511. https://doi.org/10.1007/s00330-008-1292-3

Chapter 19

Endocrine tumours

Luigi Aloj

19.1 Introduction

The endocrine system includes not only the discrete endocrine glands but also the diffuse endocrine systems of the gut, respiratory tract, heart, and endothelium. Endocrine tumours are rare, and range from well-differentiated indolent tumours to poorly-differentiated aggressive malignancies. Thyroid carcinoma, the most common endocrine gland malignancy, is discussed in separately (chapter 16). This chapter deals with neuroendocrine neoplasms, and tumours of the adrenal medulla and adrenal cortex.

19.2 Neuroendocrine neoplasms

Nomenclature of these rare tumours has been varied over time and still is somewhat confusing, with overlapping synonymous definitions for carcinoids, APUDomas, argentaffin tumours, and tumours of the diffuse endocrine system.[1] Pearse et al. first described several apparently disparate cell series in the body such as adrenomedullary chromaffin cells, enterochromaffin cells, the corticotroph, the melanotroph, the pancreatic islet B cell, and the thyroid C cell, which all share common cytochemical and ultrastructural properties including amine precursor uptake and decarboxylase (APUD) activity within the cells.[2] A generic name—APUD cells—was later proposed for these cells and its list has since expanded. The structural and chemical similarity of APUD cells to neurons suggested a neural crest origin and these cells are distributed throughout the body, where they are all prone to both hyperplasia and neoplasia. More recently the term 'neuroendocrine neoplasms' has been adopted for these tumours, which are then classified based on clinical features, histology, and proliferation into well-differentiated (low and intermediate grade tumours) and poorly-differentiated (high grade) neuroendocrine carcinomas. Most literature focuses also on anatomic subtypes (i.e. gastroenteropancreatic, pulmonary, etc.). Reference to old nomenclature is, however, still quite common in clinical practice. Currently, these tumours are usually classified on the basis of their topographical location as foregut (arising from thymus, lung, stomach, duodenum, and pancreas), midgut (jejunum, ileum, and ascending colon), and hindgut tumours (arising from distal colon and rectum).

19.2.1 Neuroendocrine neoplasms of the pancreas

19.2.1.1 Clinical background

Pancreatic neuroendocrine tumours (PNETs) are rare and typically functioning tumours, producing excessive amounts of specific hormones.[3,4] Patients may present with characteristic symptoms suggesting the possibility of a particular tumour type. Insulinoma is probably the most common tumour (incidence 1 per million per year) and usually has hypoglycaemia as the presenting symptom.

Other tumour subtypes include gastrinomas, glucagonomas, VIPomas, and somatostatinomas. Gastrinomas produce high levels of gastrin which stimulates the secretion of excessive gastric acid leading to ulcers and diarrhoea (Zollinger-Ellison syndrome). Glucagonomas produce excessive glucagon and lead to hyperglycaemia, which causes frequent urination, increased thirst, increased hunger, and a rash that spreads on the face, abdomen, or lower extremities (necrolytic migratory erythema). VIPomas produce vasoactive intestinal peptide (VIP), a hormone that plays a role in intestinal water transport and causes chronic, watery diarrhoea, low serum potassium, low gastric hydrochloric acid, flushing, fatigue, and nausea. Somatostatinomas produce somatostatin, a hormone that inhibits the secretion of several other hormones such as growth hormone, insulin, and gastrin. Thus it can produce type II diabetes, gallstones, steatorrhoea, diarrhoea, weight loss, and lower gastric hydrochloric acid secretion. Functioning tumours also include PPomas (watery diarrhoea syndrome or absence of clinical symptoms), GRFoma (acromegaly due to ectopic secretion of GH-releasing factor) and ACTHoma (ectopic ACTH, Cushing's syndrome). These are all relatively rare, and overlap with non-pancreatic gut-derived neuroendocrine tumours with and without carcinoid syndrome.[3]

Non-functioning tumours make up the majority of islet cell tumours. They produce none of the hormones and thus present with no characteristic clinical syndromes as already mentioned. As a result, they are typically diagnosed at more advanced stages of disease. Approximately 90% of insulinomas are benign, but the percentage is considerably less for gastrinomas. Between 8% insulinomas and 20–25% glucagonomas, and gastrinomas are associated with multiple endocrine neoplasia type-1 (MEN-1) syndrome, where they are multicentric and all have a capacity for metastatic spread. The prognosis and survival of patients with gastroenteropancreatic neuroendocrine tumours (GEP-NETs) are related to pathological features, including tumour differentiation, Ki-67 index, tumour size, invasion, and the presence of metastases.[3,4]

19.2.1.2 Diagnosis and staging

Diagnosis is usually established following clinical suspicion, serum tests, and imaging. Serum tests include gut hormone profile and other relevant endocrine tests, in particular plasma chromogranin A, a useful marker in all these tumours. Computed tomography (CT) or magnetic resonance imaging (MRI) and endoscopic ultrasound (EUS) play an important role in locating the primary tumour and detecting metastases.[5] Scintigraphy with radiolabelled somatostatin analogue ^{111}In-octreotide has a sensitivity of 82–95% for detecting islet-cell tumours and

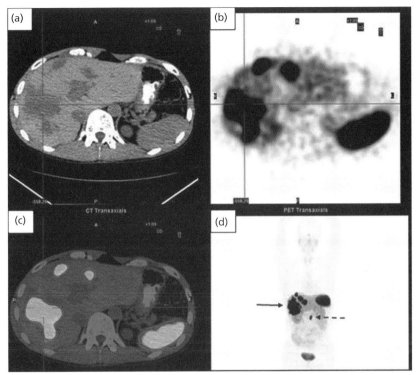

Fig. 19.1 A 35-year-old male patient with known metastatic pancreatic NET. PET/CT scan illustrates Ga-68-octreotide avid multiple liver metastases (arrow) and a pre-aortic node (dash arrow). (a), (b), and (c) are CT, PET, and PET/CT fused axial tomographic images respectively.

their metastases (80% of gastrinomas, glucagonomas, and VIPomas, and 60% of insulinomas). The introduction of Ga-68 labelled somatostatin analogues for use in positron emission tomography has markedly improved sensitivity (Figure 19.1).[6] Scintigraphy with somatostatin analogues also provides the basis for identifying candidates for targeted therapy with ^{177}Lu labelled somatostatin analogues and can also be used preoperatively to aid intraoperative localization of disease through the use of hand-held probes.[5]

19.2.1.3 Therapeutic assessment and follow-up

The primary treatment for GEP-NETs is surgical removal of all resectable primary and secondary lesions. Biochemical follow-up is far more sensitive than imaging. Gut neuroendocrine tumours often pursue an indolent course over many years, and symptomatic palliation of the sequelae of their endocrine products forms an important part of management. Most inoperable or metastatic neuroendocrine tumours express a high density of somatostatin receptors. Among treatments for these tumours, radiolabelled somatostatin analogues have been utilized. This is now an approved treatment in the UK (https://www.nice.org.uk/guidance/ta539/documents/final-appraisal-determination-document) and the first FDA and EMA approved agent for peptide receptor radionuclide therapy.[7]

19.2.2 Midgut neuroendocrine neoplasms

These are also referred to as midgut carcinoid tumours, which arise from the argentaffin cells. They may be found in any age group. About 85% of carcinoid tumours develop in the gastrointestinal tract, 10% in the lung, and the rest in various organs such as thymus, kidney, ovary, and prostate. The most common sites are the appendix, small bowel, and rectum. Carcinoids constitute about 34% of all tumours in the small intestine, but only 1% of all neoplasms in the stomach, colon, or rectum. Liver is the most common metastatic site and the metastases have one of the longest doubling times of any malignant human tumour. Despite enormous hepatomegaly, patients may remain well for a long time.

Several factors should be considered when evaluating carcinoid tumours for metastatic behaviour. These include the location of the primary tumour (approximately 70% of colonic carcinoids give rise to metastases, compared to 30–60% of ileal tumours and only 2–5% of appendiceal carcinoids), the size of the primary tumour (70% of tumours >2 cm and 6% <1 cm develop metastases). In addition, the depth of tumour penetration into the bowel wall and the histological growth pattern of the tumour are also important factors.[8,9]

19.2.2.1 Diagnosis and staging

The diagnosis of a midgut carcinoid tumour may be suspected by clinical symptoms suggestive of carcinoid syndrome or by the presence of other symptoms such as abdominal pain. Urinary 5-HIAA has been reported to have a sensitivity of around 70% and a specificity of 100% in patients with carcinoid syndrome. Plasma chromogranin A is the most sensitive marker (100%) but its specificity is lower than urinary 5-HIAA since almost all neuroendocrine tumours show increased levels of chromogranin A.

Imaging plays a crucial role in detecting and characterizing carcinoid tumours. Scintigraphy using radiolabelled somatostatin analogues such as ^{111}In-octreotide has demonstrated high sensitivity and specificity in the detection of carcinoid tumour in the past. PET with Ga-68 somatostatin analogues has been shown to be superior in this group of patients as well.

19.2.2.2 Therapeutic assessment and follow-up

Surgical treatment should be considered in every patient with a carcinoid tumour and operable disease should be resected. Although the majority of patients with midgut carcinoid tumours presenting with a carcinoid syndrome have liver metastases and cannot be cured surgically, excision of discrete hepatic metastases of this slowly growing tumour is perceived to be clinically beneficial.

Whilst external beam radiotherapy has been mostly reserved for treating painful bone metastases, radionuclide therapy is becoming of increasing importance. Therapy with the lutetium-177 labelled somatostatin analogue DOTATATE has been validated in the phase III Netter-1 study which showed significant increase in progression free and overall survival in the treatment arm and low (~20% objective response rates, complete and partial response based on RECIST criteria).[10] Treatment in this setting is approved by the FDA and EMEA. Somatostatin analogues effectively control symptoms in 40–80% patients with the carcinoid syndrome, with a reduction of biochemical markers in up to 40%. Stabilization of tumour growth has been observed in 24–57% of patients, with documented tumour progression prior to somatostatin therapy. However, partial and complete tumour response has been observed in <10% of patients. The problem of tachyphylaxis to somatostatin analogues occurs in the great majority of patients and hinders the duration of therapeutic response (median 12 months).

19.2.3 Neuroendocrine neoplasms of the lung

19.2.3.1 Clinical background

These, also referred to as bronchial carcinoids, are the most common 'benign' bronchial tumour. They arise endobronchially and frequently in the major bronchi. They usually present with haemoptysis or bronchial obstruction, and resection (lobectomy, pneumonectomy) is usually curative. Approximately 5% of bronchial carcinoids show nodal metastases and atypical carcinoids show more aggressive behaviour and could metastasize to mediastinal lymph nodes (30–50% cases), with a five-year survival rate of 40–60%.

19.2.3.2 Diagnosis and staging

The use of Ga-68 labelled somatostatin analogues for PET imaging is superior to traditional scintigraphy (Figure 19.2) and its application has been shown to impact patient management.[11] The combined use of ^{68}Ga-somatostatin analogues and ^{18}F fluorodeoxyglucose (FDG) PET/CT can be useful for lesion grading, identifying heterogeneity, and improving staging accuracy.[12]

19.2.3.3 Therapeutic assessment and follow-up

For faster-growing disease, aggressive and atypical carcinoids, the combination of cisplatin and etoposide is favoured, as for the more malignant islet cell tumours. Radionuclide therapy with labelled somatostatin analogues has been considered, but its role has yet to be completely defined.[13]

19.3 Phaeochromocytoma and paraganglioma

19.3.1 Clinical background

Phaeochromocytoma and paraganglioma (PPGLs) are catecholamine-secreting tumours arising from the adrenomedullary chromaffin cells. About 10%, arise from extra-adrenal chromaffin tissue located next to sympathetic ganglia and are classified as paragangliomas. The acronym PPGLs commonly refers to the two combined entities.

Phaeochromocytomas are rare, with a prevalence of 1:6500–1:10 000, and are reported in <0.1% of hypertensive patients. Sporadic phaeochromocytomas are often single and unilateral, whereas familial phaeochromocytomas (about 10%) are often

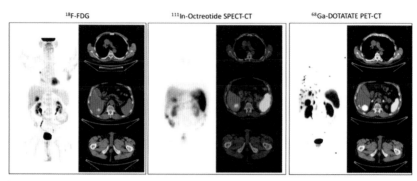

Fig. 19.2 An 83-year-old male with prior resection of an atypical bronchial carcinoid being evaluated for recurrence. Left panel: ¹⁸FDG PET-CT showing an area of intermediate uptake at the site of resection near the right mediastinal margin suspicious for recurrence. There is an avid liver lesion consistent with a metastasis. An indeterminate area of uptake in the left femur. Centre panel: ¹¹¹In-Octreotide SPECT CT shows no abnormality in the lung or bone but the liver metastasis shows high somatostatin receptor expression. Right panel: ⁶⁸Ga-DOTATATE PET CT shows widespread bone, liver, and right pleural lesions not detected with the other two methods on the maximum intensity projection image. The FDG avid lung lesion at the resection margin is not somatostatin receptor positive. This image demonstrates: (a) the superior sensitivity of somatostatin receptor PET in detecting well-differentiated neuroendocrine tumour lesions; (b) the possibility of assessing biological heterogeneity of advanced disease with some lesions detected only on FDG PET, some lesions detected only somatostatin receptor PET and some lesions positive to both tumour markers; (c) the importance of somatostatin receptor PET in helping select candidates for radionuclide therapy.

multi-centric, bilateral, have an earlier onset, and a lower risk of being malignant. About 10% of phaeochromocytomas are malignant, metastasizing to bone, lung, brain, or liver.

19.3.2 Diagnosis and staging

The diagnosis of phaeochromocytoma is based on the demonstration of increased levels of catecholamine or their metabolites. The measurement of 24-hour urinary free catecholamine has a high sensitivity for phaeochromocytoma. In a symptomatic patient, sensitivity approaches 100%. Plasma catecholamine levels are of lesser sensitivity than 24-hour urinary catecholamine levels but are useful if measured during a suspect event.

Biochemical evidence of a phaeochromocytoma should be followed by imaging for tumour localization. CT and MRI scanning can localize small adrenal, extra-adrenal, or metastatic lesions, but despite a high sensitivity (>95%), the specificity remains about 65–75%. Where there is unequivocal biochemical evidence of a catecholamine-secreting tumour, but a negative CT/MRI scan, ¹²³I-MIBG scintigraphy offers better specificity (95–100%) and reasonable sensitivity (78–83%) for tumours with catecholamine uptake. Phaeochromocytoma/paraganglioma also express somatostatin receptors and show high avidity for the glucose analogue FDG allowing for imaging with FDG-PET and Ga-68 somatostatin PET in addition to the traditional MIBG tracers.[14] PET imaging is generally regarded as more sensitive than planar and SPECT scintigraphy with 123 I or 131 I MIBG.[15] PET imaging using ^{18}F-fluorodopamine has also been shown to be effective in localizing disease.

19.3.3 Therapeutic assessment and follow-up

The treatment of phaeochromocytoma is primarily surgical resection. Annual urinary free catecholamines test is recommended in all patients for at least five years after surgical excision. In contrast to the five-year survival rate of 96% for patients with benign lesions, malignant phaeochromocytoma carries a 44% survival rate. ^{131}I-MIBG therapy is promising in advanced disease and produces partial response or stabilization of disease in more than 80% patients (Figure 19.3). In 2018 the FDA approved a high specific activity I-131 MIBG formulation for the treatment of advanced PPGL that has been recently studied.[16] The high somatostatin receptor

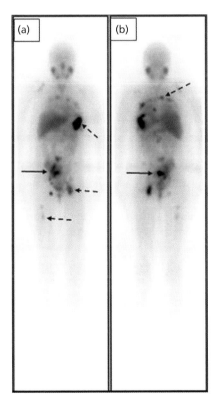

Fig. 19.3 A 34-year-old female patient with known metastatic paraganglioma. Anterior and posterior whole body views (a, b) taken three days after the administration of a therapeutic dose (11.1 GBq) of I-131-MIBG demonstrate MIBG avid pelvic retroperitoneal tumour (arrow) and multiple bone metastases (dash arrows).

positivity opens the door for radionuclide therapy with somatostatin analogues and this approach has been described in multiple small studies although it is has not been fully validated.[17]

19.4 **Adrenocortical tumours**

19.4.1 Clinical background

The majority (99%) of adrenal gland tumours are adenomas, which are benign non-functioning tumours of the adrenal cortex and usually of no clinical importance. Most functioning cortical adenomas are found in female patients. Those occurring in pre-pubertal patients tend to present with virilization, whereas those in post-pubertal patients present with Cushing's syndrome. Adrenocortical carcinoma is a rare malignancy, with an annual incidence of 4–12 cases per million population. It can be functioning or non-functioning. The left adrenal has been documented as the more common site and the disease is rarely bilateral.

19.4.2 Diagnosis and staging

Non-specific abdominal symptoms such as fullness, indigestion, nausea, vomiting, and pain are usually the most common clinical presenting features. Between one-quarter and one-third of patients with primary adrenal carcinoma have clinical evidence of endocrine dysfunction at presentation, most commonly Cushing's syndrome, often supplemented by virilism. A slightly higher fraction of the patients show evidence of abnormal hormone secretion, that is, subclinical dysfunction. Feminizing tumours due to over-secretion of oestrogens are rare (10%), as are aldosterone-secreting tumours (2%). As for suspected cortical adenomas, diagnostic tests include the demonstration of excessive and non-suppressible levels of adrenal steroids.

Imaging is an essential adjunct to clinical and biochemical findings in the diagnosis of adrenal tumours. Both CT and MRI have the capability to detect adrenal tumours <5 mm and indeed, small adrenal tumours are sometimes detected on imaging of the abdomen by CT or MRI for an ostensibly unrelated reason—the so-called 'incidentaloma'. FDG-PET/CT has been shown to detect metastases and recurrence of adrenocortical tumours with impressive sensitivity of 96%, specificity of 99%, and accuracy of 98%. PET imaging with radiolabelled cortisol analogues such as ^{11}C-metomidate have been utilized to characterize adrenal masses of cortical origin.[18]

19.4.3 Therapeutic assessment and follow-up

The treatment of an adrenal tumour depends on the size and location of the tumour. Various algorithms have been proposed to differentiate tumours that require surgical removal from those that can be simply monitored, most attempting to exclude a hypersecretory state biochemically and assess the probability of adrenal malignancy on imaging criteria. In general, small (<3 cm) lesions with 'benign' imaging characteristics can be simply observed and rescanned at intervals.

19.5 **Summary**

◆ Endocrine tumours represent a diverse group of tumours.

◆ Diagnosis is suggested by clinical presentation and usually confirmed by biochemical tests, but a variety of imaging techniques may be used to localize and stage disease, including CT, MRI, EUS.

◆ Nuclear medicine methods have an increasing role in lesion detection, biological characterization, and radionuclide therapy of advanced disease.

References

1. **Hajdu SI, Tang P** (2008). A note from history: the saga of carcinoid and oat-cell carcinoma. *Annals Clinical & Laboratory Science*, **38**(4): 414–417.

2. **Pearse AG, Polak JM, Rost FW, Fontaine J, Le Lièvre C, Le Douarin N** (1973). Demonstration of the neural crest origin of type I (APUD) cells in the avian carotid body, using a cytochemical marker system. *Histochemie*, **34**(3): 191–203.

3. **O'Toole D, Kianmanesh R, Caplin M** (2016). ENETS 2016 consensus guidelines for the management of patients with digestive neuroendocrine tumors: an update. *Neuroendocrinology*, **103**(2): 117–118.

4. **Garcia-Carbonero R, Sorbye H, Baudin E, et al.** (2016). ENETS consensus guidelines for high-grade gastroenteropancreatic neuroendocrine tumors and neuroendocrine carcinomas. *Neuroendocrinology*, **103**(2): 186–194.

5. **Tamm EP, Kim EE, Ng CS** (2007). Imaging of neuroendocrine tumors. *Hematology Oncology Clinics of North America*, **21**: 409–432.

6. **Deppen SA, Blume J, Bobbey AJ, et al.** (2016). 68Ga-DOTATATE compared with 111in-dtpa-octreotide and conventional imaging for pulmonary and gastroenteropancreatic neuroendocrine tumors: a systematic review and meta-analysis. *Journal of Nuclear Medicine*, **57**(6): 872–878.

7. **Hennrich U, Kopka K** (2019). Lutathera®: The First FDA- and EMA-approved radiopharmaceutical for peptide receptor radionuclide therapy. *Pharmaceuticals*, **12**: 114.

8. **Niederle B, Pape UF, Costa F, et al.** (2016). ENETS consensus guidelines update for neuroendocrine neoplasms of the jejunum and ileum. *Neuroendocrinology*, **103**(2): 125–138.

9. **Pape UF, Niederle B, Costa F, et al.** (2016). ENETS consensus guidelines for neuroendocrine neoplasms of the appendix (excluding goblet cell carcinomas). *Neuroendocrinology*, **103**(2): 144–152.

10. **Strosberg J, El-Haddad G, Wolin E, et al.** (2017). NETTER-1 trial investigators. phase 3 trial of (177)Lu-DOTATATE for midgut neuroendocrine tumors. *New England Journal of Medicine*, **376**(2): 125–135.

11. **Lamarca A, Pritchard D, M, Westwood T, et al.** (2018). 68Gallium DOTANOC-PET imaging in lung carcinoids: impact on patients' management. *Neuroendocrinology*, **106**: 128–138.

12. **Kayani I, Conry BG, Groves AM, et al.** (2009). A comparison of 68Ga-DOTATATE and 18F-FDG PET/CT in pulmonary neuroendocrine tumors. *Journal of Nuclear Medicine*, **50**(12): 1927–1932.

13. **Naraev BG, Ramirez RA, Kendi AT, Halfdanarson TR** (2019). Peptide receptor radionuclide therapy for patients with advanced lung carcinoids. *Clinical Lung Cancer*, **20**(3): e376–e392.

14. **Chang CA, Pattison DA, Tothill RW, et al.** (2016). (68)Ga-DOTATATE and (18)F-FDG PET/CT in paraganglioma and pheochromocytoma: utility, patterns and heterogeneity. *Cancer Imaging*, **16**(1): 22.

15. **Timmers HJ, Chen CC, Carrasquillo JA, et al.** (2012). Staging and functional characterisation of pheochromocytoma and paraganglioma by 18F-fluorodeoxyglucose (18F-FDG) positron emission tomography (2012). *Journal of National Cancer Institute*, **104**(9): 700–708.

16. **Pryma DA, Chin BB, Noto RB, et al.** (2019). Efficacy and safety of high-specific-activity (131)I-MIBG therapy in patients with advanced pheochromocytoma or paraganglioma. *Journal of Nuclear Medicine*, **60**(5): 623–630.

17. **Vyakaranam AR, Crona J, Norlén O, et al.** (2019). Favorable outcome in patients with pheochromocytoma and paraganglioma treated with (177)Lu-DOTATATE. *Cancers* (Basel), **11**(7): ii: E909.

18. **Bergström M, Juhlin C, Bonasera TA, et al.** (2000). PET imaging of adrenal cortical tumors with the 11beta-hydroxylase tracer 11C-metomidate. *Journal of Nuclear Medicine*, **41**(2): 275–282.

Chapter 20

Primary bone sarcomas

Gulshad Begum, Sarah Prewett, Gail Horan,
and Emma-Louise Gerety

20.1 Introduction

Bone sarcomas are rare tumours, accounting for 0.2% of all new cancers in the UK. They are 8–10 times less common than soft tissue sarcomas but are often more challenging to manage, with many presenting in teenagers and young adults.[1,2] They occur more commonly in males than females (59% vs. 41%), and the majority occur in the lower limb (34%), followed by pelvis (17%), upper limb (12%), and head (12%). The most common presenting symptoms are non-mechanical bone pain (typically worse at night) and swelling. Functional impairment and spontaneous fractures are usually late presentations.

Primary bone sarcomas may be bone forming (osteogenic) or cartilage forming (chondrogenic). Osteosarcoma, Ewing's sarcoma, and chondrosarcoma are the most common. Less common types include spindle cell sarcoma, notochordal tumours (chordoma), giant cell tumours of bone, vascular tumours (angiosarcoma), and adamantinomas.

Osteosarcoma is a primary mesenchymal tumour characterized histologically by osteoid-forming malignant cells. Incidence shows bimodal distribution, with a first peak at 10–20 years and second peak at 70–80 years. It is the most common bone tumour in adolescents and young adults but second most common in the older population. Osteosarcoma usually arises in the metaphysis of long bones, especially around the knee in children and adolescents. In elderly patients, the axial skeleton and craniofacial bones may be involved and it is usually secondary to malignant degeneration in chronic disorders such as Paget's disease, extensive bone infarcts, or post irradiation. There are eight different subtypes, some of which have characteristic imaging features such as parosteal and telangiectatic osteosarcoma.[3]

Ewing's sarcoma of the bone is the second most common primary bone tumour in children and adolescents. Median age at diagnosis is 15 years. The commonest sites in order of frequency are pelvis, femur, tibia, fibula, rib, scapula, vertebra, and humerus.[4]

Chondrosarcomas are malignant cartilage-containing bone tumours, most frequently seen in adulthood at 30–60 years. They are the most common bone sarcoma in this age group, ahead of osteosarcomas. Common sites include pelvis and ribs (45%), ilium (20%), femur (15%), and humerus (10%). Secondary chondrosarcoma can arise due to malignant transformation of an osteochondroma, particularly in patients with hereditary multiple exostoses. Imaging may be required to monitor potential malignant transformation of the cartilage cap, which is found to be at greater risk of chondrosarcoma if thicker than 2 cm. Chondrosarcomas may also arise in enchondromas in patients with Ollier's or Maffucci syndrome.

Chordomas account for 8% of all primary bone tumours and arise from primitive notochordal remnants. Most common sites involved are pelvis, sacrum, vertebral column, face, and skull. They show a relatively indolent course with local destruction and extension into adjacent soft tissue.

Giant cell tumours (GCT) are rare, locally aggressive bone tumours with low malignant potential, accounting for about 5% of primary bone tumours. Peak incidence is at 20–45 years of age and most commonly these occur at the ends of long bones in the lower limb. Less than 5% of GCTs metastasize, typically to the lungs.

All suspected cases of bone sarcoma should be discussed within a specialist multidisciplinary team at a specialist centre. Management of bone tumours, especially osteosarcomas and Ewing's sarcoma, involves intense and complex multi-modality treatments aiming for long-term disease control whilst minimizing late treatment toxicity.

20.2 Diagnosis and staging

Radiology has a pivotal role in the diagnosis, staging, treatment, and follow-up of patients with malignant bone tumours.[5] The age of the patient and location of the tumour are characteristics that may help initially to formulate a differential diagnosis. A radiograph is usually the first step in the diagnostic work-up, followed by cross-sectional imaging with MRI and/or CT and then nuclear medicine (Table 20.1).

20.2.1 Radiographs

Plain radiographs are usually the initial imaging modality in patients presenting with bone pain or swelling.[6] Images are acquired in two planes, usually frontal and lateral. The precise location of the lesion is described in terms of the affected bone, whether located within the epiphysis, metaphysis, or diaphysis, and whether central, eccentric,

Table 20.1 Role of different imaging modalities in the diagnosis and staging of bone sarcomas

Modality	Indication
Plain radiograph	First-line diagnosis; lung/bone metastases
MRI	Second-line diagnosis
CT	Diagnosis; surgical planning Staging/follow-up
[18F] FDG—PET/CT	Staging/follow-up
Bone scintigraphy	Bone metastases

or cortically located. The lesion is described as lucent, dense, or heterogenous and the matrix calcification classified as ground glass, chondroid, or osteoid. The zone of transition is described, ranging from well-defined and geographic to diffuse and permeative. Cortical destruction, periosteal reaction, pathological fracture, soft tissue component, and multiplicity of the lesion is also assessed. Characteristics of non-aggressive and aggressive lesions are well described, with aggressive features including an indistinct margin, cortical expansion, and periosteal reaction.

Bone has a hard outer layer of dense cortex (up to 80% of adult bone mass) and an inner, less dense layer of cancellous, trabecular, or spongy bone. Osteoblastic bone lesions appear radio-dense due to increased bone deposition resulting in thickened coarse trabeculae. Osteolytic lesions show thinning of the trabeculae with ill-defined margins and appear lucent on radiographs.

Typical features of osteosarcoma which may be demonstrated on a radiograph (Figure 20.1a,b) include a wide zone of transition, cortical breach with soft tissue mass, fluffy or cloud-like osteoid matrix calcification, periosteal elevation with a 'sunburst' appearance, and Codman's triangle. Codman's triangle represents an area of sub-periosteal bone formation due to tumour lifting off the underlying periosteum, and is usually, but not exclusively, found in osteosarcoma. Parosteal osteosarcomas arise from the outer layer of the periosteum and therefore appear pedunculated (Figure 20.1c).

Ewing's sarcoma on radiographs usually demonstrates ill-defined, permeative, moth-eaten bone destruction. Lesions can be mixed lytic and sclerotic or purely lytic. A multilayered 'onion-skin' periosteal reaction is seen in about 50% of these tumours (Figure 20.1d). There is often a much more extensive soft tissue lesion which may also be demonstrated on the radiograph as an area of increased soft tissue density.

Chondrosarcomas show a characteristic pattern of chondroid calcification, classically described as whorls and arcs with calcified cartilaginous areas (popcorn calcification) and fusiform cortical expansion (Figure 20.1e).

The location of the lesion within the bone may also provide clues as to the type of tumour. For example, giant cell tumours of bone classically extend to the articular surface in bones with a closed physis and appear as well-defined, eccentric lesions without a sclerotic margin (Figure 20.1f). Matrix calcification and reactive periosteal new bone formation is *not* seen in GCTs.

Bone destruction, new bone formation, periosteal reaction, and soft tissue mass are concerning radiographic features and require urgent investigation and referral to a bone sarcoma MDT.

Radiographs are also used to monitor progression of bone lesions and may also demonstrate pathological fracture. They are also used for follow-up after excision of bone lesions and may subsequently demonstrate metal surgical prostheses (Figure 20.2).

20.2.2 **Magnetic resonance imaging**

MRI is used for further characterization of suspicious lesions identified on radiographs as it enables assessment of the bone marrow and soft tissues and is used to stage local disease.[7] Normal bone marrow contains a high percentage of fat and demonstrates

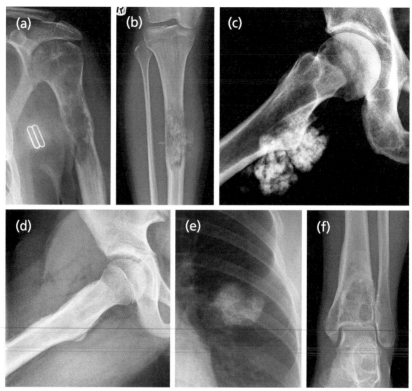

Fig. 20.1 Radiographs demonstrating: (a) aggressive, lucent bone lesion in the proximal humerus, found to be an osteosarcoma in a 22-year-old female; (b) osteosarcoma of the tibia in a 35-year-old female; (c) exophytic, ossified lesion in the right proximal femur, found to be a parosteal osteosarcoma in a 63-year-old male; (d) subtle changes of periosteal elevation and cortical irregularity in a Ewing's sarcoma of the proximal femur in a 10-year-old female; (e) chondroid calcification of a left fourth rib chondrosarcoma in a 32-year-old female; (f) aggressive, lytic lesion extending to the articular surface of the distal tibia in an 18-year-old female, characteristic of a giant cell tumour of bone.

high signal intensity on T1-weighted MRI sequences. Non-lipomatous infiltrative bone marrow lesions show low T1 signal, due to replacement of normal fatty marrow by malignant cells. On T2-weighted images, bone lesions are usually hyperintense due to high water content (Figure 20.3). Both water and fat return high signal on T2-weighted imaging so fat suppression should be used to remove the signal from the fat. High water signal may be due to intracellular water within a lesion or extracellular water such as in reactive oedema adjacent to the lesion.

Routine MRI to investigate a potential bone sarcoma should include acquisition of T1-weighted and T2-weighted, fat saturated images in two planes (Figure 20.4).

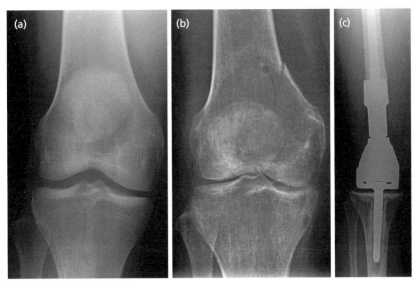

Fig. 20.2 Follow-up frontal radiographs of a giant cell tumour of the distal femur in a 40-year-old male. (a) Lucent lesion in the centre of the femoral metaphysis, extending to the articular surface. (b). Pathological fracture of the medial femoral condyle. (c) Long stem total knee replacement.

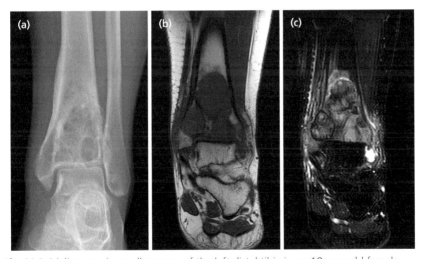

Fig. 20.3 Malignant giant cell tumour of the left distal tibia in an 18-year-old female. (a) Radiograph demonstrates a bubbly, lytic lesion extending to the articular surface of the distal tibia. (b) T1-weighted MRI with loss of fatty marrow signal due to the lesion in the distal tibia. (c) T2-weighted fat saturated MRI demonstrates high water-sensitive signal in the lesion.

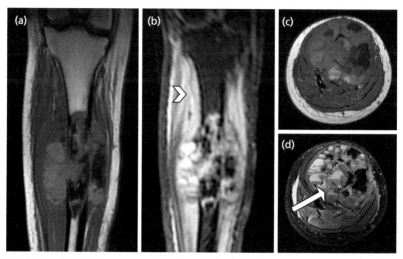

Fig. 20.4 Standard MRI sequences for characterization of an osteosarcoma in the tibia of a 35-year-old female. Imaging in two planes, coronal (a, b) and axial (c, d) with T1-weighted (a, c) and T2-weighted fat saturated (b, d) sequences. Fluid-fluid levels are noted (arrow) in keeping with haemorrhage.

Post-contrast imaging with gadolinium is rarely necessary or useful for characterization of bone lesions. However, it may in some cases help to distinguish the most vascularized part of tumour from necrotic areas and hence guide sites for successful biopsy. Post-gadolinium images are T1-weighted with fat suppression so that only gadolinium-enhanced tissues are of high signal. Recent studies have also found that the dynamic uptake of gadolinium by bone sarcomas may be able to predict chemotherapy response.[8]

MRI allows accurate assessment of the location and size of the lesion, its intramedullary extent, and any involvement of joints, muscle compartments, and neurovascular bundles. MRI also enables assessment of any soft tissue component, which may be particularly important for Ewing's sarcoma and may not be well demonstrated on radiograph (Figure 20.5).

Imaging of the affected area should include the whole of the involved bone and adjacent joints both superiorly and inferiorly, as this may identify skip lesions (Figure 20.6) and is vital for subsequent surgical planning.

Given the young age of many of the patients with osteosarcoma and Ewing's sarcoma, MRI can be challenging as it may be a daunting and scary prospect for the child and their family. It is typically necessary to keep still for 3–4 minutes at a time for acquisition of each set of images. MRI play therapists may help facilitate the imaging but younger children may still need a general anaesthetic. MRI may also be difficult in some adults due to claustrophobia and anxiety, and may be contraindicated in the presence of certain metal implants and pacemakers.

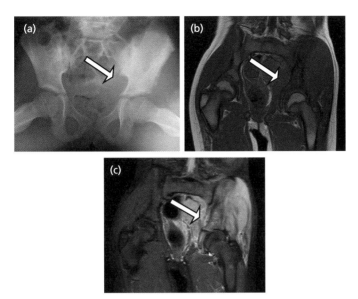

Fig. 20.5 MRI characterization of Ewing's sarcoma in the left ilium (arrow)—the soft tissue component is much more extensive than the osseous changes. (a) radiograph demonstrates density over the left ilium and subtle periosteal elevation. (b) T1-weighted MRI with loss of fatty bone marrow signal in the left ilium. (c) T2-weighted fat saturated MRI showing extensive high T2 signal in the soft tissue mass adjacent to the left ilium.

20.2.3 Computed tomography

CT is used for characterization of bone lesions when MRI is contraindicated, for image-guided bone biopsy, and for surgical planning. CT is more sensitive than MRI at demonstrating calcification, which appears black on standard MRI sequences. CT identifies areas of radiolucency, matrix calcification, and subtle cortical erosion and is better able to demonstrate bone structure. CT images are rapidly acquired in the axial plane in seconds and can then be reformatted into coronal and sagittal planes or any oblique plane as required. The axial images can also be reformatted into 3D reconstructions which may further aid surgical planning (Figure 20.7). Models may be 3D printed from the CT axial data to aid surgical planning and prosthesis design. CT also plays a vital role in the staging of tumours, and unenhanced CT of the chest is performed to look for metastatic lung disease.

20.2.4 Nuclear medicine

Bone scintigraphy for the detection of skeletal metastases is standard in the current work-up of patients with primary bone tumours (Figure 20.8). Bone scintigraphy is relatively inexpensive, convenient, and visualizes the entire skeleton, including sites that are difficult to assess on radiographs, such as ribs, sternum, scapula, and sacrum. The radiotracer technetium–99m methylene diphosphonate (^{99m}Tc-MDP) is imaged,

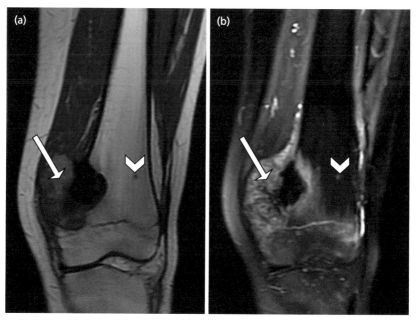

Fig. 20.6 Tiny skip lesion in a 16-year-old male with left medial femoral condyle osteosarcoma. (a) Coronal T1-weighted MRI. (b) Coronal T2-weighted fat saturated MRI. Arrow: primary osteosarcoma. Arrowhead: tiny skip lesion.

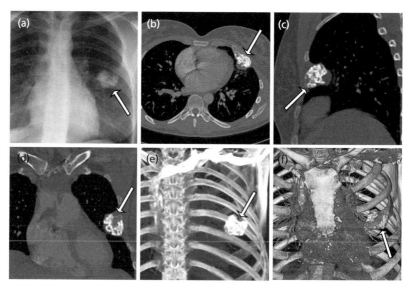

Fig. 20.7 CT characterization of a chondrosarcoma (arrow) of the left fourth rib in a 38-year-old female. (a) Radiograph. (b) Unenhanced, thin axial CT image. (c) Sagittal reformatted CT image. (d) Coronal reformatted image. (e) 3D reformatted image. (f) Virtual reality reformatted image.

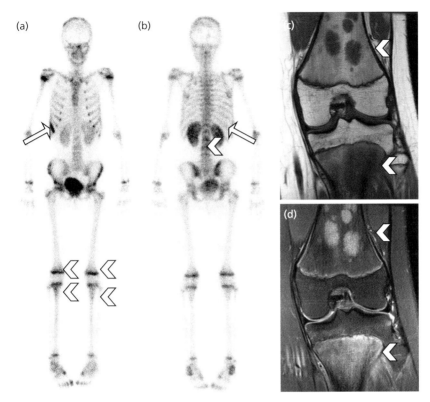

Fig. 20.8 Bone metastases demonstrated by 99 mTc-MDP bone scintigraphy (a, b) and MRI (c, d) in a 12-year-old female with a Ewing's sarcoma in the right eighth rib. (a) Anterior bone scintigram. (b) Posterior bone scintigram demonstrating uptake in the metabolically active physes as well as the primary rib Ewing's sarcoma (arrow) and bone metastases in the proximal tibiae and spine (arrowheads). (c) T1-weighted coronal MRI. (d) T2-weighted fat saturated coronal MRI of the left knee demonstrate the metastases.

which localizes to areas of new bone formation where it is taken up by active osteoblasts. Once the radiotracer has been administered intravenously, the whole body can be imaged to localize the uptake of the tracer.

Bone scintigraphy may demonstrate increased uptake of ^{99m}Tc-MDP at the site of the primary tumour, in the adjacent bone (due to increased vascularity), in bone metastases, and in bone-forming metastases in soft tissues such as osteosarcoma lung metastases (Figure 20.9). Of note, benign conditions may also show increased uptake due to degenerative or inflammatory arthritis, trauma, and infection.

Positron emission tomography (PET)/CT or PET/MRI, are being used increasingly for staging purposes (including the detection of 'skip' bone lesions), and again allow the whole skeleton/body to be imaged.[9]

18-fluoride labelled fluorodeoxyglucose (^{18}F-FDG), the most commonly used PET tracer, is a glucose analogue that concentrates in areas of high metabolic activity.

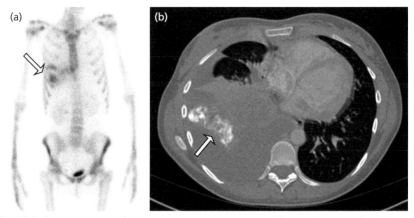

Fig. 20.9 Osteosarcoma pulmonary metastases may be positive on bone scintigraphy. (a) 99 mTc-MDP uptake in an ossified pulmonary metastasis (arrow) in a 23-year-old female with previous tibial osteosarcoma. (b) Axial CT image of ossified right lower lobe metastasis, right lower lobe collapse, and right pleural effusion.

Tumour cells show high metabolic activity with rapid cell division and an increased number of glucose transporters, therefore showing increased uptake. High uptake is also physiological in many organs, including myocardium, gastric mucosa, brain tissue, thyroid, and salivary glands, which limits evaluation of these areas. As ^{18}F-FDG is excreted within the urinary system, 'normal' uptake is also seen in the kidneys, collecting system, and bladder, which can obscure the detection of malignancy in these structures. PET images can be fused with CT or MRI images for accurate anatomical localization of tracer uptake.

About one quarter of Ewing's sarcoma patients present with metastases (40% of those are found in lung, 40% in bone/bone marrow). ^{18}F-FDG PET/CT may be sufficient for screening of bone and bone marrow metastases in Ewing's sarcoma. PET may help characterize benign versus malignant pathology, detect occult metastatic disease, identify optimal sites for tissue sampling, and assess treatment response and recurrence (Figure 20.10).[10] ^{18}F-sodium fluoride (^{18}F-NaF) is a radio-tracer that is taken up by metabolically active bone and is making a comeback as ^{18}F-NaF PET/CT has been found to have a higher sensitivity for bone metastases compared to 99mTc-MDP bone scintigraphy and ^{18}F-FDG-PET/CT. PET-CT and PET-MRI show future promise for the imaging of bone sarcomas; however, in many centres these modalities are not yet available in routine practice.

20.3 Interventional radiology

Biopsy is required for histopathological confirmation of the diagnosis and to direct further treatment. Local imaging of the affected bone allows planning of the optimal site for biopsy. Contrast enhanced MRI can reveal the most vascularized parts of the tumour and MRI guidance minimizes the risk of a non-diagnostic yield by avoiding necrotic regions. The core bone biopsy is usually CT-guided (Figure 20.11a).

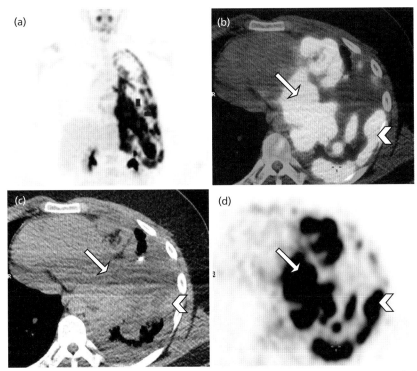

Fig. 20.10 An 18-year male with a sacral Ewing's sarcoma and left pleural (arrowhead) and lung (arrow) metastases demonstrated by ^{18}F-FDG PET/CT. (a) Coronal ^{18}F-FDG PET with uptake in the left lung and pleura. (b) Fused axial ^{18}F-FDG PET/CT. (c) Axial CT. (d) Axial ^{18}F-FDG PET.

Biopsy is ideally performed by a specialist sarcoma surgeon who will take into account possible future surgical approaches. This should minimize the risk of tumour spread to the skin or adjacent structures (biopsy tracts are marked with a small incision or tattoo to ensure that they are excised at the definitive procedure). Fine-needle biopsies are not suitable for primary diagnosis but can be used to confirm metastatic disease.

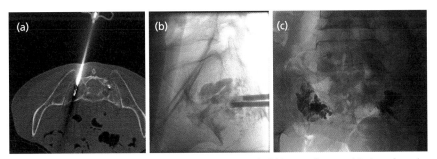

Fig. 20.11 Use of interventional radiology. (a) CT-guided biopsy of a sacral lesion, found to be a chordoma on histopathology. (b, c) Fluoroscopically guided vertebroplasty to prevent sacral collapse and to relieve pain.

Patients with spinal metastases may experience debilitating pain that significantly decreases their quality of life. Interventional radiology may aid with palliation by vertebral augmentation or radiofrequency ablation of spinal metastases.

Inoperable sacral chordomas are often treated with primary radiation and require high doses as they are relatively radio-resistant. One potential complication following radiation therapy to the pelvis is the risk of sacral insufficiency fractures in the weakened, irradiated bone. These can be incredibly painful, typically giving rise to lower back pain which may radiate down into the buttock or leg. Vertebroplasty can be performed to improve pain control and stabilize the vertebral bodies if standard analgesic measures are unsuccessful (Figure 20.11b,c).

20.4 Response to treatment and follow-up

MRI of the primary tumour may be repeated to assess response to neo-adjuvant treatment. Response may not always be demonstrated by a clear reduction in size, indeed tumours may increase in size due to tissue necrosis which may be demonstrated by changes in enhancement pattern following intravenous gadolinium.

The goal of surgery is to safely remove the whole tumour with adequate tumour-free margins and attempt to salvage the limb where possible. Limb preservation involves removing the tumour and replacing the bone defect with a custom-made artificial prosthesis (see Figure 20.2).

MRI is essential prior to definitive surgical planning to assess the degree of intramedullary extension and invasion of the adjacent soft tissues.

Contraindications to limb conservation may include poor radiological response after neo-adjuvant chemotherapy and situations where a safe complete resection is not possible, such as in the presence of extensive soft tissue infiltration and/or invasion of neurovascular bundles. In children who are not yet fully grown, careful consideration is also required of the growth plate and whether this can be spared, to reduce the risk of limb length discrepancy in later life.

^{18}F-FDG PET/CT may also be helpful in predicting histological response to neo-adjuvant therapy. Most malignant tumours have a maximum SUV>2.5 while physiological uptake is usually <2.5. Changes in SUV have prognostic value, and a 30% decrease or increase in SUV has been correlated with disease response to treatment or progression respectively.[9]

Radiographs and MRI are used for surveillance for local recurrence following curative treatment. Baseline imaging should be obtained within 3–6 months of definite surgical resection using MRI. Recommended imaging follow-up intervals vary according to whether the tumour is deemed to be low or high risk.[11]

Gadolinium is useful for distinguishing between post-surgical inflammation, infection, scarring, and recurrence. Metal prostheses may severely limit sensitivity of MRI for recurrence as the metal causes signal artefact due to distortion of the magnetic field. Metal artefact reduction sequences are possible but still may not be as sensitive in the adjacent area around the prosthesis.

Bone scintigraphy and PET/CT or PET/MRI where available, may also play a role in follow-up of primary bone sarcomas. They can be helpful in the detection of recurrence and may be of value if there is diagnostic uncertainty with other cross-sectional imaging modalities (see Figure 20.10).

With the development of novel therapeutic agents such as tyrosine kinase inhibitors and specific immunotherapies, it is becoming increasingly important to have sensitive and specific imaging for the monitoring of disease response which may induce metabolic changes before structural changes occur.

20.5 **Summary**

- Primary bone sarcomas require a multidisciplinary approach to their management.
- Appropriate imaging and the correct interpretation of this imaging is integral in the decision-making processes throughout the stages of treatment.
- As novel therapeutic drugs are developed, sensitive and specific follow-up imaging is essential for monitoring response to treatment.

References

1. **Gerrand C, Athanasou N, Brennan B, et al.** (2016). UK guidelines for the management of bone sarcomas. *Clinical Sarcoma Research*, **6**: 7.

2. **Casali PG, Bielack S, Abecassis N, et al.** (2018). Bone sarcomas: ESMO–PaedCan–EURACAN Clinical Practice Guidelines for diagnosis, treatment and follow-up. *Annals of Oncology*, **29**(Suppl 4): iv79–95.

3. **Jarmish G, Klein MJ, Landa J, Lefkowitz FA, Hwang S** (2010). Imaging characteristics of primary osteosarcoma: nonconventional subtypes. *RadioGraphics*, **30**: 1653–1672.

4. **Weber MA, Papakonstantinou O, Nikodinovska VV, Vanhoenacker FM** (2019). Ewing's sarcoma and primary osseous lymphoma: spectrum of imaging appearances. *Seminars in Musculoskeletal Radiology*, **23**(1): 36–57.

5. **Kaste SC** (2016). Imaging pediatric bone sarcomas. *Radiology Clinics of North America*, **49**(4): 749–765.

6. **Colleen M, Costelloe, Madewell JE** (2013). Radiography in the initial diagnosis of primary bone tumors. *American Journal of Roentgenology*, **200**: 3–7.

7. **Nascimento D, Suchard G, Hatem M, de Abreu A** (2014). The role of magnetic resonance imaging in the evaluation of bone tumours and tumour-like lesions. *Insights Imaging*, **5**(4): 419–440.

8. **Amit P, Patro DK, Basu D, Elangovan S, Parathasarathy V** (2014). Role of dynamic MRI and clinical assessment in predicting histologic response to neoadjuvant chemotherapy in bone sarcomas. *American Journal of Clinical Oncology*, **37**(4): 384–390.

9. **Behzadi AH, Raza SI, Carrino JA, et al.** (2018). Applications of PET/CT and PET/MR imaging in primary bone malignancies. *PET Clinics*, **13**(4): 623–624.

10. **Newman EN, Jones RL, Hawkins DS** (2013). An evaluation of [F-18]-fluorodeoxy-D-glucose positron emission tomography, bone scan, and bone marrow aspiration/biopsy as staging investigations in Ewing sarcoma. *Pediatric Blood Cancer*, **60**(7): 1113–1117.

11. **Robers CC, Kransdorf MJ, Beaman FD, et al.** (2016). ACR appropriateness criteria: follow-up of malignant or aggressive musculoskeletal tumors. *Journal of American College of Radiologists*, **13**(4): 389–400.

Chapter 21

Paediatrics

Mark Gaze, Monique Shahid, Paul Humphries, and Francesca Peters

21.1 Introduction

There are various definitions of what constitutes 'paediatric' or 'adolescent' patients, and the terms 'children', 'teenagers', and 'young people' are sometimes used loosely. In its guidance, *Improving Outcomes in Children and Young People with Cancer*, the National Institute for Health and Care Excellence regards those aged less than 15 years as children, and those aged 15–24 as young people. The Children's Cancer and Leukaemia Group reports patients aged up to 15 years separately from those 15 years and older, so in this chapter the age of 15 years will be taken as the cut-off point.

Paediatric cancer is a diverse and heterogeneous group of diseases. Table 21.1 sets out the principal categories of malignant disease, and their relative proportion, in children. Although there are cancer types which usually occur in those under 15, and other types which almost always occur in individuals aged over 15 years, there are exceptional cases when cancers occur in the 'wrong' age group, and there are other cancer types which commonly affect both children and older patients.

Paediatric malignancy is uncommon, with less than 1% of all cancers seen in children less than 15 years of age. Between 2001 and 2005, there were 21,289 registered cases of cancer (including non-malignant intracranial and intraspinal tumours) in children under the age of 15 in England, equating to an incidence of 1420 new registrations per year.

21.2 The role of imaging in paediatric oncology

Timely access to appropriate diagnostic imaging, including nuclear medicine, is essential in children and young people with suspected or confirmed malignant disease. Imaging has a number of roles which include:

- Assessment of a suspicious lesion, with the aim of providing a differential diagnosis and guiding an interventional radiology biopsy procedure which may avoid the need for an open surgical biopsy.
- Staging the local extent of disease and identifying nodal or distant metastases.
- Assessment of response to therapy.
- Target volume definition for radiotherapy.
- Management of complications and late effects.

Table 21.1 Approximate relative frequency of paediatric cancer types

Leukaemia	**30%**
Acute lymphoblastic leukaemia	25%
Other leukaemias	5%
Central nervous system tumours	**26%**
Low grade astrocytoma	12%
CNS embryonal tumours	7%
Other central nervous system tumours	7%
Lymphoma	**11%**
Hodgkin lymphoma	6%
Non-Hodgkin lymphoma	5%
Non-central nervous system solid tumours	**33%**
Neuroblastoma	6%
Soft tissue sarcoma	6%
Renal tumours	6%
Bone sarcomas	4%
Retinoblastoma	3%
Germ cell tumours	3%
Melanoma and carcinomas	3%
Liver tumours	1%
Other types	1%

There are many challenges to overcome when imaging children, particularly in the setting of malignant disease. The inherent heterogeneity of the population of 'paediatric' patients in terms of age, body size, and understanding and tolerance of imaging procedures, demands a flexible and age-appropriate approach, and reinforces the need for paediatric radiologists, trained in oncology imaging, in paediatric oncology centres.

Simply being in hospital can be bewildering and frightening for any child. It is worse if the child is unwell or in pain, or has had prior experience of distressing procedures. It is important to engage with both the child and their parents to facilitate a successful examination. Older children can cooperate with imaging investigations when the purpose and practicalities of the procedure are simply explained. In younger children, the input of a hospital play specialist and the use of distraction techniques (e.g. the use of toys, books, or videos) are particularly useful. Sometimes adopting a non-standard scanning position, for example with the child being cuddled by a parent or carer, may facilitate ultrasound (US) examinations. In younger children, especially if the scan time is long, as with magnetic resonance imaging (MRI), or when it is not advisable for a parent to remain in the room during the procedure, the use of sedation or general anaesthesia is required.

In general terms, the use of ionizing radiation investigations should be kept to a minimum. This is because of the greater radiosensitivity of children and their expected longer lifespan in which radiation effects, especially carcinogenesis, have a longer time to manifest themselves. To this end there is a greater emphasis on non-ionizing techniques, with US and MRI being utilized where possible. Where ionizing techniques (such as computed tomography (CT) or positron emission tomography (PET)) are needed, radiation dose reduction strategies are employed in order to minimize exposure.

US enables real-time evaluation and is particularly helpful with abdominal masses in assessing their relationship with solid organs and vessels. MRI provides excellent anatomical detail without the use of ionizing radiation, and although central nervous system (CNS) imaging is relatively straightforward, MRI of body tumours remains a challenge in paediatric practice.

Particular difficulties include:

♦ Relatively long scan times (compared with multislice CT), leading to motion artefact.

♦ Relatively poor signal-to-noise ratio of the images when patients are small in size, necessitating innovative use of 'adult' coils, for example using knee coils or flex coils to image abdominal tumours in infants.

♦ Inherent low image quality of chest MRI, owing to low signal generated and artefact from respiratory and cardiac motion.

♦ Issues related to patients tolerating the MRI examination, including patient co-operation, particularly in those under six years of age.

Logistical difficulties may occur in relation to radiotherapy planning and delivery as patients are often imaged in a number of separate hospitals. For example, a tumour may be imaged at presentation to a district general hospital, and further imaging may be performed at the paediatric oncology centre, whereas radiotherapy may be planned and administered at a third separate hospital. It is important for the clinical oncologist to have all relevant imaging to enable accurate target volume definition. For different cancers, treatment may be planned on the extent of disease at diagnosis or following initial chemotherapy, or on the presurgical tumour or the postoperative residual mass. Digital imaging sent in DICOM format on a disc, or by image exchange software, is preferable to hardcopy images as it can be uploaded into radiotherapy planning computers, and fused with other images. It is essential to have adequate administrative staff to locate and retrieve the required images from other hospitals in order to avoid unnecessary re-imaging of children simply because previous imaging is not to hand. Patients should be discussed at the relevant multidisciplinary team meeting; this allows patients to be considered from a range of viewpoints and expertise, and offers a greater probability of timely, appropriate treatment and better continuity of care.

21.3 **CNS tumours**

21.3.1 **Clinical background**

As a group, CNS tumours are the second most common paediatric malignancy after leukaemia. Clinical presentation includes:

- Symptoms of raised intracranial pressure, including headaches and vomiting, which is often due to the development of obstructive hydrocephalus.
- Focal neurological signs including cranial nerve palsies or a hemiparesis.
- Epileptic manifestations of various sorts including complex partial seizures and grand mal convulsions are an uncommon presentation.
- Infants may present with increasing head circumference, lethargy, and nausea and vomiting.
- Pituitary, suprasellar, and hypothalamic tumours may present with a variety of symptoms, including visual loss, appetite disturbance, precocious or delayed puberty, growth failure, or other endocrine dysfunction.
- Back pain, scoliosis, pyramidal tract signs, and flaccid paralysis may be presenting features in those with spinal tumours and metastases.

21.3.2 **Diagnosis and staging**

The first step in the differential diagnosis of a CNS tumour is to define its anatomical location. Anatomically, CNS tumours can be considered as infra- or supratentorial. Supratentorial tumours are more common in ages 1–3 years, infratentorial (posterior fossa) tumours more common in ages 4–10 years. Tumours within an infratentorial location decrease in proportion with increasing age, whilst tumours located within the supratentorial brain and meninges increase in proportion, with an equal distribution over ten years of age. Primary spinal cord tumours are very rare.

Both CT and MRI can be utilized in the investigation of a child with a suspected CNS tumour. CT, by virtue of its wider availability and shorter scanning times, is often used as the first or screening investigation. It may confirm the presence of a tumour and associated features such as obstructive hydrocephalus. CT is relatively more sensitive for the detection of calcification, which may be seen in craniopharyngiomas. Subsequent MRI is required if an abnormality is shown. MRI has the advantage of defining the location and extent of tumour more accurately, and is very sensitive to the presence of blood products. More specialized MRI techniques, such as magnetic resonance spectroscopy (MRS) and perfusion imaging may be utilized, whereby MRS can aid in differentiating normal tissue from tumour, and perfusion imaging enables identification of neovascularization associated with tumour angiogenesis. While spinal metastases are most common in medulloblastoma and other embryonal tumours, germ cell tumours, and ependymoma, MRI of the spine should be performed in all patients with brain tumours as spinal metastatic disease, although less common, can occur in almost all brain tumour types including both high-grade and low-grade gliomas.

While imaging including CT, diffusion-weighted MRI, and MRS may give a strong indication of the type of tumour, in most cases surgery or at least a biopsy is essential to define its histological type.

Possible exceptions to this general rule include:

- Diffuse intrinsic pontine gliomas which have characteristic MRI appearances and where biopsy may be hazardous (Figure 21.1), although this is being performed in clinical trials to evaluate the molecular pathology.

- Bifocal midline masses in the pineal and suprasellar regions with normal blood and cerebrospinal fluid (CSF) tumour markers which are diagnostic of germinoma.

- A midline mass associated with significantly elevated levels of the tumour markers αFP (alpha-fetoprotein) and/or βHCG (beta-human chorionic gonadotrophin) in blood or CSF, diagnostic of a secreting intracranial germ cell tumour.

For the majority of primary tumours, complete surgical resection is attempted when it is believed that this can be achieved without undue morbidity, with intraoperative MRI being increasingly used in many centres allowing the neurosurgeon to perform image-guided surgical navigation. Otherwise limited surgery such as cyst aspiration or biopsy only is indicated because of the morbidity which would be associated with radical surgery, and the effectiveness of non-surgical treatment. Where a lesion is difficult to access, MRI or CT-guided biopsy may be helpful.

Following surgery for a brain tumour, a postoperative MRI scan with gadolinium should be performed to assess the extent of residual disease. This is particularly important as a surgeon's intraoperative judgement about the completeness of removal may be wrong. It is important to image the spine at this point in time if it was not done preoperatively in those tumour types where there is any risk of metastasis. This includes gliomas of all types as well as intracranial germ cell tumours, ependymomas, and medulloblastoma and other central nervous system embryonal tumours. It is important

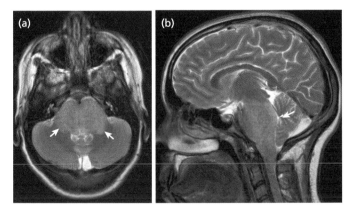

Fig. 21.1 (a) Axial T2-weighted image of a brainstem glioma, showing marked swelling and signal change of the pons, with abnormal signal extending into both cerebellar peduncles (short arrows). (b) Sagittal T2-weighted image of a brainstem glioma causing expansion of the pons and medulla, with marked effacement of the IV ventricle (short arrow).

to perform postoperative MRI within 48 hours, as beyond that time it can be more diffi-cult to distinguish between residual or metastatic disease and surgical artefact. Risk strati-fication depends on the extent of postoperative residual disease in medulloblastoma, and this affects clinical trial eligibility and the radiotherapy dose prescribed.

21.3.3 Imaging for radiotherapy planning

Patients will have a CT scan performed, usually with intravenous contrast, in the treat-ment position in their immobilization shell in the radiotherapy department. This will be of head only when localized cranial radiotherapy is to be given, or of the head and whole spine if craniospinal radiotherapy is necessary (Figure 21.2). Image fusion of pre- and/or postoperative MRI scans will help with target volume definition. Contrast

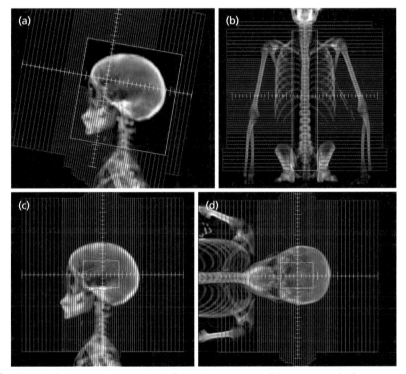

Fig. 21.2 Radiotherapy images. Medulloblastoma, germ cell tumours, and other central nervous system tumours with leptomeningeal metastases require whole CNS radiotherapy. (a) Planning DRR shows the lateral head field covering the brain and cervical spine. The clinical target volume covers the meninges and its reflections and a margin is added to define the PTV. Care is taken to ensure adequate coverage of the cribriform plate area anteriorly which means that the eyes cannot be fully shielded. (b) Planning DRR shows the field covering the whole spine. Care is taken to ensure a precise match with the cranial fields, and to ensure adequate coverage of the spinal theca inferiorly. (c) Planning DRR of the lateral phase II field covering the suprasellar intracranial germ cell tumour. (d) Planning DRR of the phase II anterosuperior field.

administration may be helpful, especially if there is an incompletely resected tumour. For localized tumours, the gross tumour volume (GTV) is usually the area of gadolinium enhancing tumour without surrounding oedema. The clinical target volume (CTV) is the GTV plus a defined margin depending on tumour type as below, or extended to the meninges. The margin for the planning target volume (PTV) will depend on the results of departmental audits of movement within the shell, but will usually be of the order of 3–5 mm.

21.3.4 Therapeutic assessment and follow-up

A baseline post-treatment MRI scan with gadolinium enhancement should be performed about six weeks after completion of treatment. This may be brain-only for tumours without metastatic potential such as craniopharyngioma, but should be of the whole CNS in tumour types which have potential for seeding through the CSF pathways such as medulloblastoma and germ cell tumours. Routine follow-up imaging is performed at 3–6-monthly intervals, usually until five years have elapsed. Interval scans will be required if new symptoms develop. The first symptoms of a recurrence or second tumour may precede imaging changes and so despite a previous normal scan a second scan after an interval of 4–6 weeks should be considered. If there is a clinical suggestion of raised intracranial pressure, a non-contrast CT scan may be adequate as an emergency investigation to confirm or exclude the development of obstructive hydrocephalus.

21.4 Renal tumours

21.4.1 Clinical background

Wilms' tumour or nephroblastoma is the most common renal tumour in childhood and arises from mesodermal precursors of the renal parenchyma. The peak incidence is between three and four years of age, with 80% of affected children being under five years of age. There is an equal sex distribution. It typically presents as an asymptomatic abdominal mass or with pain and fever. Bilateral tumours are seen in approximately 10% of cases, with two-thirds of these being synchronous. Approximately 15% of treated patients will relapse, with the majority occurring within two years after nephrectomy.

There are several associated conditions that predispose to the development of Wilms' tumour, including:

- Beckwith-Wiedemann (10–20% risk of Wilms' tumour)
- Denys-Drash
- Perlman
- WAGR syndromes

Nephroblastomatosis is the persistence of multiple immature nephrogenic rests within the kidney. These should normally involute after 36 weeks of gestation. It is thought to be a precursor to the development of Wilms' tumour and is associated with a number of conditions including trisomies 13 and 18, Beckwith-Wiedemann and Denys-Drash syndromes. It is seen in up to 40% of unilateral, and in nearly all cases of multicentric or bilateral, Wilms' tumour. In the UK, children with an associated condition having risk of developing Wilms' tumour of 5% or more are screened using ultrasound every three months until the age of seven years. The interval accounts for the doubling rate of Wilms' tumour (ten days) and the sensitivity of abdominal ultrasound.

Rarer histologies of renal tumours in childhood include clear cell sarcoma of the kidney, malignant rhabdoid tumour, mesoblastic nephroma, and renal cell carcinoma.

21.4.2 Diagnosis and staging

At US examination, Wilms' tumour typically appears as a mass with increased echogenicity, with or without cystic areas (owing to central necrosis and cyst formation). US is particularly useful in evaluating the renal vein and IVC for tumour extension. The contralateral kidney should be examined for a synchronous lesion or nephroblastomatosis. On cross-sectional imaging it is seen to arise from the kidney, classically with a 'claw' of normal renal tissue seen stretched around the periphery of the tumour. Wilms' tumour typically displaces, rather than encases, vessels in contrast to neuroblastoma (Figure 21.3). MRI may have a role in differentiating hyperplastic nephroblastomatosis and Wilms' tumour from sclerotic (regressive) nephroblastomatosis.

A percutaneous needle biopsy may be performed to confirm the diagnosis and characterize the pathological tumour type, but current guidelines developed by the International Society of Paediatric Oncology (UMBRELLA SIOP-RTSG 2016) recommend that infants under six months of age presenting with a renal mass should be considered for primary surgery, with percutaneous biopsy only recommended in instance of stage IV disease or when immediate surgery is deemed difficult.

Approximately 17% of patients with Wilms' tumours present with stage IV disease with pulmonary metastases being most common. Chest CT is now the standard

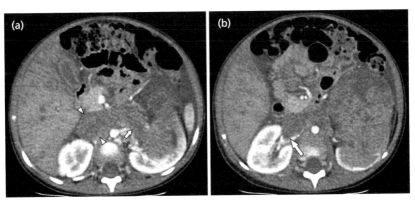

Fig. 21.3 Contrast-enhanced CT of left Wilms' tumour with: (a) left renal vein (short arrow) and IVC tumour thrombosis (arrowheads); (b) tumour thrombus also extends into the right renal vein (long arrow)—stage 2 or 3 determined by complete/incomplete surgical resection respectively.

Table 21.2 Staging system for Wilms' tumour (SIOP protocol)

Stage I	Tumour is confined to the kidney and completely excised
Stage II	Tumour extends beyond the kidney but completely excised
Stage III	Tumour incompletely excised with either microscopic or macroscopic residual disease, or with lymph node involvement within the abdomen or pelvis
Stage IV	Presence of haematogenous metastases (such as lung, bone, liver, brain) or metastases to distant lymph nodes beyond the abdomen or pelvis
Stage V	Bilateral renal involvement at the time of initial diagnosis

Source: data from Vujanić, GM et al. 'Revised International Society of Paediatric Oncology (SIOP) working classification of renal tumors of childhood'. *Med. Pediatr. Oncol.*, Vol. 38, Issue 2, pp.79–82. (2002) John Wiley & Sons.

imaging for staging and will identify small pulmonary nodules too small to be detected by chest X-ray (CXR). CT lung nodules are only treated as metastases if their transverse diameter is at least 3 mm.

Preoperative chemotherapy is utilized to reduce both tumour size and chance of tumour rupture at surgery. Pathology of the resected tumour is very important for two reasons: to determine the local disease stage (Table 21.2) and to assign the patient to a pathological risk group. The pathological risk groups are low, intermediate, or high, and together with the stage determine the details of postoperative therapy.

21.4.3 Imaging for radiotherapy planning

Radiotherapy to the flank or abdomen and pelvis is indicated in Wilms' tumour in the case of stage III intermediate or stage II or III high-risk disease (Figure 21.4), and to the thorax in patients with lung metastases which have not resolved completely with preoperative chemotherapy. The use of abdominal radiotherapy in stage IV and stage V disease is dependent on the local extent of disease.

When radiotherapy is required for the treatment of pulmonary metastases, the whole of both lungs is treated, regardless of the number and extent of metastases.

In the current era, even though treatment techniques are usually still simple anterior and posterior parallel opposed fields, CT planning is used. This allows fusion with earlier diagnostic MR or CT images for accurate target volume definition based on the preoperative tumour extent.

21.4.4 Therapeutic assessment and follow-up

Early detection of local recurrence or distant metastases is the purpose of imaging at follow-up. CXR should be obtained every nine weeks during treatment. The current SIOP surveillance protocol for localized and metastatic disease recommends CXR and abdominal ultrasound every three months for the first two years, with ongoing surveillance according to national guidance, usually repeated every 4–6 months in the third and fourth year. Follow-up should then stop five years after the end of treatment.

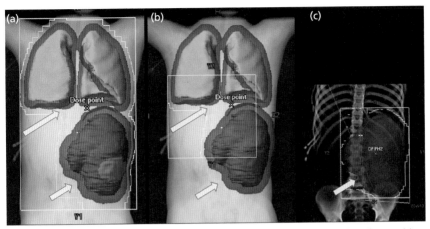

Fig. 21.4 Radiotherapy anterior beams eye view images for a patient with unfavourable histology stage IV (local stage III) Wilms' tumour, who has received pre-operative chemotherapy and surgery, requiring radiotherapy to the whole lungs and left flank. An anterior/posterior parallel opposed technique is used. The lungs and PTV margin are shown (long arrows). Target volume definition for the primary tumour and PTV margin was based on the extent of the tumour and kidney prior to operation (short arrows). Panel (a) shows the phase I main field, prescribed dose 15 Gy in 10 fractions, shaped by multi-leaf collimators, covering both the primary tumour bed and metastatic site. Panel (b) shows a segment field used to homogenise the dose distribution. Panel (c) shows the phase II field, on a digitally reconstructed radiograph showing the bone structure and the primary tumour PTV, again shaped by multi-leaf collimators, which extends medially across the midline to cover the full width of the vertebral bodies and para-aortic lymph node region, prescribed dose 10.5 Gy in 7 fractions (total dose to tumour bed 25.5 Gy in 17 fractions).

21.5 Neuroblastoma

21.5.1 Clinical background

Neuroblastoma arises from neural crest cells in the sympathetic chain. The most common primary site is in the adrenal medulla or elsewhere in the retroperitoneum, about 60%. Less commonly it arises in the posterior mediastinum (20%), or rarely in the neck, pelvis, or with no identifiable primary tumour. The median age at diagnosis is approximately 16 months with 95% of cases diagnosed by seven years of age. Rarely, it may present in teenagers and young adults. The disease shows marked heterogeneity, with age at presentation, stage of disease, and tumour biology affecting outcome. Tumour behaviour is highly variable, with some being aggressive, whilst others, typically in infancy, may spontaneously regress.

The clinical presentation depends on the site of the primary disease, loco-regional extent, and any metastatic spread (Figure 21.5). The most common presentation is with an abdominal mass. Often the tumour grows through the intervertebral foramina, forming a dumb-bell tumour which may lead to spinal cord compression or

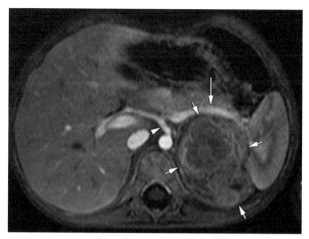

Fig. 21.5 Post-gadolinium T1-weighted axial MRI of left suprarenal neuroblastoma (short arrows) with no involvement of coeliac axis (arrowhead) or splenic artery (long arrow)—stage L1 (INRGSS).

radiculopathy. Metastatic disease may present as bone pain, symptoms of marrow infiltration, fever, and malaise. Infantile metastatic neuroblastoma can present with multiple skin lesions, the so-called 'blueberry muffin' appearance. Asymptomatic presentation is not uncommon. Adrenal masses may be found on antenatal ultrasonography or during investigation of other problems, and thoracic neuroblastoma may be detected incidentally on chest radiography.

21.5.2 Diagnosis and staging

US typically reveals a heterogeneous solid mass, separate from and often displacing the ipsilateral kidney. Further staging investigations include bone marrow trephine, CT or MRI, depending on local availability and ^{123}I labelled metaiodobenzylguanidine (mIBG) scintigraphy to evaluate the primary tumour and metastases. The classical imaging appearance of abdominal neuroblastoma is that of a large soft tissue mass encasing vascular structures (Figure 21.6), with calcification seen in approximately 80% on CT. MRI better delineates extradural intraspinal extension of tumour and bone marrow involvement than CT, with the added advantage of lack of ionizing radiation, and is becoming more widely utilized.

Staging uses the International Neuroblastoma Risk Group (INRG) staging system: stage L1 is a locoregional tumour that does not involve vital structures as defined by the list of image defined risk factors. A stage L2 tumour is a locoregional tumour where there is presence of one or more image defined risk factors. Stage M is distant metastatic disease, with the exception of stage MS. Stage MS is metastatic disease in children under the age of 18 months, with metastatic disease confined to skin and/or liver and/or bone marrow.[1]

This is based on objective radiological staging, at diagnosis, rather than previous systems which have used a post-surgical system. Disease extent is determined by Image

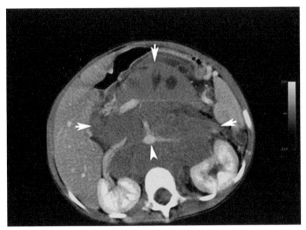

Fig. 21.6 Contrast-enhanced CT of neuroblastoma (short arrows) encasing and displacing the aorta (arrowhead), renal vessels, coeliac artery and its branches—stage L2 (INRGSS).

Defined Risk Factors (IDRF) at diagnosis. Various radiological features seen in neuroblastoma predict for incomplete resection or a greater possibility or surgical complications, and are referred to as image defined risk factors or IDRF.[1] These include:

- When disease extends across two adjacent body compartments.

- When disease in the neck: encases major blood vessels such as the carotid or vertebral arteries or the internal jugular vein; extends to the skull base; or compresses the trachea.

- When disease at the cervico-thoracic junction: encases brachial plexus roots; encases major blood vessels such as the subclavian vessels, the vertebral, or carotid arteries; or compresses the trachea.

- When disease in the thorax encases the aorta or its major branches; compresses the trachea or principal bronchi; a lower mediastinal tumour infiltrates the costovertebral junction between T9 and T12.

- When tumour encases the aorta or vena cava in the thoraco-abdominal region.

- When within the abdomen or pelvis, tumour infiltrates the porta hepatis; infiltrates branches of the superior mesenteric artery at the mesenteric root; encases the origin of the coeliac axis, the superior mesenteric artery, the aorta, inferior vena cava, or the iliac vessels; invades a renal pedicle; crosses the sciatic notch.

- When at any vertebral level, a dumb-bell tumour invades more than one third of the spinal canal in the axial plane; the perimedullary leptomeningeal spaces are not visible; or the spinal cord signal is abnormal.

- When the disease involves or infiltrates adjacent organs or structures, for example pericardium, diaphragm, kidney, liver, duodeno-pancreatic block, mesentery, and others.

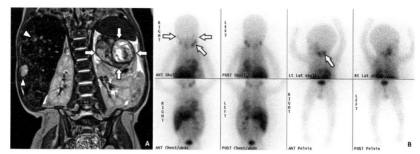

Fig. 21.7 Metastatic neuroblastoma in a 15-month-old infant. (a) Coronal T2 SPACE of left suprarenal neuroblastoma (short arrows) with liver metastases (arrowheads). (b) mIBG study demonstrated multifocal bone uptake within the left mandible, supraorbital regions and skull base (short arrows)—stage M (INRG staging system).

The presence of multifocal primary tumours, pleural effusion, or ascites, with or without malignant cells should be recorded, but these are not considered to be IDRF.

Metastatic disease is defined as any disease spread that is not in continuity with the primary tumour, including non-contiguous lymph node spread. The new stage MS (previously stage 4S) now has an upper age limit of 18 months (Figure 21.7), as the benefit of young age extends beyond infancy. Biopsy of the primary tumour is undertaken at diagnosis to evaluate the histology and cell ploidy of the tumour and determine if *MYCN* amplification is present. Approximately 20% of cases will demonstrate *MYCN* amplification, which is associated with metastatic disease and a poorer prognosis. A combination of INRG staging system, age of the patient (younger or older than 18 months), *MYCN* status, and histology define the risk group for each case, which determines the treatment received.

21.5.3 Imaging for radiotherapy planning

The treatment of neuroblastoma involves complex multimodality therapy including surgery, chemotherapy, radiotherapy, and biological treatments, and the precise treatment schedule is dependent on risk-group assignment. Radiotherapy is indicated to the primary tumour site in all patients with high-risk disease, that is to say children over 18 months of age with stage M disease, and in patients with *MYCN* amplified disease stage L2 or M regardless of age (Figure 21.8). Selected patients with intermediate-risk disease, those *MYCN* non-amplified stage L2 aged over 18 months with undifferentiated histology, should also receive radiotherapy to the primary site. Patients with low-risk disease, principally those with L1, L2, or MS disease under 18 months of age without *MYCN* amplification are managed with much less intensive treatment, surgery, or chemotherapy alone or in combination, or sometimes observation alone in the hope of spontaneous regression.

Target volume definition for radiotherapy in the local control of the primary tumour in patients with high-risk neuroblastoma and intermediate-risk disease is based on the post-chemotherapy, pre-surgery, extent of the tumour. Patients will be assessed by contrast-enhanced CT or MRI following induction chemotherapy. It is often easier to define the full extent of the disease on contrast enhanced CT, than on MRI. Subsequently patients will undergo resection of their tumour if operable and often high-dose chemotherapy also, so an interval of three months may elapse before they

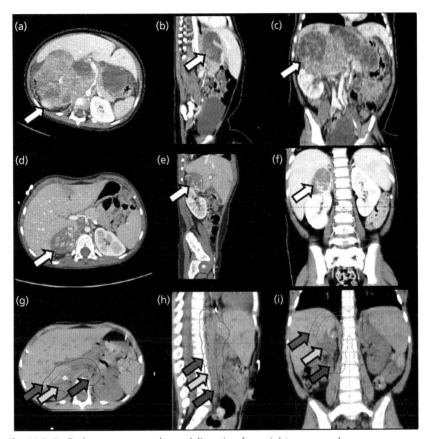

Fig. 21.8 Radiotherapy target volume delineation for a right suprarenal neuroblastoma: (a) axial; (b) sagittal; and (c) coronal CT images to demonstrate the size and location of the tumour at diagnosis. (d) axial, (e) sagittal, and (f) coronal CT images to show a much smaller tumour following induction chemotherapy prior to surgery. (g) axial, (h) sagittal, and (i) coronal planning CT scan images following surgery and high-dose chemotherapy. The bulk of the tumour has gone, but some pathological calcification remains. Virtual gross tumour volume (GTV) was based on images d, e, and f, cut back to barriers of spread where previously displaced organs had returned to a more normal position, and modified by the surgical and pathology reports (purple outline and arrows). Clinical target volume (CTV) grown from GTV by 0.5 cm except over vertebrae (pink outline and arrows). Planning target volume (PTV) grown from CTV by 0.5 cm (red outline and arrows).

are ready for radiotherapy. A planning scan done at this time may be fused with the earlier scan. The initial scan is used to define the virtual GTV, based on the extent of the primary tumour and any contiguous nodal spread. A 0.5–1 cm margin is added to define the CTV which may be modified to include whole vertebrae to avoid the development of a scoliosis and to allow for uninvolved organs such as liver which may have moved into the space previously occupied by tumour. To minimize irradiation of critical normal structures such as the contralateral kidney the CTV may be reduced again. The radiotherapy planning scan is also used to define organs at risk (OAR), including the kidneys, liver, and lungs.

The art of target volume definition in paediatric radiotherapy is to achieve the best balance between full coverage of the tumour and avoidance of OAR. Sometimes it is necessary to compromise on the recommended protocol treatment of the tumour with regard to total dose, volume, or both, to reduce the risk of unacceptable normal tissue damage.

21.5.4 Therapeutic assessment and follow-up

In addition to standard cross-sectional imaging, ^{123}I-mIBG scintigraphy is important to assess the response to therapy of metastatic disease. Semi-quantitative scoring systems are used. New criteria to assess response to therapy have been described. In these, the extent of disease, and the response, in three separate compartments: bone, bone marrow, and soft tissue, are separately evaluated. The responses seen in these three components are then combined to give an overall response (Figure 21.9).

21.6 Lymphoma

21.6.1 Clinical background

Lymphoma arises from lymphatic cells and approximately half are Hodgkin lymphoma (HL) and half non-Hodgkin lymphoma (NHL). Radiotherapy is important in the management of HL, but the treatment of NHL in childhood is almost exclusively chemotherapy. The rest of this section therefore relates only to HL.

The most typical clinical presentation is with painless cervical or supraclavicular lymphadenopathy. At least two thirds of patients will have some degree of mediastinal involvement which may be detected incidentally on a CXR taken for other reasons. Systemic symptoms such as fever, night sweats, and weight loss may also be present.

21.6.2 Diagnosis and staging

Initial imaging investigations usually include a CXR and US of both the neck and abdomen, including high-resolution US imaging of the liver and spleen to assess for small focal lesions. Cross-sectional imaging has a central role in staging, as the anatomical extent of disease at diagnosis has a profound impact on management and outcome. Imaging of the neck, abdomen, and pelvis can be performed with either CT or MRI. The chest should be imaged using CT, as current MRI techniques are not

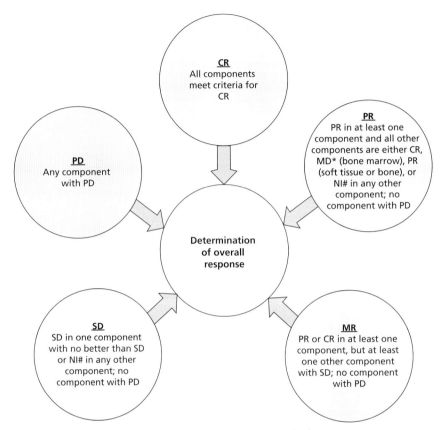

Fig. 21.9 Revised International Neuroblastoma Response Criteria
Response abbreviations: CR, complete response; MD, minimal disease; MR, minor response; NI, not involved; PD, progressive disease; PR partial response; SD, stable disease.
* For bone marrow assessment only
# Site not involved at study entry and remains uninvolved
Source: data from Park JR et al. 'Revisions to the International Neuroblastoma Response Criteria: A Consensus Statement From the National Cancer Institute Clinical Trials Planning Meeting', Journal of Clinical Oncology, (2017) Vol. 35, Issue 22, pp.2580–2587

sufficiently sensitive to detect small pulmonary nodules. HL is staged according to Cotswold revision of the Ann Arbor classification (Table 21.3).

Biopsy is essential for diagnosis either from surgical excision of a node or by percutaneous, image-guided core biopsy.

[18]F-fluorodeoxyglucose positron emission tomography (FDG PET) enables assessment of the metabolic activity of involved nodal groups and organs in addition to the anatomical evaluation obtained with CT or MRI.[2] Whole body FDG PET/CT is now a standard investigation at both diagnosis and follow-up in paediatric and adolescent HL (Figure 21.10).

Table 21.3 Cotswolds revision of the Ann Arbor staging system for lymphoma

Stage I	Single lymph node region involvement, including isolated splenic involvement
Stage II	Two or more lymph node regions involved on the same side of the diaphragm
Stage III	Lymph node groups or lymph structures involved on both sides of the diaphragm
Stage IV	Discontinuous extra-nodal involvement: Liver lesions Pulmonary lesions: nodule >1 cm or >three nodules <1 cm size Bone or bone marrow involvement CNS involvement
A	Absence of 'B' symptoms
B	Presence of at least one of: ♦ Unexplained weight loss of >10% in six months ♦ Drenching night sweats ♦ Unexplained persistent or recurrent fever >38°C
E	Involvement of a single extra-nodal site in continuity with nodal disease, except liver or bone marrow involvement—always implies stage IV disease

Source: Lister TA, Crowther D, Sutcliffe SB et al. Report of a committee convened to discuss the evaluation and staging of patients with Hodgkin's disease: Cotswolds meeting. *J Clin Oncol.* 1989 Nov;7(11):1630-6. doi: 10.1200/JCO.1989.7.11.1630.

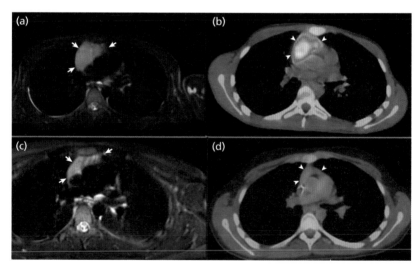

Fig. 21.10 Anterior mediastinal mass: (a) staging axial MR image of anterior mediastinal mass (short arrows) with corresponding fused PET/CT; (b) showing FDG avidity (arrowheads), restaging following two cycles of chemotherapy; (c) MR image showing reduction in size, but persistent mediastinal disease; (d) fused PET/CT image showing an excellent metabolic response to chemotherapy, with no residual FDG avidity.

21.6.3 Therapeutic assessment and follow-up

Patients are reassessed after two cycles of chemotherapy and again at end of treatment with CT or MRI of the neck, abdomen, and pelvis, with CT of the thorax if pulmonary disease was present at diagnosis, to assess anatomical response to chemotherapy (Table 21.4).

A PET scan is also performed after two cycles of chemotherapy to assess metabolic response. It is recognized that both false positive and false negative PET findings can be seen if the PET scan is performed too soon after completion of the chemotherapy cycle and hence at least a two-week gap between the end of chemotherapy and the PET study being performed is recommended. Ongoing clinical trials utilize PET response after two cycles of chemotherapy to determine if radiotherapy may be omitted. The presence of any persistent FDG PET avid nodes or organs after two cycles of chemotherapy denotes an inadequate response and therefore radiotherapy will be administered to all involved nodes, as defined by the initial staging investigations.

In the first year following end of treatment, in addition to clinical examination, it is recommended that abdominal US be performed as a surveillance tool, initially four times a year, decreasing in frequency in the third year following end of treatment.

21.6.4 Imaging for radiotherapy planning

Radiotherapy is given to patients with HL who fail to respond adequately to two courses of chemotherapy. A positive PET scan, or persistently enlarged nodes even if PET negative, is an indication for radiotherapy on completion of chemotherapy. The duration of chemotherapy is based on initial stage rather than response to treatment.

Current radiotherapy is based on CT planning (Figure 21.11). A planning CT scan is performed for target volume definition, optimization of the plan, and dosimetry of normal tissues. If it is possible to have therapy radiographers present at the reassessment PET/CT

Table 21.4 Imaging assessment of response to therapy in childhood and adolescent lymphoma

Local complete remission (local CR)	Residual tumour volume ≤5% reference volume at initial staging residual tumour volume ≤2 mL
Local complete remission unconfirmed (local CRu)	No local CR and: ◆ Residual tumour volume ≤25% reference volume ◆ Residual tumour ≤2 mL
Local partial remission (local PR)	No local CR or local CRu and: ◆ Residual tumour volume ≤50% reference volume ◆ Residual tumour volume is ≤5 mL
Local no change (local NC)	No local CR or local CRu or local PR and: ◆ No local progression
Local progression (local PRO)	Residual tumour volume >125% of reference volume or significantly increases compared with best previous response

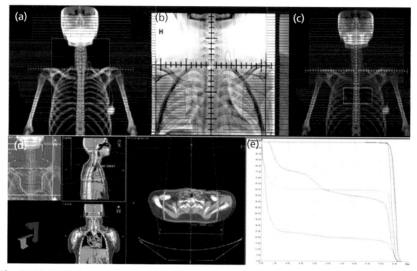

Fig. 21.11 Radiotherapy images. (a) Planning DRR to show complete anterior field covering neck, supraclavicular, and superior mediastinal nodal areas. (b) Simulator check film confirming correct field placement. (c) Planning DRR of anterior boost field used to achieve dose homogeneity. (d) Isodose plans showing dose distribution in axial, coronal, and sagittal planes. (e) Dose volume histograms confirming good coverage of target volumes and acceptable doses to organs at risk.

scan to place skin markers, and use a flat couch top with the patient in the treatment position, it is possible to use the CT component of the PET/CT scan for treatment planning rather than perform a repeat CT scan for planning purposes in the treatment department.

The current European Hodgkin trial (EuroNet: PHL C2 trial) no longer treats all involved areas at diagnosis but rather targets radiotherapy to residual metabolically active sites only. The nodal groups are identified on CT. The whole length of lymph node chains, for example down the mediastinum, are treated, but if there has been a good shrinkage of an initial bulky mass it is sufficient to use the residual width as the GTV, and not necessary to treat the whole width at diagnosis.

21.7 Primary bone tumours: osteosarcoma and Ewing's sarcoma

21.7.1 Clinical background

Osteosarcoma (OS) is the commonest malignant paediatric primary bone tumour, characterized histologically by the presence of malignant mesenchymal cells that produce immature bone or osteoid. It is rare in young children, the peak incidence of primary osteosarcoma is in adolescents between the ages of 15–19 years with 75% occurring before the age of 20. It becomes rarer again in adult life, although secondary osteosarcoma is recognized as a complication of previous radiotherapy, Paget's disease of bone in the elderly, and germline abnormalities such as Li-Fraumeni and Werner syndrome. Males are affected more frequently.

There are many histological subtypes; however, the commonest, high-grade central osteosarcoma (also known as classic or conventional OS) accounts for >90% of cases. Whilst it can affect any bone, the majority of cases arise in the appendicular skeleton, most commonly around the knee (up to 75% cases) or proximal humerus. Involvement of axial and craniofacial tumour sites increase with age. Presentation is typically delayed, patients complaining of localized pain and swelling often attributed to trivial injury. Referred pain felt in the knee may mask the presentation of a proximal femoral lesion.

The Ewing family of tumours are a rare group of paediatric small blue round cell tumours arising from primitive neural elements, which includes classic Ewing's sarcoma (ES) of bone, soft tissue ES, and peripheral primitive neuroectodermal tumours (pPNET). ES is more common than OS in young children and the second most common primary bone tumour in adolescents, with the median age at diagnosis being 15 years. Cases continue to be seen into adult life. Pain is the presenting symptom in most cases, which typically persists through the night and, as in OS, is often attributed to trivial injury or growing pains. Additional symptoms include swelling and constitutional signs such as fever.

Patients with bone tumours should be managed at designated supraregional bone tumour units. Patients should be referred to such a centre for diagnosis when the suspicion is raised, rather than being imaged and biopsied close to home in general orthopaedic units.

21.7.2 Diagnosis and staging

Plain films in two planes are the initial investigation in most cases of suspected primary bone tumour. Appearances of OS are variable, with classical OS typically having a mixed sclerotic/lytic appearance involving the metaphysis of a long bone, often accompanied by an aggressive periosteal reaction and soft tissue mass. Extension into the diaphysis and/or epiphysis is common, occasionally in association with a pathological fracture; this is associated with an increased risk of local recurrence owing to the dissemination of tumour cells into the surrounding tissues.

In ES, the extremity bones (50% of all cases) followed by the pelvis, ribs, and vertebrae are most commonly affected (Figures 21.12 and 21.13). Tumours involving long bones typically have an aggressive permeative, lytic appearance within the diaphysis, often accompanied by a soft tissue mass; however, up to a quarter of lesions are sclerotic at presentation.

For both OS and ES, further local site staging with MRI, including the whole anatomical compartment, the involved bone, and adjacent joint should be performed. MRI is used to evaluate local extent due to its multiplanar capabilities and superior soft tissue resolution, with emphasis on defining intra- and extraosseous tumour extent, and involved tissue compartments that will ultimately influence the surgical approach. MRI is also useful in the detection of skip lesions (defined as secondary tumour foci occurring simultaneously within the same bone) seen in up to 25% of OS cases, contralateral lesions, and in defining the relationship of tumour to nearby neurovascular structures. CT is routinely used in addition to MRI for pelvic tumours and is often helpful in cases of diagnostic uncertainty, allowing better

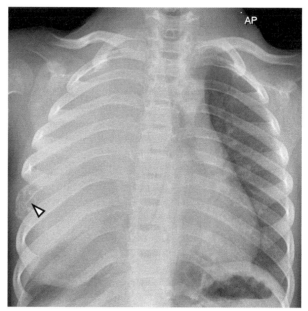

Fig. 21.12 Antero-posterior chest radiograph showing a large soft tissue mass within the right hemithorax exerting mass effect with lytic destruction of the right sixth rib (arrowhead).

visualization of microcalcification, periosteal new bone formation, and cortical destruction (Figure 21.13). Further staging includes CT chest and whole body MRI which has superseded technetium-99m (^{99m}Tc)-phosphonate bone scan. Around 20–25% of ES patients have metastatic disease at presentation, involving the lung (10%), bone/bone marrow (10%), combinations, or others (5%).

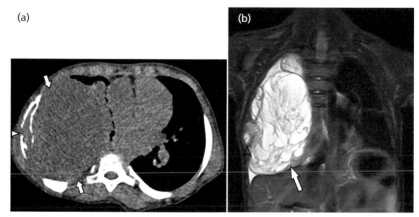

(a)

(b)

Fig. 21.13 Ewing's sarcoma. (a) Unenhanced CT chest demonstrating a large mass occupying the right hemithorax (short arrows) and destruction of the lateral sixth rib (filled arrowheads). (b) Coronal STIR MR image of the chest better depicts the nature of the soft tissue mass (long arrows) which is arising from the lateral sixth rib (empty arrowhead).

Histological confirmation requires bone biopsy, which will be performed at the designated bone tumour treatment centre and should only be done after local imaging of the affected bone. The approach taken should be discussed with the bone tumour surgeon to avoid contamination of unaffected soft tissue compartments and to ensure resection of the biopsy tract at primary surgery.

Whilst not part of routine staging, FDG PET has proven to be both sensitive and specific in detecting bone metastases, as well as being advantageous in assessment response to treatment; however, it has yet to become part of an international staging system for either OS or ES, owing to limited availability. There is also increasing evidence that whole body MRI combined with FDG PET improves the detection of bone and bone marrow metastases in children and adolescents compared with either imaging modality alone or standard skeletal scintigraphy, with earlier detection of intramedullary tumour deposits before osteoblastic responses occur which are necessary for uptake on a conventional bone scan.

Treatment of patients with ES and OS is influenced by disease stage. Several staging systems for bone tumours are in use; however, none are perfect or widely accepted. Whilst each system differs slightly, their universal aim is the identification of prognostic factors influencing both local recurrence rates and metastatic disease. Adverse prognostic factors include primary site, metastases, and age at presentation (>15 years), tumour volume or diameter >8 cm, elevated lactate dehydrogenase (LDH) levels, and poor histological response to induction chemotherapy.

21.7.3 Imaging for radiotherapy planning

Current treatment strategies rely on neoadjuvant chemotherapy with surgery for local disease control and all resectable metastases. Radiotherapy has only a limited role in the management of extremity OS, being reserved for inoperable disease or following incomplete resection. Radical radiotherapy may be used as the sole local control modality in axial OS which is inoperable. Treatment planning is based on the extent of disease as determined by MRI.

Ewing's tumours are radiosensitive. Preoperative radiotherapy is considered in borderline cases based on their response to induction chemotherapy assessed using a variety of imaging modalities including CT, whole body MRI, FDG PET, and thallium studies. Radiotherapy may be used alone in cases where only intralesional surgery would be possible or where metastatic disease is present.

Prior to radiotherapy planning, careful consideration needs to be given to the positioning of the area to be treated to allow for adequate treatment with maximum sparing of uninvolved normal tissues. Limbs should be immobilized in custom-made shells and a planning CT scan undertaken. Target volumes are defined based on the initial diagnostic MRI. The GTV is the tumour extent demonstrated by imaging. The CTV includes an additional longitudinal margin of up to 3 cm in long bones, leaving an unirradiated corridor of skin and subcutaneous tissue in the limb to prevent the development of lymphoedema. Any surgical scars or drainage sites should be included in the radiation field to ensure all potential sites of microscopic disease are treated.

21.7.4 **Therapeutic assessment and follow-up**

Local response to treatment is best monitored with MRI. Dynamic contrast enhanced (DCE) MRI is reliable in OS and allows changes in tumour vascularity to be evaluated. However, it is less reliable in ES as remaining small tumour foci may be missed. In this setting sequential FDG PET assessment may be of value. The role of diffusion weighted MRI is still under evaluation. Metastatic disease can be assessed with an array of imaging techniques dependent on the site. This will include CT chest, total body MRI, FDG PET, and isotope bone scans.

Studies report that 30–40% of patients experience recurrent disease either locally, at a distance from the primary site, or a combination of the two. Recurrence is associated with a poor prognosis, worse still if disease recurs within two years of initial diagnosis. Current guidelines recommend follow-up for at least 15 years.

21.8 **Soft tissue sarcomas: rhabdomyosarcoma and other types**

21.8.1 **Clinical background**

Soft tissue sarcomas can be classified into two main groups: rhabdomyosarcoma (RMS) and a variety of other (non-RMS) soft tissue sarcomas. RMS is the commonest childhood soft tissue sarcoma, with almost two-thirds of cases diagnosed in children aged six years or under. It is a highly malignant tumour arising from primitive mesenchymal cells prior to their differentiation into striated muscle. Histologically there are two main subtypes. About 75% are embryonal rhabdomyosarcoma (eRMS). Alveolar rhabdomyosarcoma (aRMS) carries a worse prognosis and is diagnosed on the basis of characteristic morphology and a high level of myogenin positivity on immunohistochemistry. There are many other types of soft tissue sarcoma encountered in children and young people, grouped together as non-RMS soft tissue sarcoma and including synovial cell carcinoma, fibrosarcoma, and malignant fibrous histiocytoma. As far as imaging goes, RMS and non-RMS soft tissue sarcomas can be considered together, as imaging is more dependent on anatomical site than histological type.

Clinical presentation is usually with a mass within the affected body region, in addition to disturbances in body function by an enlarging tumour, or lymphadenopathy. RMS can arise almost anywhere within the body except bone, the more commonly affected sites involve the head and neck (40%), the genitourinary system (30%), and the extremities (16%).

Within the head and neck, a distinction is drawn between those tumours confined to the orbit which carry a very good prognosis, and other sites which are divided into parameningeal (50%) and non-parameningeal primary sites (50%). Parameningeal tumours are sited near the skull base, and there is a tendency for intracranial spread to occur through the neural and vascular foramina. Such sites include the nasopharynx, nasal cavity, and paranasal sinuses, middle ear and mastoid, infratemporal fossa, and pterygopalatine fossa. Non-parameningeal sites include the oral cavity, cheek, and larynx.

Genitourinary primary sites are divided into bladder and prostate primary sites, and non-bladder/prostate sites including the vulva, vagina, and cervix in girls and paratesticular tissues in boys (Figure 21.14).

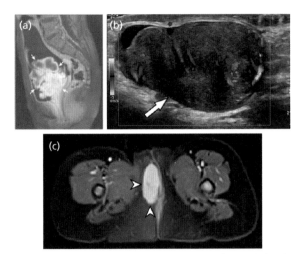

Fig. 21.14 Rhabdomyosarcoma. (a) Post-gadolinium sagittal T1-weighted MR image of a partly cystic, partly solid bladder rhabdomyosarcoma. (b) Doppler US of the left scrotum with a large, vascular paratesticular rhabdomyosarcoma. (c) Post-gadolinium axial T1-weighted MR of a homogenously enhancing, solid right labial rhabdomyosarcoma.

Age and site at presentation differ for the subtypes, eRMS typically presenting in the younger children with orbital or other head and neck or genitourinary primaries, whilst aRMS tends to affect older children and adolescents involving the extremities.

21.8.2 Diagnosis and staging

Initial diagnostic investigations will be guided by the site of primary tumour and its associated symptoms and signs. Genitourinary RMS is typically imaged with US in the first instance, followed by CT or MRI to assess extent and nodal involvement, whilst head and neck and extremity primaries are best imaged with MRI owing to its superior soft tissue resolution.

Approximately 20% of patients present with metastases at diagnosis. Evaluation for metastatic disease includes CT chest and ^{99m}Tc-diphosphonate bone scan reflecting the propensity of RMS to metastasize to lung and bone. Bone marrow aspirate and trephine are also essential to diagnose bone marrow involvement. More focused staging investigations will depend on the knowledge of spread from specific primary sites, for example CSF sampling required in cases of cranial parameningeal tumours. PET/CT is now recognized as useful in the staging of RMS, and in quantifying disease activity in non-RMS soft tissue tumours. The main staging system for risk stratification is the IRSG (Intergroup Rhabdomyosarcoma Study Group) system, which defines four categories based on the extent of spread at diagnosis and volume of residual disease following initial surgery.

◆ Group I: primary complete resection with clear margins.

◆ Group II: complete resection but positive margins on histology.

◆ Group III: macroscopic residual tumour or biopsy only.

◆ Group IV: distant metastases at diagnosis.

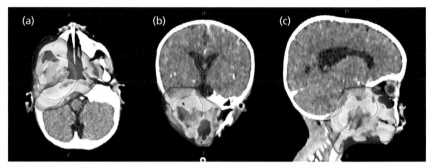

Fig. 21.15 Radiotherapy images. This patient had a parameningeal (left parapharyngeal) embryonal rhabdomyosarcoma, treated by an intensity modulated arc therapy technique with a simultaneous integrated boost. Isodose distribution in (a) axial, (b) coronal, and (c) right para-sagittal planes, showing PTV 42.5 Gy (outer margin) and PTV 50.4 Gy (inner margin). The colour wash is set at 95% of 42.5 Gy, demonstrating excellent conformality with the PTV.

Full risk stratification takes into account the size of the tumour (5 cm or less in maximum diameter, or greater than 5 cm), age, histology, site, and lymph node involvement as well as IRS group.

21.8.3 Imaging for radiotherapy planning

Radiotherapy is indicated for the majority of patients with RMS (Figure 21.15). Exceptions include very young children, IRS group I, or IRS group II or III where there is a secondary complete resection. The target volume definition is usually based on the size of the primary tumour at diagnosis. Exceptions to this include tumours which extend into a body cavity without direct invasion, and shrink back to the tissue of origin with chemotherapy. For example, a chest wall tumour may extend significantly into the pleural cavity. Following a good response to chemotherapy it is still necessary to irradiate all of the chest wall initially involved, but not the lung, which occupies the intrathoracic space previously occupied by tumour. The pretreatment T1 postcontrast MRI is usually the optimum imaging study for defining the GTV. These images can be fused with the planning CT scan performed with the patient immobilized as necessary in the treatment position (Figure 21.16). The CTV is usually the GTV plus 1 cm, but adjustments need to be made for areas of possible subclinical extension (such as the full thickness of the skull base in parameningeal cases) or if there are natural barriers to spread, and to include scars, drain sites, and biopsy tracts.

21.8.4 Therapeutic assessment and follow-up

Response to therapy in RMS is usually with the same imaging modality used at diagnosis. However, if the original imaging modality used was CT, MRI should be considered to reduce the use of ionizing radiation. The response to chemotherapy is not as important a prognostic factor as was thought previously. Imaging of the primary site

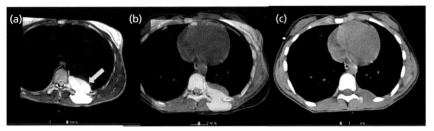

Fig. 21.16 Radiotherapy CT/MR fusion. (a) shows axial MRI left paraspinal rhabdomyosarcoma extending through the chest wall at diagnosis (arrowed). (b) shows the fused image set. (c) shows the post-chemotherapy radiotherapy planning CT scan. The original gross tumour volume can be delineated on scan (a), and then modified as necessary on scan (c).

should also include assessment of regional lymph nodes as routine lymph node sampling at surgery is not advocated in most cases. If there is a definite residual mass after therapy, FDG PET/CT imaging may be useful to identify persistent metabolic activity, or an image-guided biopsy may be undertaken to differentiate between residual active disease and fibrosis or scarring. Often there is a residual abnormality on imaging but without mass effect, in which case PET will probably be unhelpful.

21.9 Summary

◆ Malignant disease in children is uncommon.

◆ Childhood tumours are a pathologically heterogeneous group.

◆ Children with a suspected malignancy should be assessed at a designated paediatric oncology centre.

◆ An age-appropriate approach is required for both imaging and radiotherapy.

◆ Close multidisciplinary team working is vital for success.

Further reading

Arumugam S, Manning-Cork NJ, Gains JE, et al. (2019). The evidence for external beam radiotherapy in high-risk neuroblastoma of childhood: a systematic review. *Clinical Oncology* (Royal College of Radiologists), **31**:182–190. doi: 10.1016/j.clon.2018.11.031. Epub 1 Dec 2018.

Brisse HJ, McCarville MB, Granata C, et al. (2011). **International Neuroblastoma Risk Group Project.** Guidelines for imaging and staging of neuroblastic tumors: consensus report from the International Neuroblastoma Risk Group Project. *Radiology*, **261**(1): 243–257. doi: 10.1148/radiol.11101352. Epub 17 May 2011.

Casali PG, Bielack S, Abecassis N, et al. (2018). Bone sarcomas: ESMO-PaedCan-EURACAN Clinical Practice Guidelines for diagnosis, treatment and follow-up. *Annals of Oncology*, **29**: 79–95.

Cohn SL, Pearson AD, London WB, et al. (2009). INRG Task Force. The International Neuroblastoma Risk Group (INRG) classification system: an INRG Task Force report. *Journal of Clinical Oncology*, **27**: 289–297. doi: 10.1200/JCO.2008.16.6785. Epub 1 Dec 2008.

Dumba M, Jawad N, McHugh K (2015). Neuroblastoma and nephroblastoma: a radiological review. *Cancer Imaging*, **15**: 5.

Gerrand C, Athanasou N, Brennan B, et al. (2016). UK guidelines for the management of bone sarcomas. *Clinical Sarcoma Research*, **6**: 7.

Louis DN, Perry A, Reifenberger G, *et al.* (2016). The 2016 World Health Organization classification of tumors of the central nervous system: a summary. *Acta Neuropathologica*, **131**: 803–820. doi: 10.1007/s00401-016-1545-1. Epub 9 May 2016.

Matthay KK, Maris JM, Schleiermacher G, et al. (2016). Neuroblastoma. *Nature Reviews Disease Primers*, **2**: 16078. doi: 10.1038/nrdp.2016.78.

Metzger ML, Mauz-Körholz C (2019). Epidemiology, outcome, targeted agents and immunotherapy in adolescent and young adult non-Hodgkin and Hodgkin lymphoma. *British Journal of Haematology*, doi: 10.1111/bjh.15789. 6 Feb 2019. Review.

Park K, van Rijn R, McHugh K (2008). The role of radiology in paediatric soft tissue sarcomas. *Cancer Imaging*, **8**: 102–115.

Park JR, Bagatell R, Cohn SL, et al. (2017). Revisions to the International Neuroblastoma Response Criteria: a consensus statement from the National Cancer Institute clinical trials planning meeting. *Journal of Clinical Oncology*, **35**: 2580–2587. doi: 10.1200/JCO.2016.72.0177. Epub 4 May 2017. Review.

Skapek SX, Ferrari A, Gupta AA, et al. (2019). Rhabdomyosarcoma. *Nature Reviews Disease Primers*, **5**: 1. doi: 10.1038/s41572-018-0051-2. Review.

Toma P, Granata C, Rossi A, et al. (2007). Multimodality imaging of Hodgkin disease and non-Hodgkin lymphomas in children. *Radiographics*, **27**: 1335–1355.

van den Heuvel-Eibrink MM, Hol JA, Pritchard-Jones K, et al. (2017). Rationale for the treatment of Wilms' tumour in the UMBRELLA SIOP-RTSG 2016 protocol. *Nature Reviews Urology*, **14**: 743–752.

Reference

1. Monclair T, Brodeur GM, Ambros PF, et al. (2009). The International Neuroblastoma Risk Group (INRG) staging system: an INRG task force report. *Journal of Clinical Oncology*, **27**: 298–303.

Chapter 22

Imaging for common complications

Helen Addley, Katy Hickman, and
Thankamma Ajithkumar

22.1 Introduction

Patients with cancer are prone to multiple complications, whether secondary to treatment or due to the cancer itself. Imaging plays a critical role in their diagnosis and evaluation. It is beyond the scope of this chapter to present a detailed review, but the imaging appearances of the most commonly encountered complications in clinical practice are outlined.

22.2 Venous thromboembolism

Malignancy is a major risk factor with both cancer type and stage influencing the development of venous thromboembolism (VTE), notably pulmonary embolism (PE) and deep venous thrombosis (DVT). The highest incidence is seen in metastatic pancreatic, stomach, bladder, uterine, renal, and lung cancer. Other contributory risk factors include chemotherapy, radiotherapy, surgery, and immobility (Table 22.1). Cancer-associated VTE is serious and potentially life threatening, being the second leading cause of mortality in cancer patients following the disease itself.[1] Major risk factors for VTE are as follows: surgery—major abdominal and pelvic surgery, hip or knee replacement, postoperative intensive care; obstetrics—late pregnancy, caesarean section, puerperium; lower limb problems—fracture, varicose veins; malignancy—abdominal/pelvic, advanced/metastatic; reduced mobility—hospitalization, institutional care; miscellaneous—previous proven VTE.[2]

22.2.1 Pulmonary embolism

22.2.1.1 Clinical assessment of pulmonary embolism

The value of clinical judgement in diagnosing pulmonary embolism (PE) has been demonstrated by several large series including Prospective Investigation of Pulmonary Embolism Diagnosis (PIOPED) II. The British Thoracic Society (BTS) guidelines[2] require that the patient has clinical signs and symptoms compatible with

Table 22.1 Wells Score for PE

Variable	Points
Previous PE or DVT	+1.5
Heart rate >100 bpm	+1.5
Recent surgery or immobilization	+1.5
Clinical signs of DVT	+3
Haemoptysis	+1
Malignancy with active treatment	+1
Alternative diagnosis less likely than PE	+3

Source: data from Philip S. Wells et al. 'Excluding pulmonary embolism at the bedside without diagnostic imaging: management of patients with suspected pulmonary embolism presenting to the emergency department by using a simple clinical model and D-dimer'. *Annals of Internal Medicine*. Vol. 135, Issue 2, pp. 98–107. (2001) American College of Physicians.

PE, that is, breathlessness and/or tachypnoea with or without pleuritic chest pain and/or haemoptysis. In order to help standardize clinical judgement several prediction tools have been developed, with the most frequently used being the Well's score. This score consists of seven questions, outlined in Table 22.1, to establish if PE is the more likely diagnosis. The modified Well's score separates patients into a low probability group (score ≤4) or high probability (>4).

22.2.1.2 D-dimer

For patients with a low probability of PE based on the Well's score, the negative predictive value of a D-Dimer <750 µg L^{-1} is 99%. Therefore, no further testing is required for those with a normal D-dimer and a low probability clinical assessment. However, it reduces to 79% for those with a high probability of PE; as such, D-dimer assays are not recommended for patients with high pre-test probability. The utility of the D-dimer test is in a negative result which reliably excludes PE in patients with low or intermediate clinical probability.

22.2.1.3 Computed tomographic pulmonary angiography

Computed tomographic pulmonary angiography (CTPA) is the initial imaging investigation recommended by both BTS and PIOPED II for all patients except those with low or intermediate clinical probability and a negative D-dimer (Figure 22.1). This method has higher specificity for diagnosis of PE, detection of alternative pathology, wider availability, and very short scanning time. Potential disadvantages include the use of iodinated contrast and the reduced sensitivity for small subsegmental thrombus when compared to pulmonary angiography. However, the widespread use of multi-slice computed tomography (CT) scanners, means that detection rates are increasing, even on standard CT imaging follow-up. Patients with a good quality negative CTPA do not require further investigation for PE.

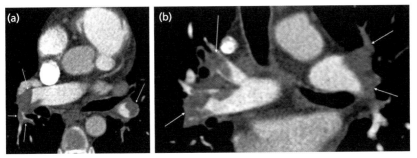

Fig. 22.1 Axial (a) and coronal (b) CTPA images demonstrating filling defects in the right and left main pulmonary arteries and all segmental branches consistent with bilateral pulmonary emboli (white arrows).

22.2.1.4 Ventilation/perfusion scanning

A ventilation/perfusion scan remains a helpful option for patients with renal impairment, in young patients, and pregnant women or women of reproductive age, to diagnose PE. A normal scan will reliably exclude PE. However, interpretation is only reliable when a current high-quality erect chest radiograph is available. Indeterminate scans are often seen in patients with an abnormal chest radiograph and therefore should not be performed unless the chest X-ray is normal. Further imaging is mandatory in patients with either an indeterminate lung scintigraphy scan or discordant clinical and scintigraphic probabilities. The BTS recommends that ventilation/perfusion scans should only be used as the initial imaging assessment when the facilities are available, the chest radiograph is normal, and further imaging is always performed following an inconclusive result.

22.2.1.5 Echocardiography

Both transoesophageal and transthoracic echocardiography can be diagnostic in massive PE but are rarely definitive in other situations. It may be useful in critically ill patients as it can be performed at the bedside, but is not recommended for the vast majority of patients who are clinically stable enough to tolerate CTPA.

22.2.2 Deep venous thrombosis

Compression ultrasonography (US) is the imaging procedure of choice in patients with suspected DVT, with high specificity and sensitivity >90% for proximal DVT. The principal criterion for diagnosis is the inability to completely compress the vein lumen, with supportive signs including distention of the involved vein and absence of flow on Doppler evaluation. Accuracy rates for the detection of thrombus isolated to the deep calf veins are lower and the evaluation of deep calf veins is more technically challenging, in addition to being more time consuming. For patients with a high pre-test probability for acute DVT, serial US testing is recommended, with at least one additional follow-up compression US study over a one-week interval. Compression

US may also be useful in the investigation of suspected PE, as 70% of patients with proven PE have proximal DVT.

22.3 Superior vena cava obstruction

Superior vena cava obstruction (SVCO) can occur either from external compression due to a mediastinal mass, or from intraluminal thrombus, usually associated with an intravascular device. Malignant causes account for approximately 65% of cases of SVCO, the most common associated malignancies being (in descending order of frequency) non-small cell lung cancer, small cell lung cancer, lymphoma, and metastases. The resultant clinical syndrome involves oedema of the affected areas, which can rarely cause airway or neurological compromise due to involvement of the upper respiratory tract or cerebral oedema respectively. Symptoms usually progress initially over a few weeks, then may improve somewhat as a collateral network develops.

Contrast-enhanced CT of the chest is the most useful initial imaging modality (Figure 22.2). CT phlebography, in which there is cannulation of veins within both ante-cubital fossae has been shown to be a useful technique for demonstration of the site of the occlusion and associated collateral vessels. Conventional venography is usually reserved for planning subsequent intervention, such as placement of a stent. Magnetic resonance venography may be helpful in patients with a severe contrast allergy.

Percutaneous intravascular stenting is currently the treatment of choice. Stent placement is associated with more rapid improvement in symptom than chemoradiation and oedema usually resolves within 48–72 hours. Stent patency has been reported as 69–94% at 12 months with secondary interventions required in 18% of patients 12–36 months post stenting due to tumour overgrowth or thrombosis.[3] Potential complications of stent placement include stent migration, pulmonary embolus, haematoma at the puncture site, and perforation. Radiotherapy is considered only if stenting is not feasible technically or patients are unfit for the procedure. For patients with chemosensitive tumours (e.g. lymphoma, mediastinal germ cell tumours, small cell lung cancer), urgent chemotherapy is the first-line treatment.

22.4 The acute abdomen

A number of conditions related to the malignancy itself or as a complication of treatment can present with acute abdominal pain and gastrointestinal symptoms in patients with cancer. Surgical oncological referrals for patients presenting with an acute abdomen whilst undergoing chemotherapy include acute appendicitis, paralytic ileus, neutropenic colitis, intestinal perforation, acute intestinal obstruction, obstructed hernia, and intussusception. Clinical evaluation, particularly in the immunocompromised patient, can be difficult as symptoms and signs may not develop until late in the course of the illness and are often non-specific.

Abdominal CT is the most valuable non-invasive and rapidly available imaging modality which provides high quality reproducible problem-solving diagnostic information as well as providing an update of the disease status. The imaging appearances of

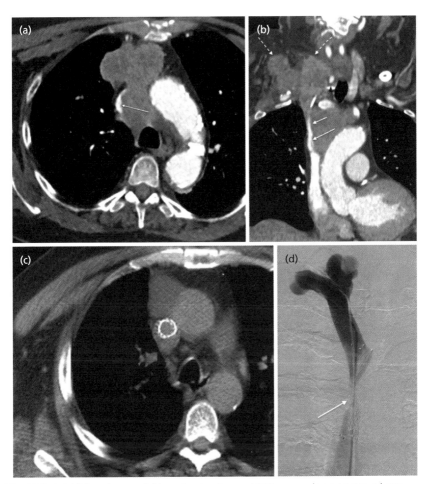

Fig. 22.2 Axial (a) and coronal (b) contrast-enhanced CT images demonstrate a large soft tissue mediastinal mass causing slit-like narrowing of the opacified SVC with likely invasion of the vessel wall (white arrow). In addition, there is soft tissue disease outside of the mediastinum with a conglomerate nodal mass in the right side of the neck (dotted arrows). Digital subtraction angiography (c) and corresponding axial CT images (d) show a metal stent placed in the SVC which is significantly narrowed due to extrinsic compression from tumour (arrow).

some of the most common causes for an acute abdomen in this population are briefly discussed in the rest of this section.

22.4.1 Colitis

There are several causes for colitis in oncology patients, the most common being neutropenic colitis (typhlitis), pseudomembranous colitis due to *Clostridium difficile*, ischaemia, infections related to immunodeficiency such as cytomegalovirus, and the direct effects of treatment, including radiotherapy, certain chemotherapeutic regimens, and, increasingly, immunotherapy-related colitis (discussed at the end of this chapter).

CT is the most sensitive method for the detection of colitis and can demonstrate concerning features for impending perforation and other associations such as mesenteric venous thrombosis which would change management. A number of findings are common to all of the causes of colitis described here, although certain appearances may help to refine the diagnosis. The hallmark appearances of colitis on CT consist of bowel wall thickening to >3 mm, mucosal enhancement, wall nodularity, the presence of air within the bowel wall (pneumatosis intestinalis), bowel dilatation, mesenteric stranding, and ascites.

22.4.1.1 Neutropenic enterocolitis

Neutropenic enterocolitis or typhlitis is a poorly understood entity but is thought to result from compromise of bowel wall integrity, with subsequent bacterial or fungal invasion. It is the most common final diagnosis in neutropenic patients with radiologic bowel abnormalities.[4] The caecum is the most common site of disease, although any segment of the small or large bowel may be involved (Figure 22.3). Pneumatosis intestinalis, the combined involvement of small and large bowel and/or disease isolated to the right hemicolon may be helpful pointers to this disease.

22.4.1.2 Pseudomembranous colitis

Pseudomembranous colitis is limited to the colon, with no small bowel involvement seen; it almost always involves the rectum and left hemicolon, with a pancolitis often demonstrated. Common features include low attenuation bowel wall thickening (creating the 'accordion sign'), mesenteric stranding, and ascites. Abnormal CT

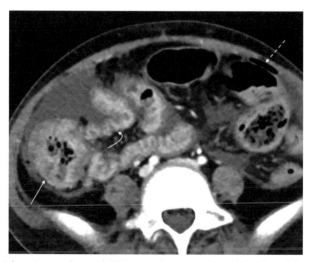

Fig. 22.3 Axial contrast-enhanced CT image demonstrating thickening of the caecum (white straight arrow) and small bowel (curved arrow) in keeping with a typhlitis, which has been complicated by perforation and pneumoperitoneum (dotted arrow).

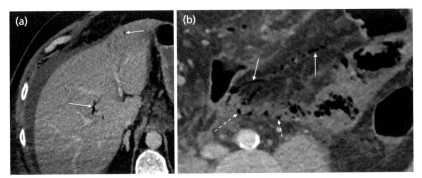

Fig. 22.4 Axial contrast-enhanced CT images of a patient with bowel ischaemia demonstrating portal venous gas (a, white arrows) and abnormal enhancement of the bowel wall (b) with mesenteric gas (white arrow) with pneumatosis (dotted arrows).

appearances were seen in 50% of a series of 152 scanned hospitalized patients with *C. difficile* colitis.

22.4.1.3 Ischaemic colitis

Ischaemic colitis is classically a disease of the elderly with arteriosclerotic disease. However, other precipitating causes include sudden hypotensive episodes, distal colonic obstruction, and vascular occlusion related to neoplasia. A segmental pattern of colitis is most commonly reported, which can be left- or right-sided, although a pancolitis can also be seen. Intramural air (Figure 22.4) is a relatively specific, but insensitive finding and may be associated with portal venous gas.

22.4.2 **Obstruction**

There are multiple possible causes of intestinal obstruction in patients with cancer. Malignant large bowel obstruction is most commonly caused by colorectal cancer, with 10% of colon cancers presenting with large bowel obstruction. Less commonly, large bowel obstruction is caused by local invasion by primary tumours arising from the gallbladder, pancreas, kidneys, and ovaries. Small bowel obstruction is most commonly caused by adhesions and peritoneal carcinomatosis, but rarer causes include metastases to the bowel wall, reported with breast cancer, melanoma, and osteosarcoma, among other tumours. Gastric outlet obstruction is most commonly caused by extrinsic compression from pancreatic cancer.

Abdominal CT is the imaging modality of choice as it enables evaluation of the site of obstruction and can determine the cause (Figure 22.5). For example, large bowel obstruction due to a polypoid tumour may demonstrate associated features such as pericolonic lymphadenopathy and extramural vascular invasion. Intussusception is seen as bowel-within-bowel with an enhancing tumour as the lead point. Obstruction due to carcinomatosis can be identified on CT as nodular peritoneal thickening or even discrete peritoneal masses. In the palliative setting malignant bowel obstruction can be alleviated by the placement of colonic stents either endoscopically or radiologically.

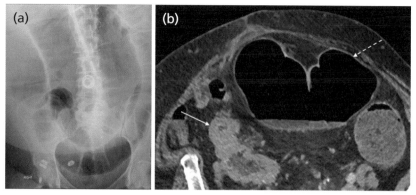

Fig. 22.5 Abdominal radiograph (a) and corresponding axial contrast-enhanced CT image (b) demonstrating dilated loops of large bowel (dotted arrow) with a transition point at the site of the luminal narrowing secondary to primary sigmoid tumour (white arrow).

22.4.3 **Pneumoperitoneum**

The presence of free intraperitoneal gas almost always indicates perforation of a viscus. Abdominal CT is the most sensitive imaging modality for the detection of free air (Figure 22.6), with up to 100% sensitivity. It may also help to localize the source of perforation often with phlegmonous changes adjacent to the perforation site. Bowel perforation can occur due to longstanding obstruction or ischaemia. Additionally, metastatic deposits can spontaneously perforate after chemotherapy, especially in lung cancer.

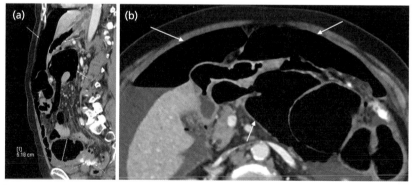

Fig. 22.6 Sagittal reformatted contrast-enhanced CT image (a) demonstrating pneumoperitoneum (arrows) secondary to large bowel perforation secondary to serosal disease from ovarian carcinoma (dotted arrows). There is large bowel obstruction proximal to the soft tissue stricture with the sigmoid colon dilated up to 5 cm. Axial imaging in the same case (b) shows free intraperitoneal gas outlining the falciform ligament and extending into the lesser sac (arrows).

22.5 **Metastatic epidural spinal cord compression**

Metastatic epidural spinal cord compression (MESCC) occurs when an epidural metastatic lesion causes true displacement of the spinal cord from its normal position in the spinal canal. It is a relatively common complication of malignancy, occurring in 5–14% of cancer patients. If left untreated, virtually 100% of patients with MESCC would become paraplegic and this is therefore considered a true medical emergency requiring immediate intervention.[5] Whilst therapy is primarily palliative, up to one-third of patients may survive beyond one year and preservation of quality of life is essential.

As multiple studies have demonstrated a correlation between neurological function at the time of diagnosis and prognosis from MESCC, diagnosis before the development of neurological deficit is particularly important. Magnetic resonance imaging (MRI) is considered the gold standard imaging modality with sensitivity and specificity >90%.[6] In particular, it has a higher sensitivity for detecting bone metastases as compared to CT, with superior depiction of soft tissues, tumour margins, neural elements, and paravertebral tumour extension. However, in patients who are unable to undergo MRI, CT provides an alternative means for assessment.

MRI typically include sagittal T1- and T2-weighted sequences with STIR fat suppression (Figure 22.7) followed by relevant axial scans of the same sequences through identified regions of interest. Osteolytic metastases display low signal on T1-weighted and high or intermediate signal intensity on T2-weighted scans. Highly sclerotic metastases such as seen in breast or prostate cancer show low signal intensity on all sequences. MRI features suggestive of metastatic compression fractures include a convex posterior border of the vertebral body; abnormal signal intensity of the pedicle

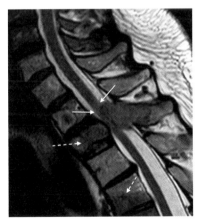

Fig. 22.7 Sagittal T2-weighted MRI imaging of a metastasis within the posterior elements of the second thoracic vertebra with extension into the epidural space. The lesion displaces the spinal cord with T2 high signal within the cord (white arrows). Additional intermediate to low signal deposits seen throughout the vertebrae in keeping with widespread bone metastases (dotted arrows).

or posterior element; an epidural mass, particularly when it is encasing the theca; a focal paraspinal mass; and other spinal metastases.

22.6 Sepsis

Fever is a common symptom among patients with cancer and may be caused by a variety of factors including drugs, infection, or due to the tumour itself. Fever is the most consistent and sometimes the only sign of infection. The most common sites of infection are the respiratory tract, followed by the urinary tract, gastrointestinal system, and soft tissues. Febrile patients are usually initially assessed with a thorough history and clinical examination, chest radiography, and routine cultures. If chest radiography shows possible infection, then broncholaveolar lavage may be performed. In patients with persistent fever, but no evidence of respiratory tract infection a CT of chest, abdomen, and paranasal sinuses is usually performed; MRI of the head and liver, transoesophageal echocardiography, and fluorodeoxyglucose positron emission tomography/CT may be considered if the source of sepsis remains elusive.

22.6.1 Respiratory tract infections

Bacteria are the most frequent cause of pneumonia in immunocompromised patients. The radiographic features of lobar or segmental consolidation usually do not differ from those in the general population, although there may be a delay in their appearance.

Fungal infections are important pathogens, particularly *Candida* and *Aspergillus fumigatus*. *Candida pneumonia* often occurs in association with other pathogens and in the presence of systemic disease with mucous membrane involvement. The radiographic findings vary from diffuse bilateral non-segmental opacities of varying sizes to a miliary pattern, or unilateral or bilateral lobar, or segmental consolidation (Figure 22.8). Cavitation is not thought to be a feature. *Aspergillus* in the immunocompromised patient may be suggested by ground glass opacification, consolidation, poorly defined nodules, and cavitation.

Pneumocystis jiroveci (formerly *Pneumocystis carinii*) is an important pathogen. Prolonged lymphopenia during or after chemotherapy increases the risk of infection. The radiologic appearances are similar to those seen in patients with AIDS, although the clinical course may be more fulminant, with a higher mortality. Radiographic features include diffuse or perihilar reticular and ill-defined ground glass opacities, which may progress within a few days to homogeneous opacification in the untreated patient (Figure 22.9).

High-resolution thin-section CT is significantly more sensitive for the detection of pulmonary disease and several studies have demonstrated the value of CT in the evaluation of febrile neutropenic patients with a normal chest radiograph.[7]

22.7 Lymphangitis carcinomatosis

Lymphangitis carcinomatosis is caused by infiltration of tumour cells into the lymphatic vessels and results histologically in thickening of the interlobular septa and of

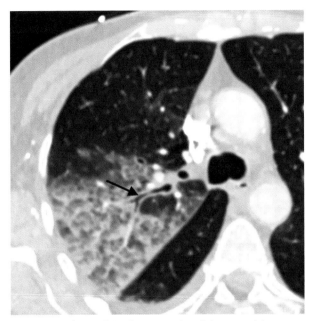

Fig. 22.8 Axial contrast-enhanced CT demonstrating right upper lobar pneumonia with air bronchogram (black arrow) seen within the consolidated lung.

the bronchovascular interstitium. The most common tumours causing this pattern of disease arise from bronchus, breast, pancreas, stomach, colon, and prostate. Approximately 25% of cases are due to infiltration of hilar lymph nodes causing peripheral lymphatic obstruction, whilst the remainder result from direct haematogenous spread to the lung interstitium.[8]

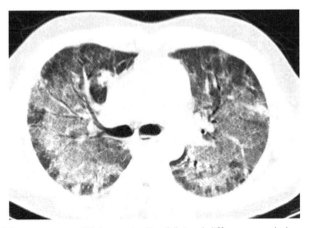

Fig. 22.9 Axial non-contrast CT demonstrating bilateral diffuse ground glass opacification seen with *Pneumocystis jiroveci* pneumonia.

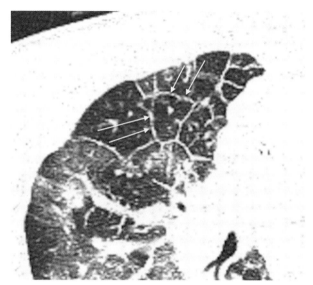

Fig. 22.10 Septal line thickening (arrows) of the right lower lobe in keeping with lymphangitis in a patient with a diagnosis of adenocarcinoma of the lung.

The chest radiographic findings are positive in approximately 50% of cases of pathologically proven lymphangitis and include Kerley A lines, peripheral septal thickening (Kerley B lines), and fine reticulonodular opacification, which may be accompanied by hilar enlargement. The appearances may be very similar to those of pulmonary oedema, particularly in the absence of lymphadenopathy, and clinical correlation in association with previous radiographs is helpful in their differentiation.

CT is significantly more sensitive than radiography, particularly thin-section high resolution CT (Figure 22.10). Common findings include thickening and irregularity of the fissures, thickening of the bronchovascular bundles and interlobular septa and often associated patchy air space shadowing. The nodularity of the septal thickening is not seen in pulmonary oedema and may be a helpful distinguishing feature.

22.8 **Complications as a direct result of treatment**

22.8.1 **Radiation-induced lung injury**

The effects of radiation therapy are commonly seen on chest radiographs and CT. The pattern of radiation injury is described in two distinct phases. The initial phase is a pneumonitis, which typically develops 1–6 months after therapy. This phase is characterized by loss of type 1 pneumocytes, increased capillary permeability, interstitial oedema, alveolar capillary congestion, and inflammatory cell accumulation in the alveolar space. CT features include ground glass opacities and consolidation.

The second phase of lung injury is fibrosis, which has a variable time course and a poorly understood mechanism of pathogenesis. More homogeneous linear or angled

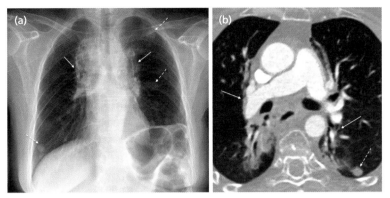

Fig. 22.11 PA Chest radiograph (a) demonstrates a well-demarcated central opacity extending either side of the mediastinum at the site of the previous radiotherapy field (white arrows). In addition there are multiple rounded opacities in keeping with pulmonary metastases seen more peripherally (dotted arrows). Axial contrast-enhanced CT image (b) of the same patient demonstrates the clearly defined central fibrosis with abrupt change to normal lung extending across anatomical boundaries (arrows). A pulmonary metastasis is seen at the apical aspect of the left lower lobe (dotted arrow).

opacities may be seen on chest radiographs, with accompanying volume loss, which can distort adjacent structures. Traction bronchiectasis may be a dominant feature on CT as well as pleural thickening.[9] Again, the appearances are usually geographically rather than anatomically distributed (Figure 22.11). If there are progressive changes beyond 18 months, an alternative diagnosis should be sought.

Other rarer manifestations of radiation-induced lung injury include hyperlucency, pleural effusions, and spontaneous pneumothorax. Second primary tumours may arise within the radiation field, particularly when radiation therapy is given in childhood. Infection and tumour recurrence should be considered as differential diagnoses in radiation-induced lung injury. Infection is not usually confined to the radiation field, although secondary infection can occur in an area of radiation injury.

Tumour recurrence may be detected by the development of focal masses or cavitation on CT. FDG PET scanning can be helpful in distinguishing fibrosis from recurrent tumour. However, false positives are likely to occur if this is performed <4–5 months post-completion of radiation therapy.[9]

22.8.2 Chemotherapy-induced lung injury

Of the standard chemotherapy agents, bleomycin and methotrexate are most commonly associated with pulmonary toxicity. Bleomycin-induced pneumonitis is dose dependent, seen at high cumulative doses, and typically presents at 1–6 months with patterns such as organizing pneumonia, hypersensitivity pneumonitis, and interstitial fibrosis. Methotrexate pulmonary toxicity also typically presents within the first year of therapy, this time with a non-specific interstitial pneumonia pattern of fibrosis being the most common manifestation.

22.9 Osteoporosis

Osteoporosis is increased in many cancer patients, in particular breast and prostate cancer patients receiving hormone manipulation therapy; oestrogen deprivation and androgen deprivation therapy (ADT) cause a reduction in bone mineral density (BMD) and are associated with a 40–50% increase in fracture incidence.[10]

BMD is assessed by dual-energy X-ray absorptiometry with measurements taken at the posterior-anterior spine, total hip, and total body. A T-score is calculated using a young adult reference group: T-score = (individual BMD – mean of young adult reference BMD population/standard deviation of young reference BMD population. Osteoporosis is defined as a t-score <-2.5.

22.9.1 Vertebral compression fractures

When a cancer patient develops an acute vertebral compression fracture then distinction between metastasis or osteoporosis is important. Radiographs are often unhelpful in this situation and bone scintigraphy will show increased activity in either circumstance. A number of studies have shown that MRI may be helpful. Several distinguishing features have been demonstrated, although no single feature should be taken in isolation given the overlap in metastatic and benign disease.

MR features suggestive of acute osteoporotic compression fractures include:

- Band-like shape of bone marrow oedema.
- Spared normal bone marrow signal intensity of the vertebral body.
- Retropulsion of a posterior bone fragment.
- Multiple compression fractures.

22.9.2 Pelvic insufficiency fractures

Pelvic insufficiency fractures (PIF) are a common complication of pelvic radiotherapy. One study investigating the rates of PIF in women who had received radiotherapy for cervical cancer found an incidence of 32%.[11] Postmenopausal patients and those with decreased bone density appear to be at the highest risk.[11] These fractures have characteristic imaging appearances and it is very important for prognosis and future treatment that they are not misinterpreted as bony metastatic disease.

The most common sites for the development of fractures are within the sacrum and ilium. These are often bilateral and symmetric. Pubic fractures have been reported also. Fractures may be visualized on radiographs, although these are insensitive. Bone scintigraphy classically shows a bilateral symmetrical pattern of increased uptake within the sacrum and ilium, giving rise to the 'Honda sign'. CT can confirm the presence of fractures by demonstrating focal cortical disruption, a fracture line, and callus formation in the absence of osteolytic lesions or a soft tissue mass (Figure 22.12). They are demonstrated on MR as focal and often multiple

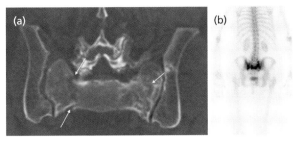

Fig. 22.12 Coronal reformatted CT image (a) demonstrates fracture lines and sclerosis in parallel to the sacroiliac joint (arrows). Bone scintigram study of the same patient (b) demonstrated increased uptake in the typical H-sign.
Images courtesy of Dr H K Cheow, Cambridge University Hospitals NHS FT, UK.

areas of marrow oedema, with low signal on T1-weighted images and high signal on STIR sequences

22.9.3 Avascular necrosis

Corticosteroids are a common cause of non-traumatic avascular necrosis (AVN). They form part of the treatment regimen for patients with haematological malignancies and can also be used in control of emesis for patients with cancer receiving standard chemotherapy. Corticosteroid-induced AVN most commonly affects the femoral head but can also occur at other sites such as the knee and shoulder. Patients present with insidious onset of pain and radiographs are the initial investigation, with findings such as cystic or sclerotic change, abnormal bone contours and collapse of the articular surface in advanced cases. MRI is the most sensitive modality to diagnose AVN, with findings such as diffuse oedema or focal low signal intensity lines separating an area of osteonecrosis, crescent sign (Figure 22.13). Bone scintigraphy is also useful to detect AVN, especially when there are multiple sites of involvement.

22.10 Imaging immune-related adverse events

A new form of targeted immunotherapy has recently been introduced; the class of drugs are referred to as 'immune checkpoint inhibitors' (ICI). Immune evasion is one of the hallmarks of cancer growth and these drugs work to inhibit the negative regulation of T-cells thereby stimulating the immune system to destroy cancer cells.

The monoclonal antibody ipilimumab, a drug that blocks cytotoxic T-lymphocyte-associated antigen 4 (CTLA-4), was the first ICI to be approved for the treatment of metastatic melanoma in 2011. Subsequently, a second class of drugs that block the checkpoint receptor cell death protein 1 (PD-1) were developed: nivolumab and pembrolizumab.

Overactivation of the immune system can lead to unique set of complications. Fortunately, immune-related adverse events (irAE) can often be managed effectively with discontinuation of the therapy and the administration of corticosteroids.

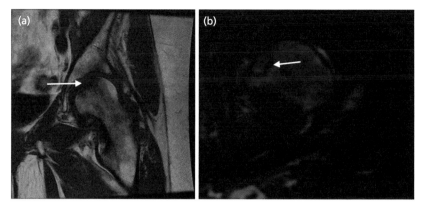

Fig. 22.13 Coronal T1-weighted image (a) of the left hip demonstrates low signal intensity in the subchondral femoral head (white arrow) with preservation of the joint space. Corresponding axial STIR image (b) demonstrates high signal intensity within the femoral head in keeping with oedema and serpiginous line (white arrow) in keeping with crescent sign.

Therefore, it is important to recognize these novel adverse events promptly with imaging.

The overall incidence of radiological abnormalities for patients with complications of ipilimumab was reported as high as 31%.[12] Whilst events can occur at any point along a patient's treatment course, it has been shown that for ipilimumab the majority of adverse events occur during the first 12-week treatment induction period.

22.10.1 Immune-related colitis

After dermatologic manifestations, colitis is the most frequent irAE, typically occurring 5–10 weeks after the beginning of treatment. A case series of 16 patients with ipilimumab associated colitis described CT findings of mesenteric vessel engorgement (83%), bowel wall thickening (75%), and colonic distension (25%). These imaging features are non-specific, with pseudomembranous colitis, inflammatory bowel disease, and ischaemic colitis all having similar CT appearances. Pseudomembranous colitis is associated with extensive colonic wall thickening, whether that be circumferential or eccentric, and this is often greater than that seen in any other inflammatory or infectious colitis, helping to differentiate this diagnosis.

A second case series described three patterns of immune-related colitis: (1) diffuse colitis; (2) segmental colitis in the setting of diverticulosis; and (3) rectosigmoid colitis without diverticulosis. Segmental colitis was associated with greater mural thickening and pericolic fat stranding compared with diffuse colitis (Figure 22.14). Segmental colitis often presents with bloody diarrhoea and responds to combined corticosteroid and antibiotic therapy; whilst diffuse colitis is more frequently associated with watery diarrhoea and can be managed by steroids alone.

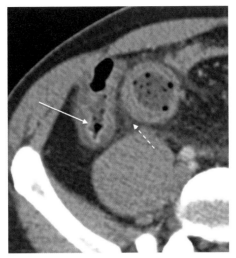

Fig. 22.14 Axial contrast-enhanced CT demonstrating marked mural thickening of the ascending colon with mucosal hyperenhancement (white arrow) and adjacent fat stranding (dotted arrow) in a patient with colitis.
Image courtesy of Dr. Ed Godfrey, Cambridge University Hospitals NHS Foundation Trust, UK.

22.10.2 Immune-related hepatitis

Patients presenting with immune-related hepatitis are often asymptomatic and so liver function testing is recommended prior to initiating an ICI, and then regularly prior to each infusion. The incidence of immune-related hepatitis is reported as 2–9%, with rates increasing for patients on combined therapy of nivolumab and ipilimumab. The average time of onset of hepatitis after the initiation of therapy is 12–16 weeks (after the third dose).

The imaging findings of hepatomegaly, periportal oedema (seen as T2 high signal on MRI, or increased periportal echogenicity on US), periportal lymphadenopathy, and reduced attenuation of the liver parenchyma are non-specific, with only clinical history able to distinguish immune-related from viral or alcohol induced acute hepatitis.

It is also important to exclude hepatic metastases in the context of deranged liver function tests. What is more, metastases may be obscured by the reduced attenuation of the liver parenchyma secondary to hepatitis or could be confused with new geographic areas of low attenuation that can mimic metastases.

22.10.3 Immune-related pneumonitis

Pneumonitis is a rare complication seen in 1–5% of patients. Evaluation of patients taking PD-1 inhibitors found the median time to develop pneumonitis was 2.6 months after initiation of therapy. There is a broad range of presentations from patients who are asymptomatic to those with life-threatening hypoxia. Given the potentially serious nature of this toxicity it is important that pneumonitis is recognized

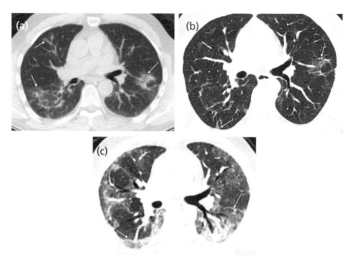

Fig. 22.15 Sequential axial CT images of the thorax each taken a month apart (a, b, c). The bilateral peripheral ground glass opacification (white arrows) improves over the first month (a, b) but then rapidly deteriorates with ground glass infiltration with associated tractional bronchiectasis throughout the lungs (c). These appearances are in keeping with an organizing pneumonia pattern of drug reaction.
Images courtesy of Dr J Babar, Cambridge University Hospitals NHS FT, UK.

promptly; however, this is difficult as its presentation on imaging is non-specific and highly variable. Ground glass opacities, reticular opacities, and consolidation (Figure 22.15) were the most common CT findings (as is also the case for standard drug-related pneumonitis).

One study followed the classification of interstitial pneumonias and applied it to describe the varying patterns seen with immune-mediated pneumonitis: 65% fit a cryptogenic organizing pneumonia (COP) pattern, 15% a non-specific interstitial pneumonia pattern (NSIP), 10% a hypersensitivity pneumonitis (HP) pattern, and 10% an acute respiratory distress syndrome (ARDS) pattern.

22.10.4 Immune-related hypophysitis

Symptoms of headache, fatigue, hypothyroidism, hypogonadism, and hypocortisolism have a median onset of nine weeks for patients who have ipilimumab treatment associated pituitary hypophysitis. It has an incidence of 2–4%, increasing to 25% for those on combined therapy. The most commonly seen MRI findings are moderate enlargement of the pituitary itself, enlargement of the stalk or infundibulum, and homogenous contrast enhancement (Figure 22.16).

Immune mediated hypophysitis can mimic metastatic disease; for example from melanoma, breast, or more rarely, lung cancer. It is also important to distinguish appearances from pituitary macroadenomas. Macroadenomas are usually seen as a focally enlarged pituitary with a normal stalk and heterogeneous enhancement.

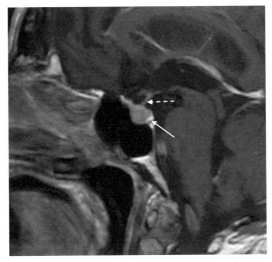

Fig. 22.16 Sagittal T1-weighted MRI following the administration of intravenous contrast medium demonstrates diffuse enlargement of the pituitary gland (white arrow) with superior displacement of the infundibulum (dotted arrow) in a patient with hypophysitis.
Image courtesy of Dr T Das, Cambridge University Hospitals NHS FT, UK.

22.11 **Summary**

- Complications either as a result of malignancy or as a consequence of treatment are common.

- Complications may mimic malignancy.

- Imaging plays a critical role in the diagnostic pathway. Final diagnosis may require the use of several imaging modalities. Comprehensive clinical information is essential to aid the radiologist with narrowing the differential diagnosis.

References

1. **Khorana AA, Francis CW, Culakova E, Kuderer NM, Lyman GH** (2007). Thromboembolism is a leading cause of death in cancer patients receiving outpatient chemotherapy. *Journal of Thrombosis & Haemostasis*, **5**: 632–634.

2. **British Thoracic Society Guidelines (2003)**. British Thoracic Society guidelines for the management of suspected acute pulmonary embolism. *Thorax*, **58**(6): 470–484.

3. **Kalra M, Sen I, Gloviczki P** (2018). Endovenous and operative treatment of superior vena cava syndrome. *Surgical Clinics in North America*, **98**(2): 321–335.

4. **Kirkpatrick IDC, Greenberg HM** (2003). Gastrointestinal complications in the neutropenic patient: characterization and differentiation with abdominal CT. *Radiology*, **226**(3):668–674.

5. **Kaloostian PE, Yurter A, Zadnik PL, Sciubba DM, Gokaslan ZL** (2014). Current paradigms for metastatic spinal disease: An evidence-based review. *Annals of Surgical Oncology*, **21**(1): 248–262.

6. **Smoker WR, Godersky JC, Knutzon RK, Keyes WD, Norman D, Bergman W** (1987). The role of MR imaging in evaluating metastatic spinal disease. *American Journal of Roentgenology*, **149**(6): 1241–1248.

7. **Gerritsen MG, Willemink MJ, Pompe E, et al.** (2017). Improving early diagnosis of pulmonary infections in patients with febrile neutropenia using low-dose chest computed tomography. *PLoS One*, **12**(2): 1–13.

8. **Stein MG, Mayo J, Müller N, Aberle DR, Webb WR, Gamsu G** (1987). Pulmonary lymphangitic spread of carcinoma: appearance on CT scans. *Radiology*, **162**(2): 371–375.

9. **Giridhar P, Mallick S, Rath GK, Julka PK** (2015). Radiation induced lung injury: prediction, assessment and management. *Asian Pacific Journal of Cancer Prevention*, **16**(7): 2613–2617.

10. **Coleman R, Body JJ, Aapro M, Hadji P, Herrstedt J** (2014). Bone health in cancer patients: ESMO clinical practice guidelines. *Annals of Oncology*, **25**(August): 124–137.

11. **Uezono H, Tsujino K, Moriki K, et al.** (2013). Pelvic insufficiency fracture after definitive radiotherapy for uterine cervical cancer: retrospective analysis of risk factors. *Journal of Radiation Research*, **54**(6): 1102–1109.

12. **Kwak JJ, Tirumani SH, Van den Abbeele AD, Koo PJ, Jacene HA** (2015). Cancer immunotherapy: imaging assessment of novel treatment response patterns and immune-related adverse events. *RadioGraphics*, **35**(2): 424–437.

Chapter 23

Imaging for treatment verification

June Dean

23.1 Introduction

In order to achieve tumour control a sufficiently large dose of radiotherapy needs to be delivered and still remain within the known maximum safe dose for the surrounding tissues. Historically, therapeutic radiographers have relied upon external reference marks on the patient's skin as a surrogate for tumour (target) position. However, this method increases the risk of missing the target for some or all of the treatment, and potentially increases the dose to the surrounding normal tissues.

With modern radiotherapy, image guided radiotherapy (IGRT) is performed to increase precision and accuracy in radiation delivery.[1] In its simplest term, IGRT requires the comparison of a reference image—the computed tomography (CT) acquired at pre-treatment planning—with a 3D image dataset acquired on the day of treatment delivery; given the goal to optimize, with minimal compromise, target coverage, and organs at risk (OAR) avoidance. IGRT can use the target itself or a surrogate (gold seed, titanium clip, bone) if the target cannot be visualized.

In order to undertake IGRT successfully a therapeutic radiographer must have a working understanding of professional guidelines and local protocols; and have an awareness of the limitations of their own knowledge and experience and when and from whom to seek advice. Robust local competency programmes must be in place to support therapeutic radiographer led practice.[2 8]

The image review process requires the radiographer to make decisions based on clinical knowledge and judgement. Clinical judgement is the ability to critically appraise an image and apply knowledge to make a considered and appropriate decision and to be aware of factors (both indications and contraindications) for the use of various imaging modalities, including the recognition of artefacts and their impact on visible anatomy, which influence any decision to repeat images or take additional views, whilst considering modality and imaging dose. Speed is also important in review and intervention;[9] it is essential in maintaining accuracy and validity of the information obtained—minimum action for maximum effect. Factors that affect validity include time and compliance of the patient, and can only really be assessed and actioned by the person undertaking image review.

The process of image review is not simply looking for and correcting inconsistencies in anatomy seen in an image. Any decision made must take into account the following:

♦ Is the image quality sufficient to be sure the structures seen are there?

♦ Has there been any internal or external contour change?

♦ Are the fields close to critical structures and how would any correctional shift affect the dose to those structures?

♦ Can we be confident in our decision?

23.2 **Verification**

It is always worth remembering when outlining that a planning CT and daily volumetric images are only snapshots at any one time point Care must be taken to account for possible target movement from day-to-day. There are three sources of geometric uncertainties:[3]

♦ Planning

♦ Delivery

♦ Verification

With single fraction imaging, the mean tumour position is unlikely to be detected and the tumour on the planning CT scan is not always an accurate representation of the tumour position during treatment.[4] With modern CT scanners rapid acquisition of planning data reduces the effect of patient motion significantly. The image acquired with cone beam (CBCT) is a composite image and demonstrates the motion of a target over a number of breathing cycles. This can be observed especially in lung and abdomen (Figure 23.1).

Treatment accuracy is affected by reproducibility, shape change during a treatment, and physiological processes, including respiration and bladder and rectal filling, will

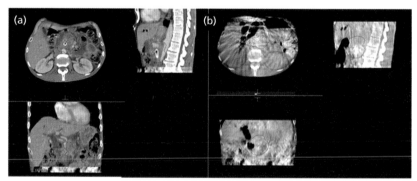

Fig. 23.1 The images on the left (a) are from the CT Planning scan. The images on the right (b) are on-treatment images. The red contour is the PTV. The images demonstrate the difference between images for outlining and images for on-treatment positional correction. The rippling noted in the coronal section on images (b), demonstrates motion, indicated by the red arrow.

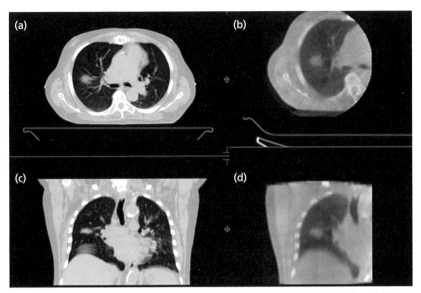

Fig. 23.2 The images in (a) and (b) are from a planning CT, the images in (c) and (d) are from a CBCT. The CBCT target appears slightly larger and more indistinct as a result of target motion with respiration. The motion in the cranial-caudal direction is greater than in the anterior-posterior direction.

move the target (Figure 23.2). For oral tumours, swallowing can occur, which will also move the larynx out of the treatment field for a portion of the delivery time. Compliance of patients is important in controlling unwanted voluntary movements during treatment. There are any numbers of reasons why patients move; some do not understand why it is important, or simply forget to keep still. Some are in too much pain or too breathless to lie down for any length of time on a hard treatment couch, others have medical conditions such as Parkinson's and are unable to remain still. There must always be a balance between efficiency and efficacy—what can or cannot be achieved.

Having two therapeutic radiographers review the same image will produce two slightly different results. There are a number of factors that can influence these differences, including variation in visual acuity and the background lighting level. The minimum contrast detection of the eye is about 2% of the background illumination. If images are viewed in a bright room, the small contrast differences on the image will be missed. Many image processing tools within the available systems are available to 'clean up' poor quality images; however, the information in an image can be stripped or stretched in the cleaning up process. Always be aware of the individual effect of filters before employing them in image processing optimization. The usefulness of the data depends on what information was used to compare the images; ideally accuracy of field positioning should be assessed using the tumour itself and where this is not possible a surrogate may be required.

23.3 **Image quality**

Technically, image quality for image review has to be optimal for target or surrogate recognition. Theoretically, it does not need to be of a diagnostic quality, although the principles of the ALARA (As Low As Reasonably Achievable) should be followed. Decisions should also be justified in accordance with IR(ME)R (Ionising Radiation (Medical Exposure) Regulations).[5,6] Modern multi-modality diagnostic imaging is utilized for outlining targets and OARs to ensure that the target is covered and that sensitive structures and healthy tissues are avoided where possible. If we optimize imaging for outlining and hence planning, should we also optimize imaging for on-treatment geometric verification? Is it better to be confident that we are delivering high dose radiotherapy where it was planned using higher dose on-treatment imaging techniques or reduce the dose and rely on larger margins? Are we too focused on stochastic risk rather than treating the target? There is a need to balance risk against benefit and we should respect dose whilst not being afraid of increasing it when optimizing imaging presets. Manufacturer presets (kilovoltage, milliamperes, number of frames and projections, acquisition range (degrees)) provide a starting point for local optimization. The arc is the acquisition range of the individual frames required to create an acceptable image. This may be a full or partial arc depending on detail required and proximity to OARs. Figure 23.3 demonstrates differing field of views (FOV) and image quality with an Elekta™ imaging system. For the first fraction it is important to assess for any change between the CT planning scan and treatment. Ideally, a complete FOV to assess for contour change is preferred; however, this may not be required daily.

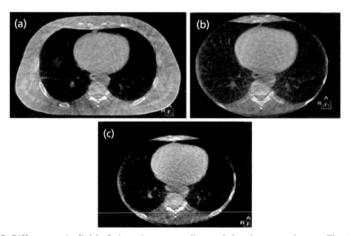

Fig. 23.3 Differences in field of view, image quality and the dose are shown. The target anatomy in (a) is clearly identifiable; (b) has a slightly higher imaging dose than (c); however, the use of this preset is justifiable in that the oesophagus (target), is more easily identifiable.

23.4 **Radiological anatomy**

A working knowledge of common anatomical references for each body site, imaging planes, and effects of positional variation will assist the therapeutic radiographer. Volumetric images (CBCT, MVCT (megavoltage CT)) acquired locally are extremely useful for therapeutic radiographer training in anatomical recognition. Figures 23.4, 23.5, 23.6, and 23.7 are examples of anatomy from common treatment sites: head and neck; thorax, abdomen, and pelvis.

23.5 **The IGRT process**

The daily process of IGRT[7] starts with positioning the patient as indicated at CT planning for treatment. A volumetric CBCT or fan beam megavoltage CT (FBMVCT) scan is acquired and registered to the planning CT. A gross error check is performed to assess for translational or rotational positional variation; and whether or not the patient needs to be re-positioned and re-scanned. If satisfactory, depending on equipment available, 3, 4, or 6 degrees of freedom can be applied and treatment delivered.

Ideally, image review will use the target for matching; however, in reality it is not always possible. In these cases, radiopaque fiducials can be employed as a surrogate. These include seeds implanted in an organ, for example prostate or titanium clips delineating the tumour bed, for example breast. It is important to not only review the target but also OARs that are in close proximity to the target itself.

It may be useful for training and decision making in online image review to categorize anatomical sites into simple and complex. Simple volumetric image review could be used to describe a level of knowledge and skill that is required in order to optimize a match for sites where there is a single planning target volume (PTV), where minimal deformation of the target will have little or no associated effect on PTV coverage, or where matching to implanted fiducials (prostate gland).

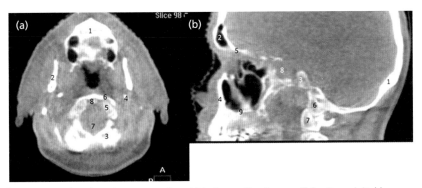

Fig. 23.4 Head and neck anatomy. Panel (a): 1. maxilla; 2. mandible; 3. occipital bone; 4. styloid process of temporal bone; 5. occipital condyle; 6. atlas C1; 7. foramen magnum; 8. odontoid peg C2. Panel (b): 1. occipital bone; 2. frontal sinus; 3. greater wing of sphenoid; 4. maxilla; 5. frontal bone; 6. occipital condyle; 7. atlas c1; 8. pituitary fossa; 9. hard palate.

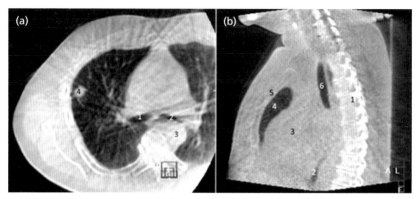

Fig. 23.5 Thoracic anatomy. Panel (a): 1. right main bronchus; 2. left main bronchus; 3. descending aorta; 4. tumour. Panel (b): 1. thoracic spine; 2. oesophagus; 3. heart; 4. lung; 5. sternum; 6. trachea.

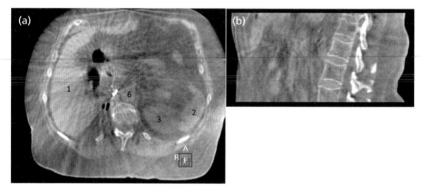

Fig. 23.6 Abdominal anatomy. Panel (a): 1. liver; 2. spleen; 3. left kidney; 4. aorta. Panel (b): vertebrae.

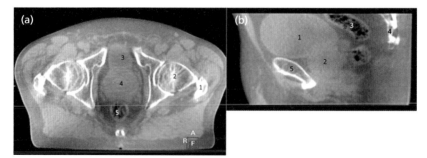

Fig. 23.7 Pelvic anatomy. Panel (a): 1. greater trochanter; 2. femoral head; 3. bladder; 4. prostate gland; 5. rectum. Panel (b): 1. bladder; 2. prostate; 3. rectum; 4. coccyx; 5. symphysis pubis.

On the other hand, complex volumetric image review would be the analysis used to describe a level of knowledge and skill that is required in order to optimize a match for sites where the data sets include multiple PTVs and/or cover long volumes (limbs, cerebral spinal axis) and/or are subject to deformation resulting in poor coverage of the target by the planned PTV.

23.5.1 Image processing for 3D image review

Prior to acquiring an image, the therapeutic radiographer will need to define the scan slice selection, region of interest, and the optimal preset for each site. These must be defined in local protocols.

Selection of a clip box (Elekta™) or a region of interest (ROI) (Varian™) is an important first step in preparing for image review. This will enable the computer software to 'focus' on an area for optimizing the matching of the reference and verification images. The region of interest should include stable bony anatomy, whilst avoiding mobile anatomy, for example femoral heads and femurs in the pelvis and mandible and clavicles in the head and neck. The PTV should always be included within the ROI. Caution must be taken when defining a clipbox or ROI, not to include areas outside of the patient contour; and not to extend the selection too far beyond the PTV as this may create false indications of pitch and yaw at review. Another method available for selecting a region for optimizing the automatic function is scan slice selection (Accuray™) similar to CT planning for pre-treatment delivery imaging. Ideally the PTV should be included within the scan selection. However, this may result in extended scan and match times or including OARs that have tight dose constraints (optic chiasm). If a reduced volume is selected, the radiographer must be confident that the selected anatomy will be sufficient for optimized matching.

Images can be magnified for review; however, as there are only a fixed number of pixels in an image, magnifying the pixel increases the size of the pixel only, reducing the apparent resolution and resulting in grainy and ill-defined anatomy. Image window and levels, controlling image brightness and contrast, should be optimized when reviewing the overlay of the planning and daily scan acquired by the operator. Adjusting the width of the window will alter display contrast; adjusting the level will change the brightness of the displayed image (Figure 23.8).

Filters enable the therapeutic radiographer to enhance contrast between soft tissues to assist in match decisions. A hard filter is useful when matching to the prostate gland;

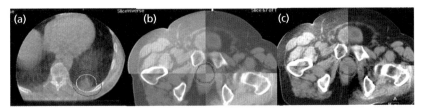

Fig. 23.8 Examples of CBCT windows available on Elekta™. (a) = Soft, (b) = Medium, (c) = Hard.

it shows up fat planes clearly and helps in identifying urine in the bladder. A lung filter 'removes' the extreme contrast, enabling a tumour to be identified. Using a low dose preset may also assist in reducing artefacts within an image, for example in single hip replacements.

23.5.2 Imaging protocols

An imaging protocol is a series of instructions that guides on the best modality to acquire an image, how to prioritize the match analysis, and what action is required at all stages of a treatment course. Protocols are developed for individual departments and include considerations of the risk of secondary malignancy induction from extra imaging dose and a potential increase in workload for that department. Any imaging acquisition and correction procedure is a trade-off between accuracy, workload, and relative risk.

Protocols include strategies for assessing gross error (GE), systematic set-up error (SSE), and random error (RE). When reviewing an image online positional translational and rotational data that is outside of local tolerances may require the radiographers to reposition and re-image the patient.

Protocols can also define which anatomy to match to, technique to match, OARs to monitor, and how to resolve common issues. Table 23.1 provides examples of a volumetric image match protocol.

23.5.3 Match techniques

There are a number of methods for reviewing images; these include chequerboard matching, which is a process whereby an on-treatment image is overlaid over a reference image (Figure 23.9), a cut view which enables the anatomy to be aligned and assessed for displacement between the planned and delivered fields.

An alternative method is using a two-colour wash (green/purple (Figure 23.10) or gold/blue). When bony anatomy or fiducials are overlaid they appear white or a spyglass (similar to chequerboard).

For all anatomical sites the anatomy is reviewed in all three anatomical planes. The therapeutic radiographers are encouraged to decide themselves which image match technique (colour overlay, chequerboard) to use when verifying images both online or offline; their preference is dependent upon their confidence in using the tools provided and how they visually process images. The sagittal view provides anterior-posterior and superior-inferior match information.

In the coronal view, the therapeutic radiographer will assess the best slice(s) for optimizing the anatomical review; this maybe a slice where the target is easily recognizable or using bony anatomy as a surrogate. The coronal plane provides translational information for left to right and superior to inferior translational corrections. Be wary of using any mobile anatomy such as ribs as an anatomical reference as these will vary with breathing. Each centre should define its own protocols based on techniques and margin data. The technique employed should be a balance of efficiency and efficacy.

When reviewing the axial/transverse planes, it is important to assess the anatomical match throughout the dataset before making any adjustments, though concentrating

Table 23.1 Volumetric image match protocol excerpt

Elekta	Site	Clip box selection	Image acquisition preset	Image matching — Match priority and check coverage	OARs to Review	Actioning issue	Resolution	Ref	Skill level
	Prostate	Include bony pelvis excluding femoral heads	First fraction Review quality of image change preset if required Prostate M10 CC	1. Match prostate gland 2. Check coverage of prostate and SVs using PTVPG and PTVSV structures	1. Bladder and rectal volume are consistent with planning volumes 2. Small bowel is not included in high dose volumes	◆ Large rectal volume (>4 cm AP) ◆ Bladder volume </> 75% of planning volume ◆ SVs not within PTVSV structure	Send patient to bathroom to empty/pass wind Send patient to bathroom to empty/refill ◆ Check rectal/bladder filling ◆ If unresolvable STOP Refer to TOL, CO, supt. or adv. pract.	Clinical protocol	2
			Prostate Seed S10 CC OR PIVOTAL S20 CC-trial only	1. Match to seeds		◆ Small bowel in high dose volume	◆ Check bladder filling ◆ Treat # only ◆ Refer to TOL, CO, supt. or adv. pract.		

(continued)

Table 23.1 Continued

Accuracy	Site	Scan slice width Coarse (C) Normal (N) Fine (F)	Scan slice selection (choose)	Match priority and coverage checks	OARs to review (check)	Actioning (if fail check) Issue	Actioning (if fail check) Resolution	Ref	Skill level
	Prostate	C	**All fractions** Whole PTV, to include seminal vesicles (SV)	**Asymmetrical PTV margins** 1. Match to the prostate gland (PG) 2. Check PG and SV coverage using isodose lines stated below: **Symmetrical PTV margins/ prosthetic hips:** 1. Centre the PG inside the PTV PG isodose stated on the plan. 2. Check PG and SV coverage using isodose lines stated below: Prescription: 60 Gy/20# PG covered by 57 Gy (95%) SV covered by 51.3 Gy (86%) Prescription: 74 Gy/37# PG covered by 70.3 Gy (95%) SV covered by 57 Gy (77%)	1. Bladder and rectal volume are consistent with planning volumes 2. Small bowel is not in high dose volume	◆ Large rectal volume (>4 cm AP) ◆ Bladder volume </> 75% of planning volume ◆ SVs not within planned isodose contour ◆ Small bowel in high dose volume	Send patient to bathroom to empty/pass wind Send patient to bathroom to empty/refill Check rectal/bladder filling ◆ If unresolvable STOP Refer to TOL, CO, supt. or adv. pract. ◆ Check bladder filling ◆ Treat this # only ◆ Refer to TOL, CO, supt. or adv. pract. before next #	Clinical protocol	2

Varian	Site	Volume of interest	Image acquisition preset	Image matching		OARs to review	Actioning issue	Resolution	Ref	Skill level
				Match priority and check coverage						
	Prostate	Include bony pelvis excluding femoral heads	**Pelvis/pelvis obese 10 cm range** **First fraction** Review quality of image change preset if required	1. Match prostate gland Check coverage of prostate and SVs using PTVPG and PTVSV structures		1. Bladder and rectal volume are consistent with planning volumes 2. Small bowel is not included in high dose volume	◆ Large rectal volume (>4 cm AP) ◆ Bladder volume </> 75% of planning volume ◆ SVs not within PTVSV structure ◆ Small bowel in high dose volume	◆ Send patient to bathroom to empty bladder/ pass wind ◆ Send patient to bathroom to empty/refill ◆ Check rectal/ bladder filling ◆ If unresolvable STOP Refer to TOL, CO, supt. or adv. pract. ◆ Check bladder filling ◆ Treat # only ◆ Refer to TOL, CO, supt. or adv. pract.	Clinical protocol	2

c = course.

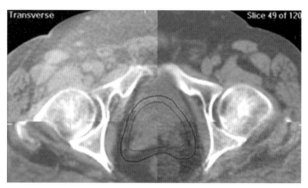

Fig. 23.9 Chequerboard for prostate online image review.

less on matching anatomy that is not included within the treatment volume or is distant from the target. If any adjustments are made the entire volume would need to be reviewed, as a small change at one level may have a more significant effect elsewhere within the volume.

23.6 **Clinical practice**

The daily process of IGRT starts with positioning the patient as indicated at CT planning. A volumetric CBCT/ FBMVCT scan is acquired and registered to the planning CT. A gross error check is performed to assess for translational and rotational positional variation and whether or not the patient may need to be repositioned and re-scanned. Depending on equipment available, 3, 4, or 6 degrees of freedom (translations and rotations) can be applied to correct for any positional variation between planning and daily treatment delivery.

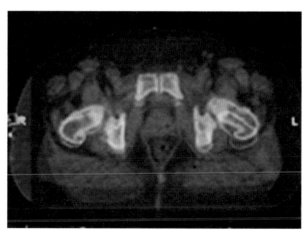

Fig. 23.10 Green/purple colour-wash for prostate online image review. The prostate is matched; however, the misalignment of bone reflects the poor correlation with bone and prostate gland position.

Image review is not a simple, easy process. As mentioned earlier in this chapter, there are factors which make the decision to treat more complicated. It is essential not just to see change but to monitor it, record it, and more importantly act upon it.

23.6.1 **Prostate**

When matching to the prostate gland, it is important to review the OARs close by, including the bladder, small bowel, and rectum (Figure 23.11). Bladder filling may not only affect prostate gland position but may also impact on small bowel dose and thereby toxicity and coverage of the seminal vesicles. If the bladder is considerably smaller than at planning, the small bowel may move into the high dose region and result in an increase in acute toxicity. In cases where there is a significant variation between the planned and imaged volume (bladder filling and presence of faeces or flatus in the rectum), action needs to be taken. For example, the patient may need to be removed from the treatment couch and instructed to wait longer or drink additional liquid if the bladder volume is significantly smaller than at CT planning. Any subsequent preparation protocol for that patient may need to be updated to reflect persistent changes. When assessing possible actions to deal with change it is important to gather information as to why the patient may not be hydrated? These questions may include:

◆ How much and what do they drink a day?

◆ Do they experience discomfort or pain, is this new or ongoing?

◆ Do they stop drinking overnight?

◆ Was the planning scan at a similar time of day to the treatment?

◆ Are they on any medication?

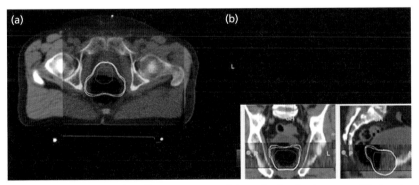

Fig. 23.11 Demonstrates the effects on expected dose distribution between CT planning and on treatment. The rectum is dilated by flatus pushing the prostate gland anteriorly. In the coronal slice, the prostate gland is now outside of the PTV; the sagittal slice clearly shows that a significant portion of the rectal wall is within the high dose volume.

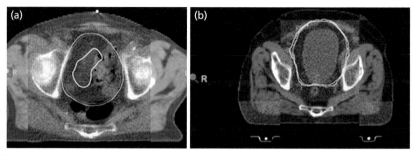

Fig. 23.12 Bladder volume is significantly smaller than planned (bold yellow contour). The red PTV indicates the bladder shape at CT planning.

23.6.2 **Bladder**

The bladder volume can alter substantially between planning and on-treatment imaging (Figure 23.12). Where a bladder volume is less than the planned volume the small bowel may receive a higher than planned dose. This may result in acute or chronic toxicity for the patient. If the bladder is outside of or touching the PTV, treatment should not be delivered as during treatment the bladder wall is likely to move outside of the PTV and hence, the high dose volume with the potential to not achieve the planned dose to the target.

23.6.3 **Pelvis**

For other pelvic sites a bone match is performed, followed by a review of the PTV coverage of the soft tissue, for example cervix or bladder. A direct soft tissue match is not always feasible as the position of gynaecological anatomy varies day-to-day and the bladder filling will vary daily, making soft tissue matching unlikely. Nodal groups are not always visible on the scans and the appropriate blood vessels are used as a surrogate, with the vessels being confirmed as included within the PTV. As with any pelvic image review, the bladder and rectal volume should also be monitored as the filling of these OARs may affect the overall planned coverage of the target (Figure 23.13).

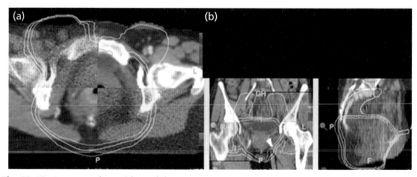

Fig. 23.13 An anus plan with nodal coverage.

23.6.4 **Breast**

Breasts can be difficult to match as the size and shape of the breast may vary day-to-day. It is crucial that the arm position at planning CT is replicated as this can introduce notable rotations in the patient position. A small change in arm position may have a significant effect on the ability to match anatomy and make the decision to treat more difficult for the therapeutic radiographer. Often a match is challenging as it is rare that the breast shape is consistent from day to day.

The match priority will vary from patient to patient and decisions on matching must include agreed departmental protocols or national guidelines. For example, a simultaneous integrated boost (SIB) to the tumour bed, becomes a priority for optimization, followed by the chest wall and the external contour, whilst ensuring that any planned nodal groups are within the PTV as indicated on the planning scan. Any external breast contour changes may be as a result of a patient being more relaxed than at CT planning, premenopausal changes, or through either weight gain or weight loss. Internally, the tumour bed post-surgery, changes shape with time, especially if there was a seroma or haematoma present either before or after planning. If a seroma (Figure 23.13) was or is present it will require careful monitoring. If any change is noted, appropriate action will need to be taken, which may include ultrasound guided drainage or in an extreme case it may be necessary to re-plan the patient's treatment (Figure 23.14).

The patient in Figure 23.15 had surgery a week before her CT planning appointment as she was going on holiday. On her first fraction five weeks after the CT planning scan, a significant change in her external contours was noted by the radiographers. The radiographers removed the patient from the treatment couch and the change was reported to the oncologist. After a review of the scan and discussion, a decision was made to re-plan the patient.

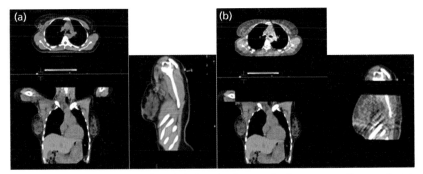

Fig. 23.14 A large seroma developed during the first week of treatment, the oncologist was consulted as to the preferred plan of action. The patient was sent to the breast clinic where 200 ml of fluid was drained, allowing the tumour bed to return to its original shape and treatment could be delivered as planned.

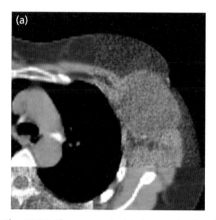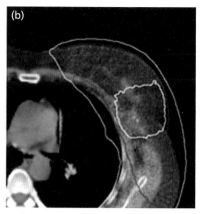

Fig. 23.15 The images in (a) denote the location of the tumour bed at planning (red outline) and the images in (b) highlight the contour changes since planning.

23.6.5 **Thoracic**

Changes are often noted on CBCT, these may result from changes in target or the differences between planning image acquisition and treatment delivery modalities. The target on a CBCT may appear different to the image of the target acquired on the CT planning scan; this may be due to a number of factors, including respiratory motion (Figure 23.16) and may result in the tumour appearing larger on the composite image.

Ongoing chemotherapy between CT and treatment can continue to shrink the target so that on the patient's first treatment fraction the target may not always be easily identifiable. Consolidation (the accumulation of material in the tissue) around

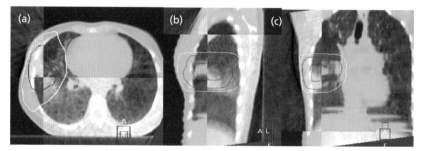

Fig. 23.16 The daily CBCT is a slow acquisition CT scan and the resultant images are a composite of the respiratory cycle; the tumour may appear larger on CBCT as this is again attributable to the speed of acquisition of the planning CT scan and the daily CBCT scan. Planning CT inhalation volume is not reproducible daily with the CBCT and may influence decision making when matching soft tissue; there may be considerable variation in the position of the diaphragm and ribs. Hence, bony matching is not a true representation of tumour position. For this patient there was a 2 cm difference between bone and soft tissue.

the target may be mistaken for target growth; consolidation may be difficult to differentiate from target change due to the image quality of the CBCT and may require the advice of the patient's oncologist. Atelectasis (partial or complete collapse of a region of the lung which can be caused by blocked bronchi or bronchioles) has the potential (depending on beam direction) to affect delivered dose and may require a re-plan. A particular patient treated in this centre had spontaneous collapse and reinflation sporadically throughout the treatment course and had two plans which were selected on each day to optimize overall delivery of the treatment course, an early case of reactive adaptive. The oesophagus is not obvious on CBCT unless there is visible lumen or the presence of a stent or nasogastric tube. The primary match is to bony anatomy as the oesophagus is closely related to the vertebral column. The aorta can also be used as a landmark for matching, especially if there are calcifications within the aorta.

23.6.6 Head and neck

All patients within this group should be treated wearing a multiple fixation point thermoplastic mask for positional reproducibility. Weight loss will impact on the ability of the therapeutic radiographer to match the anatomy on the daily scan with that from the planning scan. It is important to assess the mask fit daily, paying particular attention to gaps between the shell and the patient's skin surface. If a contour change is noted it may be necessary to use additional shims under the head and shoulders of the patient to ensure a good fit and minimize patient movement during the treatment process (Figure 23.17). When adjusting shimming be cautious of introducing pitch. Felt can also be added under the neck to extend the neck when weight loss has resulted in a loss of flexion. Strategies to cope with anatomical change will vary between centres; however, a local strategy for dealing with change

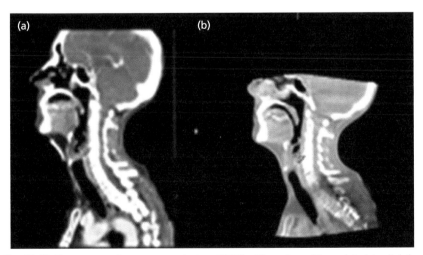

Fig. 23.17 There was a discrepancy noted on CBCT with neck position related to slightly different shaped headrests which should have been identical.

should be in place. If change is deemed to effect delivered dosimetry a re-plan may be required.

Always focus the match on anatomy close to the target. If the treatment site is close to the orbits a good match is not required posteriorly. This is a simple way of accommodating for any pitch that may be evident. Utilize any surgical scars (CNS) that are close to the target, ventricles in the brain can also be used. However, be aware that these will change shape with a change in intracranial pressure.

23.7 **Artefacts**

Artefacts caused by calcifications, metal or gas, in the patient or from the imaging modality itself have the potential to affect decision making during the match process.

♦ Metal: can be fiducials implanted to assist in automatic match techniques or prosthetic implants, for example hips (Figure 23.18).

♦ Air: can be responsible for loss of data (Figure 23.19).

♦ Rings: these are caused by a loss of a detector or from image reconstruction. Care must be taken if these are present in a data set as they may influence the radiographer to select a ring as the limits of an organ, especially with the prostate gland (Figure 23.20).

♦ *In vivo* dosimetry: the presence of diodes on the skin may affect the appearance of the external contour.

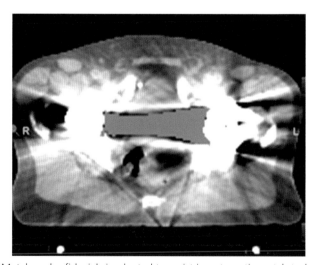

Fig. 23.18 Metal can be fiducials implanted to assist in automatic match techniques or prosthetic implants, for example hips or spinal stabilization Metal artefact can remove information from an image. The grey section is a density over-ride used to improve the accuracy of the planned dosimetry. Use of algorithms at CT planning may reduce this extreme effect. Use of specific imaging modalities (FBMVCT) or presets (reduced kV) on treatment may also reduce the effects of artefacts in images.

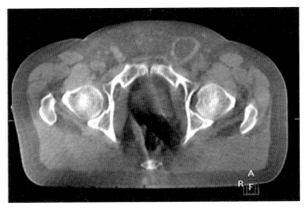

Fig. 23.19 Air artefact. The SVs have apparently 'disappeared' from the image. A flare artefact also affects recognition of the prostate gland

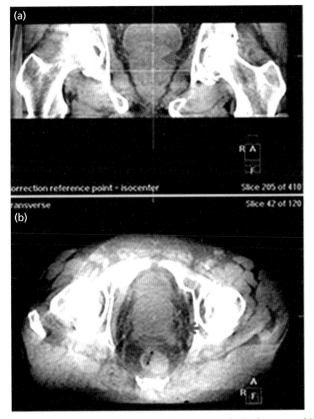

Fig. 23.20 Zipper and ring artefact. The zipper is seen as a zip in the coronal image and the concentric circles can clearly be seen in the axial slice making it difficult to identify the limits of the prostate gland.

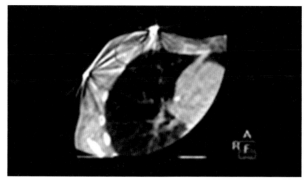

Fig. 23.21 Diodes placed on the skin surface prior to acquiring a CBCT scan. The diodes can clearly be seen in the axial slice making it difficult to identify the skin surface and clips in the tumour bed.

- Breathing motion: the speed at which planning data can now be acquired can also contribute to the difficulty in predicting the impact motion has on the target volume position. A mobile organ is unlikely to be in its exact mean position at the time of imaging, causing the treatment to be planned with as organ offset from its assumed mean position.

23.8 Summary

- Each radiotherapy centre should have protocols for defining frequency and modality of imaging requirements for each anatomical site.
- Any non-standard imaging should be recommended and annotated in the patient's record.
- Imaging outside of the planned treatment fields or PTV and through OARs (lens of the eye, liver, spinal cord) should be avoided where possible.
- Optimize images to enable visualization of match anatomy.
- If the patient moves during the time between acquiring an image and registration or during treatment, it may be necessary to re-image the patient.
- If the time between acquiring an image and initiation of treatment delivery extends beyond five minutes it may be necessary to re-image the patient.
- Review all relevant anatomy within the acquired image; including target and OA).
- When matching anatomy (soft tissue or bone) the goal is to minimize any stepping.
- Consider how any anatomical change will impact on planned dosimetry.
- For consistency in image review an audit programme is a useful tool in maintaining good practice. Where a weekly check is undertaken for each patient, a review of an imaging episode can also be undertaken. Data can be assessed for consistency in matching for both inter and intra-user variation, an important factor to be included in local margin calculations.

References

1. **SCoR, IPEM, RCR** (2008). *On-target: Implementing Geometric Verification in Radiotherapy.* London: Society & College of Radiographers, Institute of Physics in Engineering and Medicine, Royal College of Radiologists. ('On target 2: Updated for image-guided radiotherapy' 2021 is available from https://www.rcr.ac.uk/sites/default/files/radiotherapy-board-on-target-2-updated-guidance-image-guided-radiotherapy.pdf)

2. **Society and College of Radiographers** (2013). *Image Guided Radiotherapy (IGRT) Clinical Support Programme in England 2012–2013.* London: The Society and College of Radiographers (SCoR).

3. **Geometric Uncertainties in Radiotherapy** (2003). BIR Working Party The British Institute of Radiology.

4. **Erridge SC, Seppenwoolde Y, Muller SH, et al.** (2003). Portal imaging to assess set-up errors, tumor motion and tumor shrinkage during conformal radiotherapy of non-small cell lung cancer. *Radiotherapy and Oncology*, **66**(1): 75–85.

5. *Ionising Radiation (Medical Exposure) Regulations 2017 Department of Health and Social Care The Stationary office Limited.*

6. *The Ionising Radiation (Medical Exposure) (Amendment) Regulations 2018* Department of Health (2012). The Stationary office Limited.

7. **Department of Health** (2012). *National Radiotherapy Implementation Group Report Image Guided Radiotherapy.* Guidance for implementation and use. Department of Health.

8. **Dean JC, Routsis D** (2010). Training needs of radiographers for implementing tomotherapy in NHS practice. *Journal of Radiotherapy in Practice*, **9**(3): 175–183.

9. **Bates AM, Scaife JE, Tudor GS, et al.** (2013). Image guidance protocols: balancing imaging parameters against scan time. *British Journal of Radiology*, **86**(1032): 20130385.

Chapter 24

Radiation protection issues when imaging patients for radiotherapy

Simon Thomas

24.1 Introduction

The purpose of this chapter is to discuss the radiation protection implications of imaging with ionizing radiation, for patients who require such imaging as part of their radiotherapy pathway. This chapter will not consider forms of imaging, such as ultrasound (US) or magnetic resonance imaging (MRI) that do not involve ionizing radiation.

This chapter will discuss the effects of ionizing radiation on the human body. It will give guidance on radiation dosimetry, on the regulations surrounding the use of ionizing radiation, and on how to estimate the risks from ionizing radiation.

24.2 The effects of ionizing radiation on the body

Imaging is performed pretreatment (for diagnosis, staging, and treatment planning), and during treatment (for verification and image guidance). All of this adds to the radiation received by normal tissues. In most cases this radiation will be considerably less than that received from the therapy doses.

When considering the effects of radiation on the body, it is useful to distinguish between deterministic effects and stochastic effects.

◆ A deterministic effect, which will occur at high dose levels (typically tens of Gy), is an event that is predicted to occur when a dose above a certain level is given. Radiotherapy treatment planning is largely concerned with achieving the deterministic effect of killing the tumour, whilst avoiding unwanted deterministic effects in organs at risk (OAR).

◆ A stochastic effect, otherwise known as a probabilistic effect, is one that has a probability of occurring, with the probability increasing with dose. Examples of such an effect are the risk of inducing cancer, and the risk of inducing heritable effects.

The doses used for imaging are usually way below the threshold for deterministic effects, so considerations of the risks from imaging concentrate on the stochastic effects. The International Commission on Radiological Protection (ICRP) publishes guidelines on the risks of radiation to the human body; these serve as the basis for national regulations and guidance.[1,2] The data for stochastic effects are based on data from atomic bomb survivors and on epidemiological studies. Since it is hard to untangle effects for low doses from the underlying variations in non-radiation induced cancers, the data in practice are extrapolated to low doses from results at higher doses than usually seen in imaging, making an assumption that the graph of risk against dose follows a straight line through the origin. This assumption, known as the 'linear non-threshold' (LNT) model is not universally accepted; however, it forms the basis of ICRP's recommendations, and will be followed in this chapter.

The risk of fatal cancer induction varies with age and sex, and there is a latent period (5–40 years) from irradiation to clinical presentation. For whole body doses of X-rays, the data shows a risk of approximately 5% per Gy for adults. Most imaging only irradiates part of the body; in this case the risk depends on which organs are irradiated. Methods for calculating this are discussed in the next section. It should be noted that for OAR from the radiotherapy dose, both stochastic and deterministic models can be used. The QUANTEC report[3] gives thresholds for some toxicities (deterministic), but also gives Normal Tissue Complication Probabilities (stochastic) for other toxicities.

24.3 Absorbed dose, equivalent dose, and effective dose

The SI unit of Absorbed Dose is the Gray (Gy) equal to one joule per kilogram. Although this is a unit of appropriate size for considering radiotherapy doses, it is too large a unit for typical imaging doses, which are usually of a scale where the mGy (equal to one thousandth of a Gy) is the suitable unit.

Equivalent dose is a concept used to allow for the fact that different types of radiation, such as protons and alpha particles, cause greater damage for a given absorbed dose than do photons or electrons. Equivalent dose is defined as the absorbed dose multiplied by a radiation weighting factor. However, for electrons and for photons this weighting factor is equal to one, so for nearly all the imaging considered in this chapter equivalent dose is identical to absorbed dose.

Since different organs have different sensitivity to radiation, and many scenarios in which people are irradiated (including most imaging) involve irradiating only part of the body, the ICRP introduced the concept of effective dose. The effective dose is the dose to the whole body that would incur the same risk as a partial exposure of the body, when specific tissues receive an equivalent dose of H_T:

$$E = \sum_T w_T H_T$$

where w_T is the weighting factor for the specific tissue. The sum is performed over all organs and tissues of the body considered to be sensitive to the induction of stochastic effects. The value given to w_T reflects the radiation sensitivity of the tissue; it is, however, averaged over both sexes and all ages. The value of effective dose calculated using these average weighting factors therefore does not represent the characteristics of a particular individual.

The most recent values of w_T published in ICRP Publication 103, are in Table 24.1.

Table 24.1 ICRP 103 tissue weighting factors

Tissue	w_T	Sum of w_T
Bone marrow Colon Lung Stomach Breast	0.12	0.60
Gonads	0.08	0.08
Bladder Oesophagus Liver Thyroid	0.04	0.16
Bone surface Brain Salivary glands Skin	0.01	0.04
Remainder organs*	0.12	0.12
	Total	1.00

*Remainder tissues: adrenals, extrathoracic (ET) region, gall bladder, heart, kidneys, lymphatic nodes, muscle, oral mucosa, pancreas, prostate♂, small intestine, spleen, thymus, uterus/cervix♀.

Adapted with permission from CRP, 'ICRP103: The 2007 Recommendations of the International Commission on Radiological Protection,' *Ann. ICRP*, Vol. 37, pp. 2–4.

The w_T for the remainder tissue applies to the arithmetic mean dose of the 13 tissues for each sex. Effective dose is measured in sievert (Sv) rather than Gy. For an irradiation of the whole body, the effective dose and the absorbed dose are the same. In any practical imaging example, the effective dose (in mSv) will be less than the absorbed dose (in mGy). Strictly speaking, equivalent dose is also quoted in Sv. However, since we are considering only X-rays and electrons, we will ignore equivalent dose in the rest of this chapter, and regard the w_T as factors to convert absorbed dose (in mGy) to effective dose (in mSv).

It has become common practice to use effective dose when considering radiation risks from diagnostic radiology where doses are relatively low and only stochastic effects are being considered. All the values of E given in this chapter are calculated using ICRP 103 weighting factors. The uncertainties of the value of E are large (± 40%) even for a reference patient and will be much greater for the individual. Bearing in mind the above limitations of the averaging process in calculating E, the use of E does allow for comparisons of dose between different X-ray examinations, provided that a similar patient sample is considered.

24.4 Radiation protection legislation

The relevant legislation in England, Wales and Scotland is the Ionising Radiation (Medical Exposure) Regulations 2017[4] (in Northern Ireland, essentially the same regulations are the Ionising Radiation (Medical Exposure) Regulations (Northern Ireland) 2018). This legislation implements a European obligation, set out in European Council Directive 2013/59/EURATOM.

24.4.1 Ionising radiation (medical exposure) regulations (IRMER 2017)

IRMER 2017 lays down measures to protect patients and others undergoing medical exposures from unnecessary radiation. The ICRP principles of justification and optimization are incorporated into the regulations. Dose limits are not applicable to patient procedures, but the benefit to the patient (or society through research) must outweigh any detriment from exposure to radiation for the exposure to be justified.

Applied to radiotherapy the scope of the IRMER is to justify and optimize:

- The exposure of patients as part of their own medical diagnosis or treatment.
- The exposure of patients or other persons voluntarily participating in medical or biomedical, diagnostic, or therapeutic research programmes.

24.4.1.1 Duty holders

Regulation 2 of this legislation defines the roles of duty holders as:

- The employer, the referrer, the practitioner, the operator, and the MPE.

24.4.1.2 The employer

The employer as defined in this legislation is 'any person who, in the course of a trade, business or other undertaking, carries out (other than as an employee), or engages others to carry out … exposures … or practical aspects, at a given radiological installation.'

The employer as a duty holder under IRMER is responsible for providing a framework for radiation protection for patients. This framework is based on a minimum set of written procedures the 'Employer's Procedures' (EPs) (these are set out in regulation 6(1) and schedule 2 of the legislation), written protocols, and quality assurance programmes (Reg. 4).

A procedure must be in place to identify individuals who are entitled to act as referrers, practitioners, or operators and the scope of practices for duty holders must be clearly identified and documented.

The employer has a responsibility to ensure that all entitled practitioners and operators are adequately trained to perform their tasks in their defined scope of practice. A list of topics that training must cover is given in schedule 2 of the regulations, but training at local level on specific equipment, procedures, and protocols is also required. The training underpins the entitlement of the individual to act as a practitioner or operator for the range of practices for which they have been deemed competent. The employer must keep a record of all training and make it available for inspection.

The employer must also establish recommendations concerning referral criteria, including radiation doses, for medical exposures and make these available to the referrer.

24.4.1.3 The referrer

The referrer means a registered healthcare professional who is entitled in accordance with the employer's procedures to refer individuals for exposure to a practitioner. The referrer must supply the practitioner with sufficient medical data (such as previous diagnostic information or medical records) relevant to the exposure requested by the referrer to enable the practitioner to decide whether there is a sufficient net benefit to justify the exposure.

24.4.1.4 The IRMER practitioner

The IRMER practitioner's primary responsibility is to ensure that the requested medical exposure is justified. For an exposure to be justified, it must show sufficient net benefit, taking into account the total potential diagnostic or therapeutic benefits (both the direct benefits to the individual and the benefits to society), and the individual detriment that the exposure may cause. The regulations list a number of factors that need to be taken into account, including cases involving comforters and carers, and health screening of asymptomatic individuals.

24.4.1.5 The operator

The operator is any person who carries out any practical aspect of the medical exposure. The operator and practitioner must together ensure that the doses arising from the exposure are kept as low as reasonably practicable, consistent with the intended purpose. Every exposure must be 'authorized'. This authorization is primarily the responsibility of the practitioner, but in many practical cases for routine uses of radiation this is not practicable. Regulation 11(5) allows in these cases for the operator to authorize an exposure, in accordance with guidelines issued by the practitioner.

24.4.1.6 Medical physics expert

The medical physics expert (MPE) Reg. 14 (1) is defined as 'an individual or a group of individuals, having the knowledge, training and experience to act or give advice on matters relating to radiation physics applied to exposure, whose competence in this respect is recognized by the Secretary of State.' Anyone who was acting as an MPE prior to 31 December 2017 was able to be added to a list held at http://www.rpa2000.org.uk/, and to apply for transition to the formal register. Those not on the original list can apply to RPA2000 by submitting a portfolio of evidence showing they meet the requirements of the syllabus published on the RPA2000 web site.

The employer is required to ensure that a suitable MPE is appointed. They are required to be 'closely involved' in every radiotherapeutic practice, and to be 'involved' or 'involved as appropriate for consultation on optimization' in other radiological practices. IRMER lists a number of areas on which an MPE must give advice; within radiotherapy physics these largely match the areas in which physicists are routinely involved.

A member of staff may have the role of more than one duty holder if the Employer's Procedures entitle them to do so. For example the oncologist may be both the referrer and the practitioner.

24.4.2 Diagnostic reference levels

Patient diagnostic examinations are not subject to dose limits but the IRMER legislation requires that diagnostic reference levels (DRLs) be set for diagnostic examinations. The values are for the relevant dose indicator for a specific examination for a standard size patient.

The regulations require the employer to review, and make available to an operator, diagnostic reference levels; regard must be had to European and National DRLs where available.

National DRLs are in place in terms of entrance skin dose (ESD) (mGy) for individual radiographs and dose area product (DAP) (Gy.cm^2) for more complex examinations. For CT exams the DRL is given in terms of CT dose index (CTDI$_{vol}$) or dose length product (DLP).

The concept of DRLs applies only to diagnostic imaging, and is therefore not a legal requirement for radiotherapy planning images, or IGRT images. An IPEM working party is developing reference levels for radiotherapy imaging. A recently published report proposes national dose reference levels and 'achievable levels' of CT dose index (CTDI$_{vol}$), dose-length-product (DLP), and scan length.[5] These levels are proposed based on the third quartile and median values of results from a UK-wide survey of CT scanners used for radiotherapy treatment planning.

The proposed dose reference levels for CTDI$_{vol}$ and DLP are: prostate 16 mGy and 570 mGy.cm, gynaecological 16 mGy and 610 mGy.cm, breast 10 mGy and 390 mGy.cm, 3D-lung 14 mGy and 550 mGy.cm, 4D-lung 63 mGy and 1750 mGy.cm, brain 50 mGy and 1500 mGy.cm, and head/neck 49 mGy and 2150 mGy.cm. The working party will also be reporting on IGRT imaging doses.

24.4.3 Issues concerning pregnancy status (Reg. 11(1f) and 12(8d))

IRMER requires, in the case of an individual of childbearing potential, that the person carrying out the exposure has enquired whether the individual is pregnant (or breastfeeding if relevant). It is recognized that diagnostic dose levels are very much lower than those given to the patient during radiotherapy, but checking for pregnancy will be made first at the diagnostic stage for each individual patient. At diagnostic dose levels the only adverse effect of radiation on the unborn child which is likely to pose a risk is that of cancer induction. The implementation of official recommendations is discussed in the next paragraph.[6] The procedure will apply to 12–55-year-old women; the RCR has discussed the problems associated with asking teenage girls about pregnancy. It is possible, though rare, that the practitioner may proceed with radiotherapy even if the patient is found to be pregnant, in which case the MPE will be asked to make a very careful estimate of risk to the unborn child.

In the diagnostic department (X-ray, nuclear medicine, or positron emission tomography (PET) or PET/computed tomography (CT)), the referrer ascertains the pregnancy status and the operator confirms this before carrying out the exposure. If the patient is pregnant, the examination may still continue, provided further justification takes place that indicates the exposure is of net benefit. This must be documented.

In the radiotherapy department the procedure will include the following:

♦ It is the referrer's responsibility to ensure whether the patient may be pregnant and that the patient is informed about the risks of becoming pregnant (particularly if the patient is going to proceed to radiotherapy treatment).

♦ The IRMER practitioner (consultant oncologist) will reassess the pregnancy status before prescribing the RT treatment.

♦ The operator's responsibilities will include, ensuring that the patient has signed a declaration they are not pregnant and informing them that they must tell a radiographer before any ionizing radiation procedure that they may be pregnant. This declaration can conveniently be incorporated into the consent form used to give informed consent to treatment.

24.4.4 Special treatment of infants, children, and young adults

The process of justification and optimization is particularly important for infants and young children since the risk of inducing a cancer is higher. This is due partly to the increased sensitivity to radiation of bone marrow in children and for young girls the developing breast tissue. Exposure protocols used for imaging should be specific to paediatrics; this is particularly important for CT scanning where the use of techniques used for adults can lead to unnecessarily high doses. Details of the increased risk of breast cancer induction with decreasing age can be found in the BEIR VII report[7] and NHSBSP report 54.[8]

24.4.5 Reporting of incidents

Employers are obliged under regulation 8 to investigate where an incident has occurred or may have occurred involving a clinically significant unintended or accidental exposure. This includes both those incidents that are significantly greater than 'those generally considered to be proportionate', and those that are significantly lower. Guidance on what is "significant" is available on the CQC website[9], whilst guidance on what is "clinically significant" is available from the Radiotherapy Board[10].

If the investigation shows that such an exposure has occurred then the appropriate authority (in England this is Care Quality Commission (CQC); in Wales, National Assembly for Wales: Health and Social Division, for Northern Ireland the NI Department of Health, and in Scotland, Scottish Ministers: Scottish Executive Health Department) must be notified and the employer must arrange for a detailed investigation of the circumstances of the exposure and an assessment of the dose received.

24.4.6 Quality assurance

In order to maintain standards within the imaging departments and the radiotherapy department it is vital to have a quality assurance programme. This will cover all aspects of the work, staffing, and equipment within each department and will ensure that IRMER matters are covered (equipment QA is under IRR2017).[11]

Patient dose audit—it is vital that the entire procedure for a particular examination is checked routinely and that the dose given by each procedure is in line with the national guidelines. Employer's Procedures must be regularly reviewed; it should be documented how this is done, and which individual is responsible for the review being done.

Senior management must take responsibility for ensuring that procedures are reviewed at a sufficient frequency to take into account the impact of new technology and role development which will impact on ways of working.

24.5 The radiotherapy episode: justification and assessing patient dose

24.5.1 Diagnostic and staging imaging before the commencement of RT

A referral for imaging to diagnostic radiology is deemed to be a request for a professional opinion, which the radiologist as practitioner will justify and authorize if s/he thinks the exposure appropriate. Exposures which meet referral criteria, as drawn up by the radiology department, may not need individual justification; however, they need to be authorized by the person carrying out the exposure. Where imaging involves nuclear medicine or PET scanning the practitioner must be the ARSAC certificate holder.

24.5.2 Planning CT images

It is simplest to consider doses incurred during planning as included in the radiotherapy prescription. The above exposures are requested by the oncologist (IRMER referrer) in accordance with written and signed protocols drawn up by the lead specialist oncologist (IRMER practitioner). The protocols should be sufficiently flexible to allow for additional planning images but must not be open-ended. If exposures additional to those detailed in the protocol are required the exposures must be additionally justified and authorized. The protocols must be regularly reviewed.

24.5.3 Verification and IGRT imaging

These are the images taken during radiotherapy, either just before each treatment exposure is made or during the treatment exposure. They may be carried out at each fractionated treatment exposure, or less frequently in line with local protocols. Except for the exposures using the treatment field (such as MV portal imaging with no change of field size), all these verification and image guidance methods give additional dose to the patient. The treatment itself and the concomitant verification images (using portal imaging or CT as defined in the treatment protocol) will be justified by a consultant clinical oncologist.

24.5.4 Justification and dose assessment

Justification requires that the benefit and detriment of every exposure be considered, taking into account the intention of each exposure and the characteristics of the individual patient. Any exposures performed outside of protocol must be justified separately (and a note made in the patient's record). This consideration is not a simple task. The target volume must be planned optimally with as much information from the scans as possible in order to define the target and critical structures optimally. The radiotherapy delivery is checked regularly (both inter- and intrafraction), using verification imaging including the various forms of CT and cone beam CT (CBCT), to ensure that these volumes have been correctly covered or avoided respectively by the high radiation dose region. If this set of tasks is not performed optimally then the clinical oncologist is failing the radically treated patient. There is also a balance to be drawn for each patient between the potential for deterministic damage to critical structures and the risk of radiation-induced cancer. In addition, as delivery techniques become more complicated and treatment is tailored to inter/intrafractional organ movement more verification imaging will be required.

To make a full risk assessment for the individual patient, it is necessary under IRMER to understand all those doses associated with the various image procedures during a radiotherapy episode. For the diagnostic images this may be considered to be straightforward by using effective dose. For a fuller interpretation of all the doses received by the radiotherapy patient, including those doses to organs/critical structures outside the treatment volume, it will be necessary to approach the problem differently. The treatment doses to organs immediately surrounding the target volume can be very high, for example if the target dose is 70 Gy then even at levels of 1–10% the doses to surrounding organs may be 700–7000 mGy.

To estimate the risk of inducing a cancer in these organs (or damaging non-tumour tissue) it is preferable to determine individual organ doses (the most heavily irradiated organs for a particular treatment site) from all the imaging and treatment received by the patient and then to attach a stochastic risk factor to that total organ dose. This is preferable to using effective dose, since effective dose combines together all ages and does not discriminate between the sexes. This is particularly important when considering infants, children, and young adults in order to attribute the appropriate risk factor for cancer induction.

The main problem in performing such calculations is how to deal with imaging dose that covers the high dose area of the radiotherapy treatment, since cancer induction risk factors are modelled for doses where a linear response is assumed, and this is not the case at higher doses. Various models have been proposed[12] ranging from ones that plateau at a certain dose, to ones that actually decrease at high doses (on the basis that cancers induced in the high dose region of the treatment will be immediately sterilized by the treatment). There is currently no consensus on which model is correct. Calculating using several models can be useful if they all show one irradiation plan to be higher than another.

The other half of a risk calculation is to quantify the benefit that comes from image guidance. This is even harder, since evidence for the benefits of IGRT tends to be qualitative rather than quantitative. The benefits of IGRT, in avoiding an underdose due to geographic miss, or in allowing smaller PTV margins (and hence sparing organs at risk) are hard to test in a randomized trial. The CHHIP-IGRT sub-study provides some evidence for daily IGRT[13].

A risk calculation of cancer induction, even if using effective dose, is better than no calculation at all. At present the advice given by the Health Research Authority for MPEs performing risk calculations for clinical trials is to use generic risk statements such as: 'We are all at risk of developing cancer during our lifetime. The normal risk is that this will happen to about 50% of people at some point in their life. Taking part in this study will increase the chances of this happening to you from 50% to [insert estimated risk] %.' Further examples of risk statements are given at http://www.hra-decisiontools.org.uk/consent/docs/Generic-ionising-radiation-risk-statements_v4_October2020.pdf.

24.5.5 Examples of imaging exposures

Methods for making these exposures include:

◆ *Megavoltage portal imaging.* This is mainly now done using an electronic portal imaging device (EPID) attached to the gantry of the linear accelerator. Imaging is achieved either using the treatment field or using a radiation field larger than the treatment field, and often using an orthogonal pair of images. When most radiotherapy was given at fixed angles, with MLC shaped to conform to the PTV, this could be routinely used to image each field and every treatment. As rotational IMRT techniques such as VMAT take over, this has less value for geometric verification. However EPIDs have gained a new role in exit dosimetry, since they are one of the few devices that can be used for *in vivo* dosimetry of VMAT.

◆ *Kilovoltage imaging.* Most conventional linacs are now sold with a kilovoltage unit attached to the gantry; the X-ray set and imaging plate (digital) are mounted orthogonally to the megavoltage beam (for Varian and Elekta models). Other manufacturers (e.g. Accuray and BrainLab) install ceiling and floor mounted combinations of X-ray sets and imaging plates. Either form of kilovoltage unit can be used for routine imaging of the radiotherapy patient.

◆ *Megavoltage CT.* Helical tomotherapy units (Accuray Inc.) image with megavoltage spiral CT (the energy of the imaging beam is slightly lower than the treatment beam).

◆ *Kilovoltage cone beam CT (CBCT).* When a kV set is mounted on the linac gantry (Varian and Elekta) it can be used to take CT images with cone beam; a volume CT is achieved by using the cone beam and rotating the gantry through 360° in 1 min.

In order to illustrate the above points a few examples have been taken from the various examinations required for the following tumour sites: prostate, breast, and lymphoma (Tables 24.2, 24.3, and 24.4). The list of examinations is included in these tables, together with various illustrative doses—effective dose; CTDI; isocentric dose (which gives a typical value of dose in the central region of the examination for organs close to this region,); and a dose to the most critical organ.

The values given in Tables 24.2, 24.3, and 24.4 are an indication only. These values will depend on the geometry of the equipment used, the technique factors selected, the volume of the patient irradiated, and the size of the patient. The value of effective dose from a CT scan is also very dependent on the image length scanned, the image quality required, and the pitch of the scan (couch movement per rotation/X-ray beam

Table 24.2A Prostate patient with the approximate dose per examination

Examination	E (mSv)	Typical CTDI (mGy)	Typical isocentre dose (mGy)	Bladder dose (mGy)	% of bladder included
Pre-treatment images					
CT (kV)	10	22	11	21	100
Diagnostic PET (400 MBq FDG)	11	NA	NA	68	100
Verification images					
Tomotherapy image (3MV)	0.6		11	11	50
CBCT (kV)	6	30		30	50
CBCT (kV), low mAs for use with seeds	0.8	4		4	50
Portal imaging, using wide fields	1		2	2	100
Portal imaging using treatment beam	0	0	0	0	NA
Portal kV image	0.1	1	0.2	0.4	100

width). If CT is used in an over sampling mode (pitch 0.1) to remove motion blurring and to define movement related margins (e.g. for 4D CT imaging of the lungs) there is a possibility that a dose 5–10 times the conventional CT dose may be given. The medical physics expert in a cancer centre will be able to provide more specific doses for a particular equipment and image technique.

A number of verification imaging regimens have been considered for each treatment site, to indicate the variation of effective and critical organ doses with imaging modality and frequency of imaging. These doses have been multiplied by the relevant risk factor to give a possible induced fatal cancer risk (lifetime) expressed as a percentage.

Table 24.2B Prostate patient. The approximate dose and risk per imaging regime (assume 20# treatment)

Protocol: verification imaging only	Typical E (mSv)	% Risk of fatal cancer (rf of 5%/Sv)	Critical organ: bladder dose x (mGy)	% Risk of fatal bladder cancer (rf of 0.12%/Gy)
1) Daily MVCT imaging (Tomo)	12	0.06	220 (to 50%)	0.013
2) CBCT kV	120	0.6	600 (to 50%)	0.036
3) CBCT kV with seeds	16	0.08	80 (to 50%)	0.005
4)1# CBCT + 20# kV planar pairs	4.8	0.02	16 (to 100%)	0.002

Table 24.3A Breast patient with the approximate dose per examination

Examination	Typical E (mSv)	Critical organ contralateral breast mGy	Lung mGy
Pre-treatment images			
Mammogram	0.3	0	0
CT (kV) full chest	6	9	15
Verification images			
CBCT (6MV)	10	20	30
Lat portal imaging with treatment field	0.0	0.0	0.0
Lat portal imaging with 2 MU non-treatment field	1.2	3.3	5.4
Lat portal imaging kV/image	0.04	0.15	0.1

A risk factor (rf) of 5% per Sv has been taken from ICRP 103[2] to estimate the number of fatal cancers induced when adults (aged 18–64 years) are irradiated with an effective dose of E mSv.

A few examples of risk calculations have been given here, but it must be recognized that this is a developing subject.

Risk factors for inducing a cancer in an individual organ for adults have been taken from ICRP 103. The risk factors used are for irradiated adults aged 18–64, are gender specific, and are for the product of risk coefficient and lethality factor.

For lymphoma the values given in Table 24.4 are approximate but have been included because of potential risks to young patients. For example, PET/CT has become an issue with ethical committees for young people involved in clinical trials since multiple scans are given. However, in general this additional imaging dose may be more than offset by the reduction in radiotherapy dose with the use of involved fields instead of mantle fields. The evidence of second cancer risk for these patients is dramatic. Most

Table 24.3B Breast patient. Approximate dose and risk per imaging regime

	Typical E (mSv)	% risk of fatal cancer (rf 5%/Sv)	Critical organ: contralateral breast (mGy)	% risk of fatal cancer induction in breast (rf 0.34%/Gy)	Critical organ: lung (mGy)	% risk of fatal cancer induction in lung (rf 1.55%/Gy)
1) High (1 planning CT +15 CBCT)	156	0.78	306	0.10	465	0.72
2) Low (1 planning CT + PI using treatment fields)	6	0.03	6	<0.01	6	0.01

Table 24.4A Lymphoma (upper body), age ten years

Examination	E (mSv)	Critical organ		
		Breast dose (mGy)	Red bone marrow dose (mGy)	Lung dose (mGy)
Pre-treatment images				
Bone scan 355MBq Tc^{99m}	5	0	7	0.9
PET	13	5	6	6
PET with CT	17	22	10	18
CT (kV)	4	17	4	12
Simulator fluoroscopy for 1 min(AP)	1.5	7	0.5	3.3
Verification images				
AP portal kV/image	0.04	0.15	0.01	0.1
AP portal 6MV/image/MU	2	10	0.5	7

of the research work on this appears to demonstrate that the second cancers induced in breast and lung are in the margins and high-dose regions of these organs.

24.6 Discussion

24.6.1 Prostate

The effective dose from daily IGRT is strongly dependent on the technique and equipment used. The lowest doses will be given in centres that implant fiducial markers in the prostate, and use a treatment technique with static conformal fields. By imaging the seeds using the first few MU of each of the treatment fields, it is possible to do image guidance with no additional dose. Cone-beam CT doses can be considerably reduced if fiducial seeds are used. However, the reduction in dose needs to be set against

Table 24.4B Lymphoma patient (upper body) aged ten. Approximate dose and risk per imaging regime

Protocol	E (mSv)	% risk of fatal cancer (rf 10%/Gy)	Critical organ: breast dose (mGy)	% risk of cancer in breast (rf 4.3%/Gy)
1) High (1 CT + 20 portal pairs 6 MV of 1 MU + 5 PET with CT)	169	1.7	527	2.3
2) CT based (1 CT+ 10 kV portal pairs)	4.4	0.04	20	0.1

the risks involved with seed insertion, and the cost of the seeds. Volumetric imaging techniques that allow the region imaged to be closely tailored to the target volume (such as TomoTherapy) can give lower effective doses than those that have standard length imaging beams.

24.6.2 Breast

The use of CT for verification images leads to a higher contralateral breast dose than the use of a lateral portal image. The use of organ dose rather than effective dose gives a more detailed description of the cancer risk. For the regimes shown in Table 24.4B, the risk of cancer from the doses to lung alone is essentially the same as the nominal risk calculated from the effective dose.

24.6.3 Lymphoma

The total imaging doses under the 'high dose' regimen above are significant. The breast doses (approximately 0.5 Gy) by themselves give a theoretical risk for second cancer of 2.3% (for a 10–15-year-old girl). It is interesting to compare this dose with the various levels used in modern radiotherapy for these patients. The rate of induction of lung and breast cancer in patients treated for Hodgkin disease, mainly with mantle fields, is now well understood.[14–15] This risk should now be reduced by the use of involved fields where less of each critical structure is irradiated, so potentially reducing the impact of the increased imaging.

24.7 Summary

- Imaging in radiotherapy is very extensive and takes place throughout the patient journey, with images being taken for diagnosis, treatment planning, and verification of treatment.
- The control of these imaging processes is governed by IRMER 2017.
- The doses received by the patient from pretreatment imaging are relatively small, the highest effective dose being from a PET with CT examination.
- Verification and IGRT imaging doses are higher, but are still generally only a few per cent of the leakage and scatter dose. However, when frequent verification images, particularly CT, are taken the dose can become comparable to the leakage and scatter dose.
  - The critical organ typically receives a range of dose from scatter and leakage (depending how close it is to the PTV) of 1–90%.
  - A typical imaging dose to this organ will be about 0.1%, although this could increase to 1%.
- Imaging regimens need to be carefully reviewed in every radiotherapy department and this may be achieved by:
  - Where possible using imaging techniques that do not involve ionizing radiation.
  - Reducing the field of view of the image to the smallest required.

- Using image technique factors that are commensurate with the image quality required for treatment decisions to be made.

◆ It is vital to give special consideration to children and young adults who are exposed to radiation. This group of patients has a longer period of time over which they may express a radiation induced cancer and they may have more exposures to radiation during that period. It will be of great value to these patients, and the scientific community, to keep records of all these exposures for each individual.

◆ When considering risk to the individual patient the use of effective dose and a general risk factor of 5% per Sv for cancer induction may underestimate the risk. This is particularly true when the breast area is irradiated. The evidence for induction of radiation-induced cancer is sparse but suggests that the second cancers appear in the high-dose regions around the treatment area. This is also the volume that receives the verification imaging dose. Generally, the increase in dose due to this area from imaging is relatively low, but in the cases where frequent imaging, particularly (CT), is used these doses can become significant. However, the clinical oncologist has to weigh up all these issues for each patient when balancing the tumour control, morbidity, and second cancer risks.

Acknowledgements

Thanks go to the authors of the previous edition of this chapter, Jane Shekhdar and Edwin Aird. Much of their valuable contribution has been retained in this version.

References

1. **ICRP** (1991). ICRP 60: Recommendations of the International Commission on Radiological Protection. *Annals of ICRP*, **21**: 1–3.
2. **ICRP** (2007). ICRP103: The 2007 Recommendations of the International Commission on Radiological Protection. *Annals of ICRP*, **37**: 2–4.
3. **Bentzen SM, Constine LS, Deasy JO, et al.** (2010). Quantitative Analyses of Normal Tissue Effects in the Clinic (QUANTEC): an introduction to the scientific issues. *International Journal of Radiation Oncology*, **76**(3): S3–S9.
4. *The Ionising Radiation (Medical Exposure) Regulations 2017* (2017). Queen's Printer of Acts of Parliament.
5. **Wood TJ, Davis AT, Earley J, Edyvean S, et al.** (2018). IPEM topical report 2: the first UK survey of dose indices from radiotherapy treatment planning computed tomography scans for adult patients. *Physical Medicine Biology*, **63**(18): 185008.
6. **Health Protection Agency, Royal College of Radiologists, and College of Radiographers (2009).** *Protection of pregnant patients during diagnostic medical exposures to ionising radiation: advice from the Health Protection Agency, the Royal College of Radiologists and the College of Radiographers.* UK: Health Protection Agency.
7. **BEIR VII** (2006). *Health Risks from Exposure to Low Levels of Ionizing Radiation: BEIR VII Phase 2.* Washington, DC: The National Academies Press.
8. **NHSBSP** (2003). *Review of Radiation Risks in Breast Screening.* NHSBSP Publication No 54.
9. **Care Quality Commission (2020).** Significant accidental and unintended exposures under IR(ME)R. Version 2, August 2020. https:/www.cqc.org.uk

10. **Radiotherapy Board (2020).** Ionising Radiation (Medical Exposure) Regulations: Implications for clinical practice in radiotherapy. https://www.rcr.ac.uk

11. **The Ionising Radiation Regulations 2017 (2017).** Queen's Printer of Acts of Parliament.

12. **Ruben JD, Davis S, Evans C, et al. (2008).** The effect of intensity- modulated radiotherapy on radiation- induced second malignancies. *International Journal of Radiation Oncology,* **70**(5): 1530–1536.

13. **Murray J, Griffin C, Gulliford S et al. (2020).** A randomised assessment of image guided radiotherapy within a phase 3 trial of conventional or hypofractionated high dose intensity modulated radiotherapy for prostate cancer. *Radiotherapy and Oncology,* **142**, 62–71.

14. **Travis LB, Hill DA, Dores GM, et al. (2003).** Breast cancer following radiotherapy and chemotherapy among young women with Hodgkin disease. *Journal of American Medical Association,* **290**(4): 465.

15. **van Leeuwen FE, Klokman WJ, Veer MB, et al.** (2000). Long- term risk of second malignancy in survivors of Hodgkin's disease treated during adolescence or young adulthood. *Journal of Clinical Oncology,* **18**(3): 487–497.

Further reading

The DHSC has published guidance to the regulations. https://assets.publishing.service.gov.uk/government/uploads/system/uploads/attachment_data/file/720282/guidance-to-the-ionising-radiation-medical-exposure-regulations-2017.pdf This is not intended to be binding, but is a guide to help explain how the regulations should be interpreted.

The Royal College of Radiologists, Society and College of Radiographers, Institute of Physics and Engineering in Medicine (2008). *A Guide to Understanding the Implications of the Ionising Radiation (Medical Exposure) Regulations in Radiotherapy.* London: The Royal College of Radiologists.

Index

Tables and figures are indicated by *t* and *f* following the page number.